Whole Food Facts

Whole Food Facts

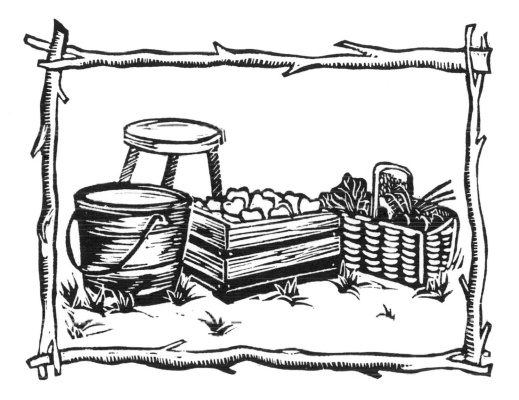

Evelyn Roehl

Illustrations by Mary Elder Jacobsen

Healing Arts Press
Rochester, Vermont

Healing Arts Press
One Park Street
Rochester, Vermont 05767
www.InnerTraditions.com

Healing Arts Press is a division of Inner Traditions International

Note to the reader: This book is intended as an informational guide. The remedies, approaches, and techniques described herein are meant to supplement, and not to be a substitute for, professional medical care or treatment. They should not be used to treat a serious ailment without prior consultation with a qualified health care professional.

LIBRARY OF CONGRESS CATALOGING-IN-PUBLICATION DATA
Roehl, Evelyn.
    Whole food facts / Evelyn Roehl ; illustrations by Mary Elder Jacobsen.
      p.   cm.
    Originally published: 1988.
    Includes bibliographical references and index.
    ISBN 0-89281-635-X
    1. Natural foods.   I. Title.
TX369.R64   1996
641.3—dc20
                              96-3961
Printed and bound in the United States   CIP

10 9 8 7 6 5

Text design and layout by Charlotte Tyler
This book was typeset in Stempel Schneidler with Bodoni as a display typeface

CONTENTS

INTRODUCTION

Food is such a basic part of our lives that we may only think about it when we feel hungry. Since that happens quite regularly in the normal course of the day, it is helpful to realize what foods provide the most nutrients to help us grow and stay healthy.

Whole Food Facts provides information on *foods as a whole,* for people who—for dietary, health, ecological, or sociopolitical reasons—want to know more about *whole foods.*

What, you may ask, are *whole foods?* The term may bring to mind a sunny outdoor market with baskets of fresh apples, squash, and other harvest delights; or of bins full of pinto beans, peanuts, and brown rice. It encompasses a *whole cuisine*—a diet consisting of whole foods, and the ways of preparing them to gain the most nutritional and culinary benefits.

Basically, whole foods are found in as close to their whole, natural state as possible. The difference between whole foods and what I'll call non-whole foods is the degree to which the foods have been processed or altered. An orange, for example, is usually peeled or juiced before it is consumed. Orange juice may be diluted with water and have sweeteners and artificial color or flavorings added to make it a "citrus beverage."

Other Definitions for "Food"

The term *natural foods* generally means the same as whole foods—foods obtained from natural, not artificial or synthetic, sources. Here, however, one can debate the question, *how* whole is whole? White sugar, for example, is derived from a natural source (sugarcane or sugar beets), but it is a 99.9 percent pure chemical: sucrose. *Natural* has become a marketing buzzword—if packages proclaim natural ingredients, people buy the goods.

Health foods are foods that provide optimum nutrition or enhance the health of people who consume them. They may include whole foods, but often they are particular food substances derived from whole foods. Bee pollen, for instance, is obtained by placing a screened barrier in the opening of a bee hive. This forces bees to crawl through it, and it scrapes the plant pollen from their legs. Given this process, bee pollen is not exactly something I would call a "natural" or "whole" food, but it *is* high in protein. *Health food,* when used as a catch-all term, sometimes connotes an association with high prices and questionable claims of miracle cures.

Less commonly used is the term *nutritional foods.* Its definition is probably the most open ended, as it can include just about any food that provides *some* nutrients, whether it is whole or highly refined, or derived from a natural or artificial source. A vitamin-fortified, chocolate-covered granola bar may be considered a nutritional food when compared with a nougat-filled candy bar, though I personally wouldn't rely on it as a major source of sustenance. But it *is* eaten by some as the sole food of both breakfasts and lunches.

You may also be familiar with references to *organic foods.* From one scientific viewpoint, any living organism is an organic substance, whereas any inanimate object, such as a rock, is inorganic. But from an ecological perspective, *organic* refers to foods that are grown without herbicides or pesticides that could cause the food to become toxic. (I remember my own naiveté back in 1974 when I donated a book on organic chemistry to the Organic Food Co-op in Saint Cloud, Minnesota, thinking it would prove to be an invaluable reference.)

Then there are *junk foods*. Junk foods generally have little or no nutrition to begin with or have been processed to the point of having minimal amounts of nutrients. Some foods have too much of certain kinds of nutrients—salt, sugar, or fat—and are therefore considered junk foods. Items often placed in this category include soft drinks, candy bars, angel-food cake, and potato chips. Others are borderline junk "health foods"—ice cream pies made with honey, carob-coated peanuts, and corn chips made with organically grown corn fall into this category.

Last—and definitely least— are *fake foods,* or fabricated foods. Concocted in the laboratories of pharmaceutical companies, food industries, and universities, these foods are synthetic imitations of real foods. Besides nondairy creamers and imitation cheese, there's tomatolike paste for pizza parlors and pseudosausage for breakfast. One agricultural commissioner claimed artificial foods to be far less nutritional and to cost 40 percent more than real foods.

The natural/health foods industry has, like most things, changed considerably in the past twenty years. Bulk foods and organic produce are now found in many supermarkets, while prepackaged and preprocessed natural food products have grown by leaps and bounds. Nutritional supplements jam the store shelves, demanding an educated clientele who can determine the validity of claims for potency, assimilability, and dosages for the myriad substances of plant or animal origin thought to have health-promoting attributes. I personally find it rather absurd that "certified broccoli tablets" are marketed as a nutritional supplement right next to fiber laxatives. Chemists are, of course, trained to isolate and analyze individual compounds; we, as consumers with other occupations and specialties, can choose to unite and experience a more wholistic, interactive life by simply eating *whole* broccoli, fiber intact.

This revised edition of *Whole Food Facts* is actually the fifth metamorphosis of the original publication.

Its genesis was a series of eleven articles published in the *Great River Review,* a newsletter for the Great River Wholesale Co-op of Winona, Minnesota, in 1975–76. These Great River Food Sheets, written by Michael Doyle and myself, soon gained notoriety throughout the Midwest food co-op network, with requests for copies coming from co-ops as far away as New York. After the Great River Co-op closed in 1977, people were still hungry for information about the foods being sold in other co-ops and food buying clubs. In Minneapolis, a food research committee was formed out of the All Co-op Assembly (ACA), a federation of co-ops in Minnesota and western Wisconsin. This committee published two handouts, "Food Talk: The Story about Butter, Margarine and Oils," and "Life Is Sweeter Than You Think." More Food Talks were planned but never materialized, as the committee of volunteers moved on to other projects. Meanwhile, I continued to research and write about food and food producers for *Faminews,* the monthly newsletter of Famine Foods Co-op in Winona, Minnesota, and a regional magazine entitled *North Country Anvil.* With the help of other co-op members, I also established the Food Learning Center in an office above the Famine Foods storefront.

In 1978–79, the members of ACA voted to make food education a priority and to reestablish the Food Research Committee. Annie Young and I proposed that the committee office be located in Winona, since we had a library and an active education committee. I was unanimously chosen to be the coordinator of the ACA Food Research Committee/Food Learning Center. During this same period, the ICC Education Project, a branch of the Intra-Community Cooperative warehouse in Madison, Wisconsin, was planning to publish informational handouts for their membership. In the spirit of cooperation, we decided not to duplicate efforts but to work together to co-publish Co-op Food Facts sheets as well as signs for bulk-food bins.

From 1979 to 1981, two women from the ICC Education Project and I wrote packets of fact sheets for what have since become the chapters "Grains," "Fats and Oils," "Legumes," "Sweeteners," "Nuts and Seeds," and "Other Foods" in *Whole Food Facts.* I also wrote information packets on fruits, vegetables, and dairy products. However, at the time many co-ops sold dry goods only, and ICC did not sell fresh fruits, vegetables, or dairy products. So ICC chose not to co-produce information packets on those foods. They were printed under the auspices of the ACA Food Research Committee, and remained as the seed for those same chapters in this book. The Co-op Food Facts sheets were written as handouts for people who wanted to know about specific kinds of foods (such as brown rice, aduki beans) and so forth, and were designed for compiling in a three-ring binder for reference. Beginning in 1982, after all of the Co-op Food Facts sheets were written, the Food Learning Center sold bright yellow imprinted binder-books to co-ops and individuals all over North America.

As part of the All Co-op Assembly, a larger non-profit organization, the Food Learning Center received continually more requests for information and materials from natural foods vendors, marketers, and consumers not affiliated with food co-ops. We decided that having a more user-friendly book with a generic title would appeal to a broader group of people. So the third generation of this book was just that—a paperback—entitled simply *Food Facts.* *Food Facts* was published in 1984.

In February of 1987, after I had moved to Seattle and brought the Food Learning Center with me, I received a call from a publisher interested in buying the rights and publishing *Food Facts.* At that time the Food Learning Center office was located above another co-op storefront, the Greenlake Puget Consumers' Co-op, in much smaller quarters than the office in Winona, Minnesota. Boxes of *Food Facts* were stashed in every conceivable space, and repeatedly scraping together several thousand dollars to pay for the next print run was getting rather wearisome. I had to check with the Food Learning Center's Board of Directors first before signing a publishing contract and selling the rights. The Board approved.

In June of 1987 a contract was signed. Healing Arts Press released the fourth metamorphosis of this book, entitled *Whole Food Facts,* in the fall of 1988. I disbanded the Food Learning Center that same year, donating the books and files to Puget Consumers' Co-op, Puget Sound Co-op Federation, Seattle Tilth, and the John Bastyr College of Natural Medicine library. Bonnie Fish, formerly with Associated Cooperatives of Berkeley, California, became the honorary custodian of numerous boxes of co-op newsletters and magazines, which she added to her existing barn of archives from California co-ops.

Healing Arts Press now brings you an updated and expanded *Whole Food Facts.* In addition to keeping you current with changes in the whole-foods marketplace, I have added new chapters on "Diets" and "Nutrients," including information on recommended intakes and food sources for vitamins and minerals.

Whole Food Facts takes the approach of answering your questions about whole foods in a clear and understandable manner, as if somebody were actually explaining what you want to know. It is a compendium—a mini-encyclopedia—telling you just enough about the foods to whet your inquisitive appetite.

Learning is a lifelong process, and eating nutritious foods is just one aspect of maintaining a healthy body. Exercise, relaxation, stress reduction, and having friends and fun are also important. *Whole Food Facts* is meant to help you learn about what you eat and make the best choices for personal well-being. Stay tuned!

EVELYN ROEHL

DAIRY PRODUCTS

What are they?

Dairy products are foods derived from the milk of cows and goats or, less commonly, from mares, sheep, buffalo, and camels. Many North Americans consume fresh milk, ice cream, cheese, yogurt, or butter as a daily part of their diets.

Fluid cow's milk is a whitish, translucent beverage with a slightly sweet taste. Present in the liquid are fat, carbohydrates, protein, and water. If it is allowed to stand in a container for several hours, the fat of *raw* or *unhomogenized milk* will rise to the surface. This is the cream. Whole milk has a minimum of 3.25 percent milkfat. Skim milk has had the cream skimmed off and contains little or no fat.

Cream can be whipped for a dessert topping, but if it is whipped long enough it will become *butter,* a semisolid fat, and *buttermilk,* a watery liquid. (See page 21 for more details on butter.)

The carbohydrate, or sugar, in milk is called *lactose.* It is 15 percent as sweet as white sugar *(sucrose).* Milk or cream that is allowed to ripen or that has special bacterial cultures added becomes sour or tart. This is the result of bacteria converting the lactose to lactic acid. *Yogurt, cultured buttermilk,* and *sour cream* are dairy products with a high lactic acid content. A cultured dairy beverage that has undergone an acid and alcoholic (yeast) fermentation is called *kefir.*

Milk that has some of the water removed is called *evaporated milk. Sweetened condensed milk* is evaporated milk with sugar added. When milk has nearly all of its water removed, it becomes *dry milk powder.*

The main protein in milk, casein, can be separated from the liquid by heating milk at a low temperature until a surface layer forms. With the addition of a coagulant (such as rennet or lactic acid), the casein will form a curd, which then becomes *cheese.* The liquid that remains after curds form is called *whey.*

How do I use them?

Drink, spoon, or slice dairy products. They can be eaten alone or with other foods.

Milk is consumed as a beverage and as an ingredient of baked goods, soups, and other foods. Cheese is eaten in sandwiches, as a topping for casseroles, or plain with crackers. Sour cream dips are tasty with vegetables or chips. Yogurt blended with fruits or other sweeteners becomes a refreshing milkshakelike drink called a smoothie. Ice cream can be eaten plain, with special toppings, or as a garnish on pies.

You can substitute dairy products in some recipes. Instead of ricotta, use cottage cheese. Buttermilk or sour milk can be replaced by fresh milk to which a small amount of vinegar or baking soda has been added (1 teaspoon per pint of milk), respectively. No sour cream? Try using plain yogurt with or without cream cheese. You can whip instant dry milk powder and ice water as you would whipping cream for a low-fat dessert topping.

Dairy products are highly susceptible to contamination by bacteria that can cause foodborne illnesses, so be sure to handle the products with clean utensils and washed hands. Heating raw milk to 145°F for 30 minutes, or 161°F for 30 seconds, then quickly cooling it to 40°F will kill or prevent the growth of unwelcome bacteria. This process is called pasteurization, named after the scientist Louis Pasteur, who discovered it.

How nutritious are they?

Dairy products are excellent sources of high-quality protein and calcium, a mineral necessary for strong teeth, bones, and muscles. Other minerals present in dairy products are phosphorus, potassium, magnesium, and sodium.

Vitamins A, B-complex, C, and D are found in dairy products. Fluid milk is often fortified with vitamins A and D. Pasteurization and exposure to ultraviolet light—from sunlight or fluorescent lights will reduce the amount of vitamin C.

All dairy products naturally contain fat. Butter, cheese, and cream are especially high in fat, most of which is saturated.

✦ Nutritive Value: Appendix, 1–91.

Lactose Intolerance

All dairy products supply carbohydrates. To be able to utilize these carbohydrates, the body must produce an enzyme called lactase, which breaks down the lactose (milk sugar) into two readily assimilable sugars, glucose and galactose. Some people—notably Native Americans and people of African and Asian descent—do not have this enzyme in their biochemical makeup, and so have a tendency to develop lactose intolerance. Consequently, the lactose does not break down in the small intestine but instead passes into the lower intestine where it can cause digestive upsets, cramps, or diarrhea.

Milk Allergy

Another potential problem is milk allergy. People who are sensitive to the milk proteins lactalbumin and lactoglobulin may have respiratory ailments such as sneezing, asthma, nasal congestion, and coughing; or digestive ailments such as diarrhea, colic, or vomiting. This allergy is believed to affect between 0.5 and 0.7 percent of the populace, although it is most prevalent in children, most of whom outgrow it by the age of six years.

BOVINE GROWTH HORMONE

In February of 1994, after the U.S. Food and Drug Administration granted its approval, a genetically engineered hormone was available for sale to dairy farmers. Recombinant bovine growth hormone (rBGH), also known as BST (bovine somatotropin) and by its commercial name Posilac, has the ability to increase the total milk production of cows by up to 20 percent. The rBGH hormone is also intended to increase the profits of its sole manufacturer, Monsanto Corporation of St. Louis, Missouri.

Dairy farmers and consumers have expressed concern about the unknown dangers of rBGH, and some have tried to stop the marketing of it. After the disasters of the 1960s and 1970s with the hormone diethylstilbestrol (DES), people feared adverse health effects that could be connected with consuming milk or meat products from rBGH-fed cattle. Due to the fact that many cows were slaughtered during the 1980s because of a glut of milk on the market, the present use of a milk-producing hormone seems absurd at best.

While conclusive results are not yet available, it appears that cows given rBGH have a slightly higher rate of illness and mortality than other cows. An estimated thirteen thousand farmers in the United States were using the hormone in early 1995, even though 80 percent of all U.S. consumers were opposed to this practice.

If you are concerned about consuming trace amounts of this recombinant drug, contact the companies that bottle or manufacture dairy products in your area to find out their policy on accepting milk from farmers who use rBGH.

How do I store them?

With the exception of dry milk powder and frozen foods, keep all dairy products refrigerated between 33 and 40°F to prevent spoilage or mold growth. Dry milk powder will keep in the cupboard if stored in a tightly sealed container away from light and excess moisture. Ice cream, ice milk, and frozen yogurt should be kept in the freezer at 0°F until ready to use.

Because of their high perishability, fresh milk products should be used within a week after purchase. Cultured, aged, or frozen dairy foods will keep for two weeks or longer under proper storage conditions.

CHEESE

What is it?

There are between 1,200 and 2,000 different cheeses known throughout the world, from the soft fresh curds of cottage cheese to the hard-ripened blocks of Parmesan. All of them have one thing in common: milk.

The use of cheese dates back to the time when, as the story goes, a traveler set out on a journey and put some milk in a common storage vessel of the day—a goat's stomach. A while later the traveler discovered that the milk had turned into curds and whey.

How is it made?

Cow's milk is typically used in making cheese, although goat, sheep, or buffalo milk is used in some countries. It is often pasteurized to kill any undesirable bacteria. Raw milk is used in cheese that is aged over sixty days.

Casein, the main protein in milk, separates and coagulates when milk is heated. This forms the curd. The liquid that remains after this separation is the whey. One hundred pounds of milk will yield 10 to 16 pounds of curds and 84 to 90 pounds of whey.

Coagulation

To cause the separation of curds and whey, heated milk is first inoculated with a starter. A lactic acid

PROCESSED CHEESE

Processed cheese is made by mixing different lots of natural cheese and an emulsifier, then heating the mixture to not less than 150°F, until it becomes plastic and free flowing. It is then poured into containers or molds.

Young cheese—less than 10 days old—is typically used for processed cheese. But sometimes natural cheese that does not meet retail standards or that has not sold by the expiration date is returned to the cheese plant to be incorporated in small amounts into processed cheese.

Emulsifiers are added to prevent fat separation and to help maintain desirable slicing and melting properties. Sodium citrate, disodium phosphate, guar gum, alginate, and carboxymethylcellulose are some of the emulsifiers used.

Sweeteners such as sugar and corn syrup are sometimes added, as well as herbs, spices, fruits, nuts, vegetables, or meat for flavoring. Processed cheese is often artificially colored and may have artificial flavor added, such as "hickory-smoked" cheese.

Nutritionally, processed cheese has less protein, vitamin A, calcium, and iron than natural cheese. It usually has a higher sodium content.

Processed cheese has a longer shelf life than natural cheese. That which has been heated or melted will keep longer than cold-pack cheese, however. Keep all cheese refrigerated.

culture is used for fresh cheeses, as it is for making yogurt and cultured buttermilk. For most aged cheeses, milk is ripened with a culture, then inoculated with an enzyme called rennet. True rennet is the dry remains of the fourth stomach of slaughtered suckling calves or the stomachs of sheep or pigs (called pepsin). Microbial rennet (vegetable rennet) is derived from laboratory-synthesized cultured molds. Cheese can also be coagulated with lemon juice, nettles, wild artichokes, or thistleheads. If pasteurized milk is used, calcium chloride is also added to enhance curd formation. Pasteurization causes the natural calcium in milk

Processed cheese was developed in the United States, where it is most widely consumed. There are five different types:

Pasteurized process cheese—Cheddar, Colby, Swiss, and/or expired cheeses are heated to stop the natural aging, then blended. Water and dry whey can also be added. Except for American cheese (which is always a pasteurized process product), labels will list the types of cheeses used in pasteurized process cheese. If it has an artificial color, the label need not specify it. The product has a minimum of 47 percent fat.

Pasteurized process cheese food—Same as above, except there is more liquid added, such as milk, cream, or whey. Artificial color, if it is present, will be listed among the other ingredients on the label. Cheese food must have a minimum of 51 percent cheese by weight, a minimum of 23 percent fat, and a maximum moisture content of 44 percent.

Pasteurized process cheese spread—Also has more liquid than the above—more than 44 percent but not exceeding 60 percent moisture content. A water-retaining stabilizer such as alginate, guar gum, or gum tragacanth is usually added, but not more than 0.8 percent by weight. It has a minimum of 20 percent fat. The label will list any artificial color or flavor.

Cold pack cheese and cheese food—Blends of cheese that were made from pasteurized milk. They are mixed cold, without heating. The moisture and fat contents are about the same as for pasteurized process cheese and pasteurized process cheese food. Any artificial color or flavor must be listed on the label. This type of cheese is sometimes called *club cheese* or *comminuted cheese.*

Imitation cheese—It looks like cheese, smells cheesy, melts like cheese, and may even taste like it. But in an effort to save money (and make money), food manufacturers have produced imitation cheeses.

There are several types of imitation cheese on the market. Some are made with dairy by-products (particularly casein, the protein in milk), emulsifiers, enzymes, and artificial flavorings and colors. These are frequently used in frozen pizzas and may not be noted on the labels. Other imitation cheeses are made from soybean derivatives, such as tofu and soy protein, or from almonds. These soy or nut cheeses often contain casein and may claim to be made of all-natural ingredients. They may have a denser, more rubbery texture than real cheese and may also taste rubbery or overly salty.

Imitation cheeses are highly processed products, so be sure to read the labels carefully and be aware of the deceptive labeling that may be found on frozen pizza packages.

to be bound, whereas free calcium is needed for curd formation.

Developing the Cheese

Once the curd forms, the processes used thereafter will determine the type of cheese. These processes include how the curd is cut, how it is treated in the whey and after the whey is drained, and how it is ripened. Ripening techniques include control of temperature and humidity, the appropriate storage time for aged cheeses, and the addition of mold—either injected as in blue cheese or applied to the outside (surface ripened) as in Limburger.

Cheese that is artificially colored usually contains annatto, an extract of a plant that grows in Mexico. It is considered to be a safe, natural vegetable coloring.

How do I use it?

Cheese has nearly as many uses as there are varieties—for sandwiches, cakes, soufflés, quiches . . . you name it.

Delicious appetizer cheese balls can be made with a blend of cheddar, blue, and cream cheese rolled in

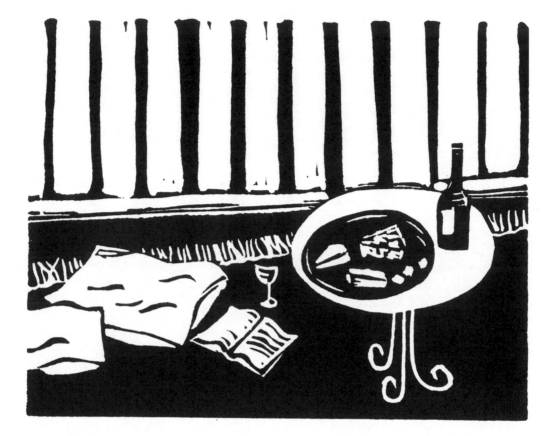

chopped nuts or parsley flakes. With or without crackers, this spread is fine fare for holidays.

Mozzarella and Parmesan are popular on pizza, but have you tried aged brick, feta, or caraway cheddar? They melt their flavor right into the sauce. Caramel-like Gjetôst will delight the tastebuds of children.

When melting cheese for sauce, be sure to use low heat or a double boiler to prevent scorching. Heat it only long enough to melt it. Excessive or prolonged heat may cause it to separate or become stringy and plastic. It melts faster if it is grated, shredded, or cut into small pieces. Use wooden utensils, and stir in only one direction.

For the best flavor, serve cheese (except fresh types such as cottage and cream cheese) at room temperature or cooler—about 55°F. Remember to remove it from the refrigerator 30 to 60 minutes before serving—2 hours for Camembert, Brie, or

other soft cheeses. Long exposure to warm temperatures, however, can cause the cheese to sweat and become rubbery. Do not cut or slice the cheese in advance, as the pieces may dry out.

How nutritious is it?

Cheese is a very good source of protein and is even better when it is eaten with grain proteins such as bread, crackers, and pasta, or with beans or nuts and seeds.

Cheese is 20 to 50 percent milkfat depending on the type. Of that, about 40 percent is saturated and 60 percent is unsaturated fatty acids. Cheese is high in calories.

The cheesemaking process causes the loss of most B-complex vitamins. It also converts the lactose (milk sugar) to lactic acid, so people who are lactose intolerant can eat cheese.

There is an ample supply of vitamin A, calcium,

phosphorus, and potassium in cheese. Most types are also high in sodium, due to the salt used for curing and flavoring. Salt and lactic acid act as preservatives in natural cheese. This is why low-salt or no-salt cheese is more susceptible to mold.

✦ Nutritive Value: Appendix, 1–26.

How do I store it?
Cheese keeps best at 35 to 40°F, and at a relative humidity of 70 to 80 percent. Excessive heat and moisture can enhance mold growth.

If your cheese is moldy, simply cut the mold off. Mold can be prevented by sponging the surfaces with a salt and water solution.

If the cheese has dried out or has become hard, you can still grate or crumble it and use it in cooking and baking. A quarter pound of cheese yields 1 cup of grated or shredded cheese. Dryness can be prevented by buttering the surfaces or keeping the cheese tightly wrapped. Crumbly cheese has a tendency to dry out. This can be prevented by drawing the flat blade of a knife across the cut surface of the cheese.

Freezing cheese is possible but not usually recommended because the texture can become mealy, pebbly, or rough. For best results, cut the cheese into half-pound pieces (or less) no more than a half-inch thick. Tightly wrap them in plastic film, then in aluminum foil, and seal the seams with tape. Freeze the pieces individually—not piled up—at a constant 0°F or below, until the pieces are frozen solid. You can then stack them, and they will keep for up to six months. Be sure to thaw them slowly in the refrigerator (not at room temperature) before using.

Where does it come from?
Of the many cheese varieties made in the world, about four hundred are from France. The vast majority of other types were developed in Italy, Switzerland, England, and other European countries. The cheeses made in North America are mostly attempts to duplicate "Old World" cheeses. Only four natural cheeses were developed in the United States: cream cheese, Monterey Jack (from Monterey County, California), Colby (from Colby, Wisconsin), and brick (another Wisconsin discovery).

The consumption of cheese in the United States has steadily increased, from sixteen pounds per person in 1977 to twenty-six pounds per person in 1993.

CREAM

What is it?
Nothing makes an upside-down cake quite so tantalizing as a plump dollop of whipped cream.

Cream is the part of milk that will rise to the top if the milk is not homogenized. There are a number of cream products available, mostly differentiated by the amount of fat present:

Sweet cream is fresh and has a subtly sweet taste. Because of its high perishability, sweet cream is available only in specialty markets or direct from dairies.

Half-and-half is homogenized with milk to prevent cream separation. It contains from 10 to 12 percent milkfat.

Light cream (also called *table cream* or *coffee cream*) is used in baking or cooking and as a beverage. The milkfat is 18 to 30 percent.

Light whipping cream has 30 to 36 percent fat content.

Heavy whipping cream has a minimum of 36 percent milkfat. It is sometimes referred to as pastry cream or double cream.

The fluid types of cream available in retail stores are pasteurized (heated to at least 161°F for 30 seconds) to destroy germs and undesirable bacteria. Whipping cream is often ultra-pasteurized, a process whereby the cream is heated to 200–210°F for several seconds. Ultra-pasteurized cream has a shelf life of thirty to forty days, compared to regular pasteurized cream, which has a shelf life of ten to twenty days. There is no nutritional difference between the two, but the flavor of ultra-pasteurized cream may be altered and the product may not whip as well as regular whipping cream.

To make it appear richer and creamier, cream is sometimes homogenized. It may also contain a thickening agent such as xanthan gum. Another technique used to increase the viscosity of cream is to keep it cooled to 40°F for one or two days after its arrival at the creamery and before it is processed or packaged.

Sour cream is a food similar to yogurt, although it is made from cream instead of milk. To make it, sweet cream with 18 to 20 percent milkfat is pasteurized at 180°F for 30 minutes, then slightly cooled and homogenized. When the cream cools to 70°F, it is mixed with a lactic acid culture and incubated for 12 to 14 hours—until a 0.6 percent level of acidity is reached. Stabilizers such as sodium alginate, carrageenan, locust bean gum, or gelatin are sometimes added to make the product thick and smooth.

How do I use it?

Fluid cream is a rich beverage that can be poured lightly on a bowl of fresh strawberries or sliced peaches, or on dry cereal. It gives cream of potato soup the essence to live up to its name.

In baking, you can add cream to cakes, pies, and casseroles for extra richness and flavor. Stove-top confections are smooth when cream is added to the recipe.

Whipped cream is a quick and easy dessert topping to make. If you want 2 cups of whipped cream, use 1 cup of cream, preferably more than a day old. Make sure you use whipping cream (that which contains at least 30 percent fat), otherwise it may not whip. Chill the bowl and beaters for about one-half hour, then take them out and pour the cream into the bowl. Whip it at the highest speed on your mixer or as fast as you can by hand until peaks form. Add sweetener and/or vanilla extract to taste, and whip again until blended. Use honey or maple syrup for the sweetener if you wish. Be sure not to over whip the cream; if you do it will harden and begin turning to butter.

Although you can keep whipped cream refrigerated for up to an hour, it is best to add the sweetener right before serving so the mixture will not fall. For a less fattening dairy topping, try instant milk powder and ice water (see page 17 for directions).

Ice cream fanciers will enjoy making this dessert at home, using fresh sweet cream and their favorite fruits or flavorings. A special ice cream freezer or machine is needed for most recipes.

Butter can be made at home: simply whip cream until it becomes thick and separates into butter and

NONDAIRY CREAMERS AND TOPPINGS

Today, artificial coffee "whiteners" and synthetic dessert toppings are sometimes substituted for cream.

Coffee creamers or whiteners are concoctions of coconut oil, palm kernel oil, or other highly saturated and hydrogenated vegetable oils, plus a list of chemicals to flavor and control the texture or effect of the whitener. Both liquid and powdered forms of artificial creamers are sold. Some contain casein and lactose—the protein and sugar of milk, respectively—so they are undesirable for people who are allergic to or must avoid dairy products.

Nondairy whipped toppings are made of the same substances as coffee whiteners, but they contain more corn syrup solids or other sweeteners. Those in aerosol cans are pressurized with propellants such as nitrous oxide. The products are also available in plastic bowls and in powdered form, to which water must be added.

Because these imitation products are made of vegetable oils with a higher saturation level than milk or cream (coconut oil and palm kernel oil are more than 80 percent saturated fats), they are not suitable substitutes for people who must avoid saturated fats.

a watery liquid (buttermilk). Then squeeze out as much of the buttermilk as you can with the back of a spoon, and add a small amount of salt if desired.

Sour cream is favored as a topping for baked potatoes. You can make a delicious dip for parties by mixing herbs and seasonings with sour cream. For a slightly tangy taste in cakes and breads, use sour cream instead of milk.

How nutritious is it?

Cream is high in fat, so it provides lots of calories. The fat is about two-thirds saturated and one-third unsaturated.

There is a high amount of vitamin A present in cream, as well as small amounts of B-complex vitamins.

Like other dairy products, cream is high in calcium, phosphorus, potassium, and sodium. It provides some protein.

✦ Nutritive Value: Appendix, 27–47.

How do I store it?

Cream should be refrigerated. It will stay sweet for about a week. Cream that has soured can still be used in baked goods. Commercial sour cream will keep for up to two weeks under refrigeration. If watery whey appears on the surface, simply stir it back in.

FROZEN DAIRY PRODUCTS

What are they?

Ice cream is the favorite dessert of people in the United States—especially vanilla or vanilla mixed with other flavors. Chocolate- and strawberry-flavored ice creams follow in popularity. The average annual consumption of ice cream per person in the United States is over fifteen quarts; in Canada it is over thirteen quarts.

Frozen dairy products also include ice milk, sherbet, popsiclelike ice cream bars, and frozen yogurt. They are all made from cream, milk or milk products, water, sweeteners, flavorings, coloring, stabilizers, and emulsifiers.

Imitation ice cream, usually called *mellorine,* is also manufactured with vegetable fat and nonfat milk solids rather than milkfat derived from cream or other milk products.

How are they made?

First, the liquid ingredients (milk and cream) are mixed with the dry at 110°F; then the mixture is pasteurized and homogenized. After being cooled to 23°F, it is whipped to incorporate air, which increases its volume—up to 150 percent in hard ice cream, or 40 to 80 percent in soft ice cream used in cone dispensers. This is called the overrun. Ice cream is then frozen at –20° to –50°F.

Ice milk is made in the same manner, except the fat content is 2 to 7 percent instead of the legally required 10 percent for ice cream. The levels of sugar and flavoring are higher in ice milk, however, to compensate for the difference. The overrun is about 90 percent.

Sherbet (also called sorbet) is made mostly of water and sweetener, and it has only a small amount of milk or milk solids. Citric acid or other acids, fruit flavoring, and coloring additives are present in small amounts. Sherbet has an overrun of 30 to 45 percent.

Ice cream bars are made the same way as ice cream, although chocolate coatings or cookielike crackers (for ice cream sandwiches) are added after the mix is frozen or partially frozen.

Frozen yogurt is made with milk that has been fermented with a lactic acid culture. It is less creamy, tastes slightly tart, and usually contains less fat and calories than ice cream.

How do I use them?

Commercial frozen dairy products are quick and easy desserts that just need to be scooped into a dish or cone and eaten. Children find it fun to create new flavors by adding syrups, fruits, nuts, or cookies.

Cold, sweet beverages such as milkshakes and floats certainly satisfy the thirsty sweet tooth on hot summer days.

An intriguing dessert called Baked Alaska is made by covering a block of frozen ice cream with whipped

FLAVORINGS AND COLORINGS

About 1,200 different chemicals can be used in the manufacture of ice cream and related products for emulsifying, stabilizing, flavoring, and coloring. The majority of these chemicals are for flavoring.

If the ice cream has natural flavoring, the label will simply state: "vanilla," "strawberry," and so forth. If it contains mostly natural but some artificial flavoring, the label will read "vanilla (or other) flavored." If it contains both natural and artificial flavoring and there is more artificial, or if all the flavoring is artificial, the label will say "artificially flavored." Products must also list if there is any artificial coloring added. At this time the specific flavoring and coloring chemicals do not have to be listed on products sold in the United States, although some manufacturers are voluntarily listing them.

One flavor that generally needs no artificial color or flavor is chocolate because the cocoa provides enough brown color and flavor. However, some of the chocolate ice cream on the market was formerly a light-colored ice cream that did not sell by the expiration date or that began to spoil. This old or inferior ice cream is returned to the plant to be reworked into chocolate ice cream.

Because so many different chemicals can be found in frozen dairy products, they should be avoided by people who are sensitive to additives or by those who are concerned about potential risks from consuming unknown substances.

egg whites, then baking it. Amazingly, the egg whites act as insulation, and the meringue turns brown but the ice cream stays frozen instead of melting.

If you want ice cream and frozen yogurt with really natural flavor, try making them at home in a hand-cranked or electric ice cream churn. Mix real cream, yogurt, or milk; eggs; honey or other sweetener; ripe sliced or pureed fruits; and chopped nuts in the ice cream vat. Keep mixing until it is thick. Be sure to keep plenty of ice cubes and salt in the bucket surrounding the vat.

How nutritious are they?

Ice cream is high in carbohydrates (sugar) and fat, so it contains a lot of calories. Protein is also present. Vitamin A, calcium, phosphorus, potassium, and sodium are found in high amounts. Soft ice cream usually contains less sugar than hard ice cream.

Ice milk is lower in fat and calories but provides essentially the same level of other nutrients as ice cream. Sherbet is nearly as high in calories as ice cream but has lower levels of most other nutrients.

Don't be misled by so-called all-natural ice creams—they usually contain sugar, emulsifiers, and

stabilizers, and they aren't necessarily any better or worse than other commercial ice creams. They may be even higher in fat and cost considerably more than other commercial brands.

✦ Nutritive Value: Appendix, 77–86.

How do I store them?

Always keep frozen dairy products in the coldest part of your freezer. Most refrigerator freezers are about 0°F, which will keep ice cream hard and usable for about a week. If stored below 0°F, ice cream and other frozen dairy products will keep for a month or more.

For easier serving, move the ice cream or ice milk from the freezer to the refrigerator 10 to 20 minutes prior to scooping it out.

Ice Cream Substitutes

In the last several years many nondairy frozen desserts have hit the market. Instead of milk, the new products contain soybean derivatives or rice that has been specially treated.

The soybean-derived frozen desserts contain either soy milk, made by blending soaked soybeans and water and then cooking the mixture, or tofu, a bean curd made from soy milk. Other ingredients include water, fructose or other sweeteners, vegetable oil, and flavorings. Some companies, trying to profit from the tofu ice cream trend, use little or no tofu, so be sure to read package labels carefully.

The rice-based frozen desserts are made with rice cultured with koji, a grain inoculated with *Aspergillus oryzae*. This culture produces enzymes that break down the protein and starches and enhance the sweetness of the rice. Additional sweeteners, if any, are fruits used for flavors or maple syrup. Other ingredients include water, vegetable oil, lecithin, carob bean or guar gum, carrageenan, and salt.

Nondairy frozen desserts are usually lower in calories than dairy-based desserts and have no cholesterol. The prices are comparable to regular ice cream.

MILK

What is it?

Milk is a liquid secreted from mammary glands to provide nourishment for young animals. Mother's milk is nature's perfect—and often the only—food for young babies, containing all the nutrients necessary for infants until about age six months. Baby calves and kid goats likewise need their mothers' milk for survival.

It is the milk of cows—and to a lesser extent goats—that becomes a beverage and the source of all other dairy products for human consumption in North America.

Types of Milk

Raw whole milk is that which comes straight from the cow or nanny goat. For the most part consumers

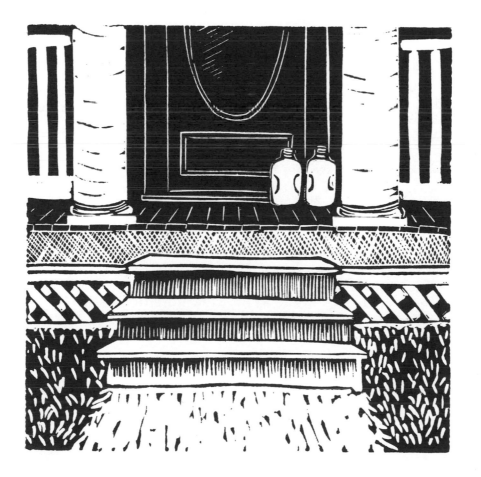

are unable or are not allowed to purchase raw milk today. The two biggest milk-producing states, Wisconsin and Minnesota, prohibit the sale of raw milk except directly by the producers from their farms. In other areas people may obtain raw milk produced by a certified milk dairy, of which there are only a few in the United States. Certified milk dairies must meet stringent standards of sanitation; the milk must have a bacteria count of less than 10,000 colonies per milliliter. (Pasteurized milk can be sold with up to 30,000 colonies of bacteria per milliliter.) Raw milk is considered to be a carrier of several diseases, including tuberculosis.

To kill or stop the growth of bacteria, milk is pasteurized by heating it to 145°F for 30 minutes or to 161°F for 15 seconds. It must be quickly cooled to 40°F after this heating process. Pasteurized milk has a few days' longer shelf life than raw milk.

Whole milk, as marketed, has a minimum fat content of 3.25 percent, which gives the beverage a creamier flavor. Both 2% and 1% milk have a reduced fat content—to 2 percent and 1 percent respectively. Skim milk contains virtually no fat (the fat is skimmed off) and is more watery than whole milk.

Because milkfat (cream) rises to the surface of milk when it is allowed to stand for several hours, a technique called *homogenization* was developed. Milk is forced through very small openings at high pressure, which causes the fat globules to become very small and dispersed throughout the milk. This prevents the fat from floating to the top. Goat's milk does not need to be homogenized, as the fat globules are naturally small and dispersed.

Evaporated milk is made by evaporating off 60 percent of the water in whole milk. It takes about 2¼ pounds of milk to make 1 pound of evaporated milk. The United States federal standard requires evaporated milk to be not less than 7.9 percent milkfat and not less than 25.9 percent milk solids.

Sweetened condensed milk is basically evaporated milk that has sugar added. Between 40 and 45 percent of the product is sugar. The federal standard requires sweetened condensed milk to be not less than 8.5 percent milkfat and not less than 28 percent milk solids.

Both evaporated and sweetened condensed milk may contain stabilizers, such as sodium citrate, sodium bicarbonate, carrageenan, and calcium chloride. The products are sealed in cans and are then sterilized to prevent bacterial spoilage and to extend shelf life.

Two other popular milks are also manufactured. Chocolate-flavored milk is whole or skim milk with about 1 percent cocoa and 5 to 7 percent sweetener added. To prevent cocoa from settling, a stabilizer such as sodium alginate or vegetable gum is added. *Malted milk* is a dried product made by mixing ground barley malt and whole milk, then drying it to 3.5 percent moisture content.

How do I use it?

Milk is typically consumed as a beverage, poured over dry cereals, and used in cooking and baking. It is a major ingredient in puddings, cream soups, and eggnog. Milk makes cookies, breads, and cakes moist and helps form soft crusts.

To prevent curdling or the formation of scum during cooking, use low heat. It is helpful to mix milk with a small amount of already cooking soup stock or gravy in a separate bowl before adding it to the mixture.

You can reconstitute evaporated milk by adding an equal amount of water. Use it as a replacement for fresh milk. At full strength, evaporated milk is a rich and creamy ingredient for casseroles, pies, cookies, and confections. Try it instead of cream in coffee and coleslaw.

Sweetened condensed milk is favored for rich desserts, icings, and candy. Remember to use less sweetener in recipes when substituting this milk product for evaporated milk.

How nutritious is it?

Milk contains high-quality protein and is deficient in only one amino acid, methionine. It is high in the amino acid lysine, which makes it an excellent food for complementing grains, flours, nuts, and seeds (see Protein Complementarity, pages 71, 112).

Lactose, the carbohydrate in milk, is found only in dairy products. The body breaks lactose into two sugars: glucose and galactose. These can then be utilized by the body. However, certain people cannot digest this sugar because they lack a digestive enzyme called lactase. They can become ill if they consume too much milk.

Whole milk provides fat, of which 60 to 70 percent is saturated and 30 to 40 percent unsaturated. Fat is necessary, among other reasons, for the body to utilize vitamins A, D, E, and K, which are also present in milk. Milk also offers B-complex vitamins and vitamin C.

Calcium, magnesium, phosphorus, potassium, and sodium are abundant in milk. Only a small amount of iron is present.

Raw milk has a high nutritive value, since nothing is taken out or destroyed by heat. Pasteurized, evaporated, and sweetened condensed milks have lower quantities of vitamin C, thiamine (B_1), and B_{12}. The heating process for these types of milk also causes 10 to 20 percent of the calcium to be bound and therefore less available to the body.

Pasteurized and evaporated milks are often fortified with vitamins A and D. In Canada, evaporated milk is also enriched with vitamin C. The fortification with vitamins A and D is to provide these nutrients in the diet as it has been thought that many people do not receive adequate amounts. These vitamins are not destroyed by heat but are fat soluble—fat must be present for these vitamins to be utilized by the body—so you may have to consume other foods that contain fat if you drink lowfat and skim milks. This is generally not a problem for North Americans, however.

Lacto-vegetarians who abstain from fish products might be interested to know that the vitamin D added to milk is usually obtained from fish oil. If this is of concern to you, contact the plant from which your milk comes to find out exactly what type of vitamin D is added.

✦ Nutritive Value: Appendix, 49–76.

How do I store it?

Fluid milk should always be refrigerated and used within a week. Raw milk is particularly susceptible to spoilage, so be sure to use it before it sours.

Canned milk—evaporated and sweetened condensed—will keep for a year or longer if stored in a cool, dry place. To prevent jellying or thickening, turn cans of evaporated milk upside down every two months or so.

CULTURED MILKS
Acidophilus Milk

Acidophilus milk is made by inoculating sterilized low-fat milk with *Lactobacillus acidophilus* culture. It tastes similar to whole milk and is thought to be beneficial for people with digestive problems. Reportedly, *L. acidophilus,* unlike other bacteria, is implanted in the intestine, where it creates an acid condition and destroys putrefactive bacteria. Research on its claims is still being conducted.

Acidophilus milk has essentially the same nutrients as yogurt or lowfat milk. Like other dairy products, keep it refrigerated. Use it within a week.

Cultured Buttermilk

Cultured buttermilk, a thick, pourable beverage, is *not* made from the liquid left over from butter making (true buttermilk). Instead, pasteurized skim milk is used—often that which has gone out-of-date and is reclaimed from retail stores.

The milk is inoculated with a lactic acid culture and is incubated at 70°F until a .7 to .9 percent level of acidity is reached. Cultured buttermilk may also have butter granules added for simulated authenticity. Stabilizers may be added to prevent separation and to keep it thick.

You can use buttermilk in pancakes and baked goods or as a beverage. For convenience, use buttermilk powder. Buttermilk powder is made in a manner similar to dry milk powder.

Buttermilk provides protein, carbohydrates, and a small amount of fat. Vitamins A, B-complex (including B_{12}), and C are present in fair amounts. The minerals calcium, phosphorus, potassium, and sodium are quite high in buttermilk.

Store liquid buttermilk in the refrigerator where it will keep for a week or so. Use older buttermilk for baking rather than as a beverage. Buttermilk powder should be kept in a tightly covered container in a dry place.

Kefir

Kefir (pronounced **kee**-*fur*) is a delicious, creamy, yogurtlike drink made by introducing special fermenting organisms called kefir grains to milk. These gelatinous particles consist of lactic acid cultures *(Streptococcus lactis* and *Lactobacillus bulgaricus, L. acidophilus,* and *L. caucasicus)* and special yeasts that cause the product to undergo both an acid and alcoholic fermentation. It is the creation of alcohol/carbon dioxide gas that causes the bubbly effervescence of kefir.

Plain kefir has a tart taste similar to that of plain yogurt. Flavored kefir is also available, including maple, strawberry, pineapple, and other fruit flavors.

Use kefir as a drink or in creamed soups, pancakes, casseroles, desserts, pies, and salad dressings. To make it at home, heat a quart of milk until scalding (180°F), then pour the milk into a hot, sterilized jar with a lid. Allow the milk to cool to room temperature (70 to 75°F) and add a packet of kefir grains or 2 tablespoons plain kefir as a starter culture. Put the sterilized lid on and wrap the jar in a large towel or blanket. After about 18 hours, a curd will form. Stir it to make a smooth product.

Kefir provides protein, fat, carbohydrates, B-complex vitamins, calcium, and other minerals. Flavored kefir usually has sweetener added, which increases the amount of carbohydrates and calories.

Because of its high perishability, kefir should be used within a week after purchase. Out-of-date kefir becomes too sour and gaseous to be consumed as a beverage, but it can be added to the batter of baked goods or pancakes.

DRY MILK

What is it?

Milk that has had almost all of the water removed becomes a powder. Most of the time the fat is also removed, thus resulting in nonfat dry milk.

Initially, the milk is condensed to about 35 per-cent solids, then prewarmed to 190 to 200°F for high-heat powder, or not over 170°F for low-heat powder.

How is it made?

Two main methods are used to dry milk. One method is roller or drum drying, for which the condensed and prewarmed milk is piped to a container next to a drum or trough formed by two rollers that are steam-heated at 200 to 300°F. As the drums rotate, milk sticks to the surface, and upon a complete revolution the water in the milk will have evaporated, leaving dry milk solids. The milk solids are mechanically scraped off the drums and ground into a powder. This milk is called high-heat nonfat dry milk. Most of the high-heat dry milk is used by bakeries and food manufacturers. It will have lost over 30 percent of both the amino acid lysine and vitamin B_6.

The other common drying method is spray drying. Condensed and prewarmed milk is sprayed as a mist into a heated dryer with an air temperature of up to 350°F for nonfat milk and 150°F for whole milk. (The milk itself stays at 110 to 120°F.) The heated air removes the moisture, thus allowing milk particles to settle to the bottom of the dryer. This powdered milk is called low-heat nonfat dry milk. It is usually marketed to consumers or is added to ice cream or other dairy products.

How do I use it?

Instant nonfat dry milk has undergone an additional step after being spray dried. The particles are moistened by steam and are agitated, causing them to form clusters. The clusters are then dried to 3.5 percent moisture, followed by sifting or pelletizing to a uniform size, which results in a flaky product. This process enables the dry milk to dissolve instantly in water.

Instant dry milk can be used as a nutritious addition to breads, cookies, soups, and desserts. Mix it with granola for a camping trip, then add water when you are ready to eat. As a replacement for fresh milk, use about 6 tablespoons instant dry milk per cup of water, or about $1^1/_2$ cups dry milk and $3^1/_2$ cups water to make a quart.

Instant dry milk can also be whipped into a dessert topping. Mix equal amounts of dry milk and ice water in a chilled bowl and beat until foamy. Add a small amount of sweetener, vanilla extract, and lemon juice according to taste, and beat until soft peaks form. Serve immediately or chill for up to 1 hour.

Noninstant dry milk is more economical to use than instant dry milk, but it does not readily dissolve in water and therefore has limited uses. It is an excellent food for fortifying pancakes, baked goods, omelettes, and sauces. To reconstitute noninstant dry milk, use about 3 tablespoons per cup of water, or 1 part noninstant dry milk to 4 parts water, and blend or shake vigorously. Agitate it long enough—or use a blender— to get the lumps out. If you are cooking with it, use low heat and stir it often to prevent scorching.

How nutritious is it?

Nonfat spray-dried milk is nutritionally comparable to skim milk. It provides protein, carbohydrates, minerals, and some B-complex vitamins. For proper utilization of calcium, eat reconstituted nonfat dry milk with a food that contains fat.

How do I store it?

If tightly sealed, dried milk can be stored for six months at room temperature, and up to two years if it is refrigerated at 40°F. Be sure to keep it in a moisture-proof container and away from light. Too much moisture will cause it to become lumpy and can encourage the growth of harmful bacteria.

YOGURT

What is it?

Yogurt is milk to which certain strains of bacteria have been added—notably *L. bulgaricus* and *Streptococcus thermophilus,* or *L. acidophilus*—and held at a constant temperature of 100 to 120°F for 3 or more hours. These bacteria cultures convert the lactose (milk sugar) to lactic acid, which causes the milk to become tart and to thicken.

The bacteria cultures used in yogurt making are all live during the incubation process. They can become inactive at temperatures of less than 90°F. If the yogurt is pasteurized after incubation (heated to 145°F or higher), the bacteria culture will be dead.

Plain yogurt can be made from whole milk, which has at least 3.25 percent milkfat, or from skim milk, which has little or no fat. It is usually slightly sour tasting and unsweetened. Yogurt is also available sweetened with sugar, honey, or fruit preserves, and flavored with nuts or other flavorings. *Natural*

HOW TO MAKE YOGURT

To make a quart of yogurt, use:
　　1 quart fluid milk
　　(heat raw milk to 185°F to kill
　　any undesirable bacteria)
or
　　3½ cups warm water (100–
　　110°F) blended with
　　2½ cups instant nonfat dry milk

Mix in:
　　1–2 tablespoons honey
　　1 packet yogurt culture or
　　3 tablespoons fresh, plain
　　　yogurt

Mix all ingredients by hand or with a blender until smooth. Pour into clean, prewarmed containers, then put them in your yogurt maker or other device where a constant temperature (about 105°F) can be maintained (see below).

After 4 hours or so, check containers by gently tipping them to see if the yogurt is thick. If not, let it sit a bit longer. If it is, put it in the refrigerator.

Flavored yogurt—Before pouring the milk into the containers, add fruit, nuts, maple syrup, or other foods and flavorings. Incubate as above.

Tips on Making Yogurt

If you use plain yogurt as the starter culture, remember that the yogurt you make will have similar characteristics (tart, thick, and so forth). The older the yogurt is, the more tart it will be. Do not use yogurt that is more than a week old.

Don't bump or jiggle the yogurt while it is incubating, as that may cause it to become lumpy or watery, or cause it to not thicken. The longer you incubate the yogurt, the thicker it becomes. If there is whey at the top, either too much yogurt starter was used or it was incubated too long.

Use clean utensils and containers. It helps to prewarm everything—the spoons (not wooden), bowls, and especially the glass jars or containers in which the yogurt will incubate.

Incubating Devices

You can use a wide-mouth thermos bottle. You can also set sealed jars in large pots of hot water (a pressure cooker works well) wrapped in blankets or towels, or you can set jars in a bowl of hot water and put the bowl in a gas oven with the pilot light on.

yogurt will have fruit at the bottom of the cup, which you then stir into the yogurt. *Processed* or *Swiss-style yogurt* has the fruit mixed in and usually contains stabilizers to keep the yogurt thick and the fruit from settling.

Yogurt drink is similar to kefir (see page 16), although different bacterial cultures may be used, such as *L. bulgaricus* and *L. bifidus.* Yogurt drinks often contain fruit or fruit juice for flavoring. They commonly have thickening or stabilizing agents added, such as carob bean gum and pectin.

How do I use it?

Yogurt is ready to eat from the container. All you need is a spoon.

Plain or flavored yogurt can be mixed with dried fruits and nuts for a textured, chewy breakfast. Smoothies are refreshing and easy to make: Blend yogurt with fresh fruit or fruit juice, other sweeteners, and spices if you wish, for a thick, milkshakelike beverage.

For a sour cream substitute with about half the calories, try plain yogurt on baked potatoes, for salad dressings, and in dips with herbs and seasonings. Desserts can be topped with sweetened plain yogurt as a substitute for whipped cream.

Casseroles, cookies, and confections all can be made using yogurt instead of milk or other liquids. Experiment!

Frozen yogurt is a suitable replacement for ice cream or sherbet. Eat it in cones or scooped into a baked pie shell.

How nutritious is it?

Plain yogurt provides protein, fat, carbohydrates, calcium, phosphorus, potassium, vitamin A, vitamin C, and B-complex vitamins, including B_{12}. If it is made from commercial milk, it will also contain vitamin D.

Yogurt made with skim milk will have less fat and therefore fewer calories than that made from whole milk. Fruit-flavored and sweetened yogurts are higher in calories than plain yogurt.

Nutritional and medicinal claims about yogurt as a special food or healing agent are for the most part unproven. The bacteria strain *L. bulgaricus,* if it is live, reputedly aids in digestion, although a contrary theory is that the bacteria would die in the intestines from the acidity present there. *L. acidophilus* is also attributed to be a digestive aid that could, unlike *L. bulgaricus,* become implanted in the lower intestine and create an acid environment that would destroy putrefactive bacteria. Again, there is no conclusive evidence—and this culture is not widely used in commercial yogurt making. The claim that yogurt eaters live longer is also disputed.

♦ Nutritive Value: Appendix, 88–91.

How do I store it?

Keep yogurt refrigerated at 33 to 40°F, and use it within a week to ten days. It can still be eaten after the expiration date or after lengthy storage (over ten days), but it will have become very sour and would then be best to use in cooking or baking.

Where does it come from?

The use of yogurt dates back to early civilization, when people in what is now Greece, Turkey, and Bulgaria discovered that soured milk could be kept longer than fresh milk and that the tart taste was pleasantly palatable.

Yogurt has been popular in the Middle East and in Europe for centuries. It has many different names besides the Bulgarian term *yogurt;* it is known as *dahi* or *lassi* in India and *leben* in Lebanon, and also carries various spellings such as *yoghurt* and *youghurt.*

In North America yogurt has been known for about fifty years but became popular in the mid-1960s. It was the fastest growing food category in the United States during the mid-1970s.

FATS AND OILS

What are fats and oils?

Fats and oils are a necessary part of our diets. They conserve body heat, form certain hormones, and carry fat-soluble vitamins A, D, E, and K (vitamins that need fat or oil to be absorbed by the body) to all the cells of the body.

Our bodies need, on the average, at least one tablespoon of fat or oil per day. North Americans consume an average of eight tablespoons of fat or oil daily, and most of it is saturated fat.

When fats are eaten, they are broken down during digestion to fatty acids, which make up 95 percent of fats, and monoglycerides, which become glycerol. There are more than twenty different fatty acids, of which all but two can be manufactured by the body from sugars. These two, linoleic and linolenic, are called essential fatty acids. If linoleic acid is supplied in the diet, then linolenic acid can be synthesized from other substances.

What is saturation?

Fatty acids are defined as *saturated, monounsaturated,* or *polyunsaturated,* according to chemical composition.

A saturated fatty acid is composed of a complete carbon chain saturated with hydrogen atoms:

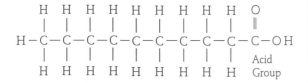

A fat or oil is called *saturated* if most of the fatty acids it contains are saturated. Saturated fats and oils are usually solid at room temperature. Some of the foods that contain saturated fats are lard, shortening, butter, meat, cheese, coconut oil, and palm oil.

Monounsaturated fatty acids are made of a carbon chain with one double bond, and there is room for more hydrogen atoms:

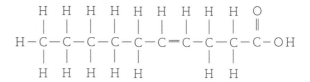

Polyunsaturated fatty acids are similar, except there are two or more double bonds and therefore room for many hydrogen atoms:

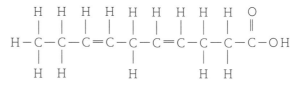

Monounsaturated and polyunsaturated fats and oils contain, respectively, mostly monounsaturated or polyunsaturated fatty acids. Some of the foods that contain polyunsaturated fats are oils extracted from safflower, sesame, and sunflower seeds, corn germ, soybeans, peanuts, and most nuts. Olive oil is a monounsaturated oil.

How do I use them?

Fats and oils are used for baking, cooking, frying, and sauteing. They are the main constituents of salad dressings and mayonnaise. Butter and margarine are often spread on breads and crackers.

Typical uses of the more common types of fats and oils are:

Butter—sauteing, baking, as a spread
Corn oil—baking, cooking
Margarine—baking, sauteing, as a spread

Olive oil—salad dressing, sauces

Peanut oil—popcorn, salad dressings, cooking, baking

Safflower oil—baking, sauteing, salad dressing, frying

Sesame oil—sauteing, salad dressing

Shortening—baking, frying, cooking

Soybean oil (unrefined)—baking

Soybean oil (refined)—baking, cooking, frying, sauteing

Sunflower oil—sauteing, baking

Besides these obvious uses, oil can be rubbed on the jackets of potatoes before baking to keep them tender. For easier and neater measurements of honey and sorghum, brush or rub a bit of oil on the measuring cups and spoons; this prevents the sweeteners from sticking to the utensils.

Most processed oils tend to be pale, clear, bland, and virtually odorless. Bland oils are favored by those who want certain flavors of foods (other than the oil) to come through.

Natural and unrefined oils, however, may contain a little sediment or cloudy material, which is made up of minerals, phosphatides, and other trace elements. They also have a distinct aroma and taste, which may seem strong at first if you are accustomed to refined oil. Unrefined corn oil, for example, has a pleasant corn smell.

Freshness and Taste

The quality of fats and oils is greatly affected by their freshness. Fats and oils become rancid (spoiled) when exposed to light, warmth, and air for long periods of time. Rancid fats and oils will usually smell and taste bad. Learn to identify such a smell and taste so you can avoid any fats and oils that are rancid—that is, if the product smells or tastes slightly bitter, acrid, or otherwise "off."

All fats and oils are subject to rancidity, though at different rates, depending on their type and the way they are processed. Unsaturated fats and oils will generally become rancid sooner than saturated fats and oils.

Most unrefined vegetable oils are rich in vitamin E, which acts as an antioxidant and natural preservative. The refining process destroys some of

the oil's natural vitamin E, and it can chemically alter the oil as well. Manufacturers of refined oils often extend their products' shelf life by adding preservatives such as BHA, BHT, and citric acid. See page 31 for more information on these additives.

How nutritious are they?

The nutritional value of fats and oils varies considerably, depending on the level of saturation, the degree of freshness, and the amount of processing or refining. Unsaturated, fresh, and unrefined fats and oils—when properly stored—are generally more nutritious than saturated and refined fats and oils.

Generally speaking, the more saturated a fat or oil is, the more likely it is to contribute to the buildup of fat and cholesterol deposits in the bloodstream. Studies have shown that many people who have a high intake of saturated fat have high levels of cholesterol in their blood—a condition frequently associated with heart disease and other arterial diseases. Most physicians agree that eating less saturated fat reduces the chance of developing arteriosclerosis. However, despite warnings by health professionals to reduce consumption of fats, people in the United States, on average, increased their consumption of all fats (butter, margarine, lard, shortening, and salad and cooking oils) from fifty to fifty-five pounds per year during the 1970s to the current annual rate of sixty to sixty-five pounds.

It is good to monitor the level and kind of fat intake in your diet. One suggested guideline is to reduce the amount of total fat to no more than three or four tablespoons a day. Do not eliminate solid fats, but do increase the ratio of unsaturated liquid fats to saturated solid fats. You can do this in several ways:

- Substitute liquid oils for butter, lard, and shortening
- Choose margarine made from mostly liquid (not hydrogenated) vegetable oil
- Eliminate or severely reduce your intake of deep-fat fried foods, as well as pies and pastries
- Replace pork, beef, and lamb with chicken, turkey, or fish

- Use lowfat milk, yogurt, and cheese instead of whole milk, full-fat yogurt, and full-fat cheese

✦ Nutritive Value: Appendix, 99–131, 465.

How do I store them?

Heat and oxygen promote rancidity, so the best place to store fats and oils is in a tightly closed container in your refrigerator. Dark or amber colored bottles will protect oil longer than clear glass bottles. Foods that contain natural oils—such as wheat germ, whole grain flours (especially corn and soy flours), and shelled raw nuts—should also be refrigerated.

Natural or unrefined oils will keep from four to six months or longer if stored properly. Refined and heavily processed oils will keep at least twice as long.

Did You Know . . .

Some of the major oil manufacturers have their oil packaged in hourglass-shaped bottles. This is to give the subtle suggestion of slenderness, to distract the consumer from the prevalent bias against fats or foods that might make people fat.

BUTTER

What is it?

Almost everyone is familiar with butter. It's nice to spread on toast, it's great for sauteing vegetables, and it makes wonderfully rich pastries and desserts.

On the average, people in the United States eat four to five pounds of butter every year—about one-half as much as margarine. This trend was the other way around in the early 1900s, however, when margarine was considered an inferior product.

Butter is made by agitating whole milk or cream until the fats separate into a solid mass. The milk is usually pasteurized (heated to destroy microorganisms), then ripened with the aid of a special culture. Salt and yellow coloring are often added as well. The yellow coloring used is annatto, derived from a plant that grows in Mexico.

Salt is added to butter to enhance the taste, but it can also be added to mask any "off" flavor or poor quality and to help preserve the butter. Unsalted butter is also marketed and is preferred by some nutrition-conscious consumers, particularly those on low-sodium diets.

Most butter sold in the United States is graded

FATS & OILS

Kind of Oil	Percent Saturated*	Percent Unsaturated*	Percent Polyunsaturated
Canola Oil	5.4–6.8	88.8–90.2	23.8–33.3
Coconut	86.5	7.6	1.8
Corn	12.5	82.9	58.7
Olive	13.5	82.1	8.4
Palm kernel	81.4	13.0	11.4
Peanut	16.9	78.2	46.2
Safflower	9.1	86.6	74.5
High oleic safflower	6.1	89.5	14.2
Sesame	14.2	81.4	41.7
Soybean	14.4	81.2	57.9
Sunflower (Northern)	10.3	85.2	65.7
Sunflower (Southern)	10.1	85.5	40.1
Wheat germ	18.8	76.8	61.7

*Values are for fatty acids expressed as grams (F.A./100 grams fat) so values will total approximately 95 percent, with remainder being glycerol.

Source: USDA Handbook 8–4.

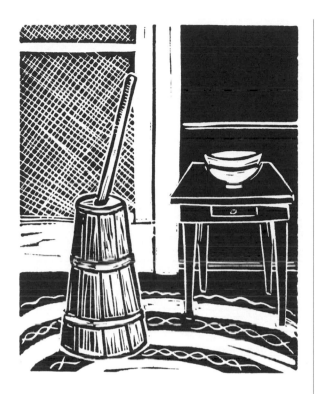

and given numerical scores based on its flavor, keeping quality, butterfat content, purity, and other characteristics. Grading is done by the U.S. Department of Agriculture. U.S. Grade AA is scored 93 and is 80 percent butterfat or higher; Grade A must be scored at least 92; other butters are scored lower (90, 89). The lower-scored butters are usually made from cream that has less butterfat content than grades AA and A, such as whey cream, a by-product of cheese making. Some butter may not be graded, as the program is optional.

How do I use it?

Butter is a favored topping for popcorn, and it adds a special taste to breads and rolls fresh from the oven. It can be used in almost any recipe that calls for an oil or fat, especially for sauteing, frying, or baking.

Homemade Butter

You can make your own butter at home. Although you probably won't want to go out and buy a butter churn like those used a hundred years ago, the method employed to make the butter is essentially the same.

Pour heavy cream into a bowl and whip it as if you were making whipped cream. Once the cream forms peaks, however, keep whipping it until it becomes butterlike or hard, or until it can no longer be whipped. Now take a spoon and press out the liquid; this is buttermilk, and it can be saved for use in baking or cooking. After you have pressed out as much liquid as possible, add a small amount of salt, a few shakes at a time, until the butter tastes right to you.

Clarified Butter

Clarified butter (drawn butter), or *ghee,* is often used in the Far East. To make it, slowly heat 1 pound of butter in a small, heavy pan until it melts and begins to froth. Make sure it doesn't turn brown. Then take it off the stove and let it sit for a few minutes. The little white particles—the curds—will sink to the bottom.

To use it immediately, put the pan in the refrigerator or in an ice-cold bowl of water for several minutes. The golden oil can then be poured off, leaving the hardened white solids in the bottom of the pan. Take what you need, then pour the rest into ice cube trays to be used later. Scrape off the residue from the frozen cubes before using. Clarified butter will have lost any salty flavor the butter may have had, and it will also be less likely to cause food to stick to the pan when cooking with it.

How nutritious is it?

Butter is an animal fat and is therefore a saturated fat. It also contains a notable amount of vitamin A and small amounts of calcium, magnesium, phosphorus, and potassium. Salted butter will, of course, contain sodium.

✦ Nutritive Value: Appendix, 99–101.

How do I store it?

Butter will keep at room temperature for several days, but for maximum freshness—especially in the summer—keep butter refrigerated. It may be frozen for long-term storage. Butter that is old or that

---

OMEGA-3 FATTY ACIDS

Omega-3 fatty acids are found in certain vegetable seeds and fish. Chemically, they are fatty acids that have eighteen to twenty-two carbon chains with three double bonds. Alpha-linolenic acid (ALA)— found in soybean, canola, flax, walnut, evening primrose, hemp, borage, black currant, and other vegetable seed oils—has eighteen carbon chains. Omega-3 fish oils have twenty or twenty-two carbon chains and are thus higher in polyunsaturated fats than omega-3 vegetable oils.

When ALA is metabolized with another essential fatty acid (EFA) known as linoleic acid, they become "derived EFAs." One of those derived EFAs is called gamma-linolenic acid (GLA); another one is called dihomogammalinolenic acid (DGLA). The labels on packages of flax seed oil and evening primrose oil sold as nutrition supplements often list these fatty acids to help promote sales of those products. Many studies have been conducted on GLA and DGLA to assess whether health claims about them are valid. These claims include aiding in recovery from and/or assisting in reducing premenstrual syndrome, atopic eczema, diabetic neuropathy, and alcoholic liver disease.

The role of omega-3 fatty acids in the body is to assist in regulating the immune system and response to infection or injury. They are also important for the formation of blood clots and regulating blood pressure and blood lipid levels. Omega-3 fatty acids are thought to help lower blood serum cholesterol and have an anticlotting action that could help prevent hypertension, stroke, or heart disease. They may also reduce the risk of developing multiple sclerosis, rheumatoid arthritis, and breast cancer.

---

has not been stored properly may become rancid.

Where does it come from?

Most of the butter sold in the United States is from milk produced in the dairy states of Wisconsin, Minnesota, and New York. If you want to know specifically where the butter was made, look for the plant number on the carton or wrapper and then contact your state Department of Agriculture or the USDA to find out the factory location from this number.

New Kinds of Butter

Researchers at the University of Wisconsin at Madison have developed processes to remove cholesterol from butter and to make butter that can be spread as soon as it is removed from the refrigerator.

The low-cholesterol butter reportedly has the same characteristics as regular butter except that it has 95 percent less cholesterol. The cholesterol is removed by a supercritical fluid extraction process, the same process used in Europe to make decaffeinated coffee.

The spreadable butter research was funded by Land O'Lakes, a large farmers' cooperative.

COCONUT OIL

Coconut is a plant native to the tropics. The oil is pressed from the boiled nut meats of either fresh or dried coconut. It is subjected to the same refining processes as other oils, namely bleaching, deodorizing, and hydrogenating.

Coconut oil is used in ice cream, salad dressings, confections, as a spray oil on crackers, and especially for nondairy coffee whiteners and whipped toppings.

This vegetable oil has an astonishingly high percentage of saturated fat—nearly 90 percent, which is even higher than the animal fats butter and lard. Coconut oil is also quite resistant to oxidation, so rancidity is not a great problem.

Most coconut comes from the Philippines, Indonesia, and other countries in the South Pacific. About three million metric tons of coconut oil is produced worldwide every year; one-half million metric tons is imported to the United States. Some is used for cosmetics such as suntan oil and other nonfood purposes.

COTTONSEED OIL

Cottonseed oil is derived from the small, pea-sized seeds of the cotton plant. About fifty seeds are found in each cotton boll (the fluffy white puff that becomes fiber for clothing). One hundred pounds of cotton seeds will yield approximately 16 pounds of oil. The remaining 84 pounds becomes lint and cottonseed meal, the latter used as livestock feed.

From 250 to 300 million pounds of cottonseed oil is used in the United States every year, most of that as salad oil, margarine, or shortening. It is usually blended with safflower oil, soy oil, or other vegetable oils in those foods. The comparatively low cost of cottonseed makes this a popular oil for processed foods.

Cotton is generally not considered a food crop, and residues from pesticides—which are heavily used in its cultivation—may be present in the oil, thus rendering it potentially unsafe for consumption.

FLAX SEED OIL

Flax seeds are shiny, brown, oval-shaped seeds that contain up to 38 percent fat. While most of the flax grown throughout the world is for linen making, some is grown specifically for the high-yielding oil seeds. Flax seed oil is also known as linseed oil and used industrially with wood products.

The flax seed oil sold by natural food and health food stores is intended as a nutrition supplement rather than for cooking purposes. In comparison to other vegetable oils, it is two to five times more expensive. In Eastern Europe, however, flax seed oil constitutes an estimated 1 to 2 percent of the edible fats and oils. (For more information, see flax seeds, page 117.)

Because of its high susceptibility to rancidity, keep flax seed oil and capsules refrigerated.

MARGARINE

What is it?

Margarine, now more popular than the butter that it imitates, is eaten at the rate of about ten to eleven pounds per person annually in the United States. Most margarine sold today is made of vegetable oils—especially soybean, corn, cottonseed, palm, and safflower oils—but some may also contain beef fat or lard.

Any margarine that is semisolid at room temperature has been made from either hydrogenated oils or animal fats. A margarine in which liquid vegetable oil is listed first in the label means the product is made of an oil that has not been hydrogenated, and it is considered more polyunsaturated than one that contains no liquid oil. The advertisement of oils as "partially hydrogenated" (or "partially hardened") refers to the fact that some of the oil has undergone hydrogenation, a process whereby hydrogen gas is bubbled through oil to chemically alter it by saturating it with hydrogen atoms (see page 26).

Regulations controlling the manufacture of margarine require that it be at least 80 percent fat from edible vegetable oils or animal carcass, either natural or hydrogenated. The U.S. Food and Drug Administration requires that margarine labels specify the type of oil used and if (and to what degree) the oils were hydrogenated.

To equate it with butter, vitamin A must be added to margarine. Salt or potassium chloride, fatty emulsifiers, natural sweeteners, preservatives, antioxidants, acids and alkalis, flavorings, vitamin D, and edible food coloring are also allowed in margarine. Some of these additives are:

Sodium benzoate, citric acid, benzoic acid— preservatives

Mono- and diglycerides—emulsifiers

Lecithin—for imitating the frying quality

Diacetyl—butter flavoring

Isopropyl or stearyl citrates—flavor protectors

OIL PROCESSING

There are two basic ways in which manufacturers extract oil from a seed or bean: the expeller (or pressure) method, and the solvent extraction process.

In the expeller method, ground or flaked seeds are fed into a large cylinder and are driven against a back plate by a screw. Tremendous pressure squeezes out up to 95 percent of the oil in the seeds.

In solvent extraction, ground seeds are bathed in a solution of hexane or other petroleum solvent. The resulting oil-solvent solution is then heated to 160°F to evaporate the solvent. This method is preferred by most oil processors because it extracts about 99 percent of the oil from the seed.

HOT- AND COLD-PRESSED

The terms hot-pressed and cold-pressed refer to the expeller method of extraction, although hot-pressed sometimes refers to a higher pressure, more efficient process. These terms are essentially meaningless, however, unless you know the exact temperature at which the oils were pressed. The term cold-pressed is especially misleading because it suggests that the oil is not exposed to heat in the extraction process.

In fact, all commercial oil extracting processes involve a fair amount of heat—at least 120° to 150°F. Furthermore, many "cold-pressed" oils are refined, bleached, and deodorized after extraction, and thus are exposed to even hotter temperatures.

REFINING

The part of processing that has a significant effect on the nutritional value of oil is the amount of refining it goes through after extraction.

An unrefined or crude oil is extracted (by expeller or solvent method), settled or filtered, and bottled. Nothing else is done to it. Unrefined oils

that are expeller extracted are sometimes called *natural oils*.

Refined oil, on the other hand, undergoes a number of processing steps after extraction. The main purpose of these additional processes is to remove all extraneous materials whose strong flavors or colors may affect the character of the oil. The major processing steps are:

1. Degumming—The oil is mixed with water at a temperature of 90 to 120°F and is centrifuged (placed in a cylindrical container and rotated at high speeds) to separate out various substances, including phosphatides, which cause oil to darken at high temperatures. One of these phosphatides is lecithin, a substance added to commercially prepared baked goods and also sold as a dietary aid.

2. Alkali refining—An alkali (a substance that can neutralize acid) such as lye or caustic soda is added to oil, followed by one or two water washes. It is then agitated and heated to remove unwanted substances by chemical reaction and centrifuged to separate the oil. A by-product of this process is called soap stock. Almost all oils that have passed through the alkali refining stage are also bleached and deodorized.

3. Bleaching—The oil is mixed with specially treated clays, called activated earths, to which unwanted particles of pigment will cling. The oil is then heated, agitated, and finally filtered to remove the activated earths and any particles they have picked up. One commonly used activated earth is Fuller's earth.

4. Hydrogenating—For certain purposes, hydrogen gas is bubbled through oil to stabilize it, that is, to change the liquid oil to a semisolid or solid fat. This process raises the melting point of the fat or oil, allows

for air to be incorporated into baked goods, prevents oil separation, and extends shelf life. But hydrogenation chemically changes many of the oil's unsaturated fatty acids to saturated fatty acids. Margarine, shortening, imitation cheese products, and some commercial peanut butters contain hydrogenated fats.

The advertising of hydrogenated fat products may be misleading. Margarine, for example, may be advertised as being made from polyunsaturated oils, while it is never mentioned that the fatty acids in those oils have been hydrogenated and that the margarine has thus become a saturated fat. Some products may be labeled as "partially hydrogenated" or "partially hardened," which is better than completely saturated or hydrogenated fat, but its nutritional value is still compromised. Be sure to read the labels on all products containing fats or oils.

5. Deodorizing—During this final stage, the oil is processed by steam-stripping it at temperatures above 400°F. This removes all odors, objectionable flavors, some of the remaining pigment, and peroxides in the oils that contribute to rancidity. From 30 to 40 percent of the vitamin E that was present in the oil is removed in this process. Some vitamin manufacturers use the distillate to make their vitamin E supplements.

The end product after all this processing is a bland-tasting and odorless oil that contains mostly triglycerides (fatty acids). According to Bailey's *Industrial Oil and Fat Products,* "Well deodorized oils of different kinds, when still fresh, are virtually indistinguishable from one another by odor or taste, and merely give a sensation of oiliness in the mouth."

How nutritious is it?

Since margarine is made to be as much like butter as possible, the vitamin A, salt, and calorie content of the two products are the same. Butter has small amounts of some B-complex vitamins and minerals that are lacking in its imitator, while margarine—if it is made with liquid oil—may contain less saturated fat. So-called low-calorie margarine is simply whipped—it contains more air and is therefore lower in calories than the same volume of unwhipped margarine.

✦ Nutritive Value: Appendix, 106–117.

Where does it come from?

Margarine was developed in 1869 by a French chemist, Hippolyte Mége-Mouriés, who won the prize offered by Napoleon for finding a cheap formula for imitation butter. He mixed lard and the drippings from meat packing with milk and water, and colored it with annatto, a yellow vegetable dye still used today for the same purpose. This mixture really didn't taste like butter, but its low price was appealing.

For a long time the sale of margarine was strongly opposed by United States dairy farmers and manufacturers, who feared its competition with butter. They helped instigate legislation that levied state and federal taxes on margarine sales and that prohibited commercial coloring of margarine. For years it was sold in a white block along with a packet of yellow dye that could be stirred in to make it look like butter.

Margarine became popular during World War II when food was rationed and butter was scarce. Sales also increased after the war ended. In the 1960s, the regulations for taxing and banning the coloring of margarine were abandoned.

SHORTENING

What is it?

What margarine is to butter, shortening is to lard.

Shortening was developed in the early 1900s, before refrigeration. It can be kept at room temperature for a fairly long time, unlike lard which hydrogenation (see page 26). This changes the oil into a solid, or saturated, fat. The final product is a mixture of partially hydrogenated oil and a small percentage of crystallized, very hard hydrogenated fat that is evenly dispersed to give the substance a solid look. Shortening is often fluffed by whipping in an inert gas, such as nitrogen, to improve its appearance and baking qualities.

How do I use it?

Shortening is used mostly for baking, especially in pie crusts, cookies, cakes, and pastries. Mono- and diglycerides are often added to shortening to make it easy to mix, but they also reduce the smoking point (the temperature at which fat starts to smoke and deteriorate). Shortening is not recommended for frying because of this low smoking point, which is usually in the range of 335 to 420°F for an animal and vegetable blend, and 345 to 395°F for an all-vegetable shortening. Most liquid vegetable oils have a smoking point of about 465°F.

How nutritious is it?

Shortening is nutritionally inferior to other fats and oils. The only nutrient it offers is fat, most of which is saturated or hydrogenated.

✦ Nutritive Value: Appendix, 102, 103.

How do I store it?

Because most commercial shortenings have been hydrogenated and contain preservatives, the shelf life is quite long—several months or more. Store shortening on any shelf in your kitchen or pantry.

can become rancid quickly whether it is refrigerated or not.

Over five billion pounds of shortening are manufactured each year in the United States, where consumption has steadily increased from eighteen pounds per person in 1976 to twenty-two pounds per person in 1992.

Today, shortening is generally made from vegetable fats, particularly soybean and cottonseed oils but also palm oil and coconut oil. It may also be made of a combination of animal and vegetable fats. If the oil that is used is liquid, or unsaturated, it undergoes

CORN OIL

What is it?

Corn oil is extracted from corn germ, the inside of a kernel of corn. About 200 million pounds of the corn oil produced every year in the United States is made into margarine. The rest is processed as salad or cooking oil or is used in mayonnaise, salad dressings, and shortening.

To make corn oil, corn germ is kiln-dried and preheated. Then the oil is extracted by either the solvent or expeller-pressed method. Unrefined corn oil is generally dark gold to amber in color, usually has a popcorny smell, and is fairly dense. Refined corn oil is pale amber, although it is not as pale as most other refined oils.

How do I use it?

Corn oil is great for baking, as it adds extra corn flavor to corn bread, muffins, or pancakes. It can also be used for frying, although unrefined corn oil has a tendency to foam and has a low smoking point (the temperature at which oil begins to smoke and break down). Refined corn oil has a high smoking point—465 to 490°F—which makes it acceptable for deep-fat frying.

Corn oil can also be used as a salad oil, if you prefer its taste over that of other common salad oils.

How nutritious is it?

Corn oil is high in polyunsaturates (about 60 percent) and fairly low in saturated fatty acids (13 percent). The vitamin E content is high, and there are trace amounts of B-complex vitamins and a few minerals.

Corn oil has a high level of the essential fatty acid linoleic acid, which makes up over 50 percent of the fatty acids in the oil.

✦ Nutritive Value: Appendix, 118, 119.

Where does it come from?

Native Americans, especially in the central region of North America, have used corn oil for centuries.

Today, most corn oil comes from domestically grown corn that has been grown with commercial fertilizers, herbicides, and pesticides. However, to-

LIPOPROTEINS

Just when you think you've grasped the concept of saturated and unsaturated fats, there is another factor to be considered: lipoproteins. These water-soluble fat-protein complexes are formed by the body to carry lipids (cholesterol, triglycerides, and phospholipids) via the bloodstream and are therefore responsible for how much cholesterol is brought from or cleaned up and returned to the liver for processing and removal.

The four lipoproteins and their main functions are:

- *High-density lipoproteins (HDL)*—These complexes are higher in protein and carry serum cholesterol out of the blood and into the liver. The body's level of HDL depends on diet and activity level. People who eat less fat, do not smoke, exercise aerobically, and maintain adequate body weight have a higher level of HDL; people who are obese and sedentary have a lower level of HDL.
- *Low-density lipoproteins (LDL)*—These lipoproteins are lower in protein and are responsible for transporting cholesterol from the liver into the bloodstream. Increased levels of LDL have been linked with atherosclerosis, as cholesterol deposits in the lining of the walls of arteries clog the pathways. Sedentary people who eat a lot of saturated fat often have more LDL than HDL and are therefore at risk for heart disease.
- *Very low-density lipoproteins (VLDL)* and *chylomicrons*—These complexes have even less protein and are mainly responsible for transporting triglycerides.

Genetic makeup also plays a significant role in cholesterol levels. The rates of cardiovascular disease increase proportionately to serum cholesterol levels, so periodic cholesterol tests are recommended by health professionals.

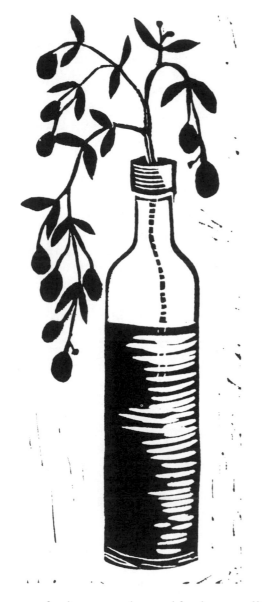

the same black olives you may eat as an appetizer. Olive trees are evergreens that love the sun and prefer a fairly dry climate. They grow quite slowly but are known to live for fifteen hundred to two thousand years. The trees reach heights from twenty to forty feet and tend to become gnarled and storybook-like in appearance as the branches spread out and curve in various directions.

Tree-ripened olives are picked when their color changes from green to purplish-black and the skins look oily but are not too soft. They may be allowed to dry slightly, then the fruits are crushed and the liquid is extracted. The oil that is skimmed off after the pulp settles is called *virgin* olive oil; it is one of the few true cold-pressed oils.

Virgin olive oils are available in four different grades. In descending order of quality, they are *Extra, Fine, Unnamed grade* (the most common grade sold in the United States), and *Lampante.*

Most of the olive oil sold in the United States, however, is not virgin olive oil. Two other kinds are more widely available. The more common of these two kinds is "pure" olive oil. It is extracted from pulp residues and ground up pits by the solvent method and is further refined by bleaching or deodorizing. The other kind is an olive oil blend, which may be only 10 percent olive oil and 90 percent soybean oil or cottonseed oil.

Fresh, high-quality olive oil should have a sweetish, nutty flavor and a golden or straw color. A greenish tint indicates a less refined oil, closer to virgin quality.

How do I use it?

Olive oil is frequently used for salads, especially in oil and vinegar dressings. It is also popular as a base in sauces for pasta dishes such as spaghetti or lasagna.

The smoking point of olive oil is 375 to 390°F, which makes it unsuitable for deep-fat frying.

How nutritious is it?

Olive oil differs from all other vegetable oils in several ways. It contains mostly monounsaturated fatty acids and is therefore low in both polyunsaturates (8 percent) and saturated fats (14 percent). This high

day some food co-ops and natural food stores offer unrefined corn oil that has been extracted from organically grown corn.

OLIVE OIL

What is it?

Used in the Middle East since earliest civilization, olives were probably the first nonanimal source of oil in the human diet.

Olive oil comes from the fruit of the olive plant—

level of monounsaturates causes the oil to become semisolid when it is refrigerated.

Olive oil also contains small amounts of calcium, copper, and iron. It has less vitamin E than most other oils.

✦ Nutritive Value: Appendix, 120, 121.

How do I store it?

Rancidity is less of a problem with olive oil than other oils, but it is wise to refrigerate it. Excessive exposure to heat will cause olive oil to become rancid, and too much light may cause its color to fade. Buy it in small quantities to maintain a fresh supply.

Avoid storing olive oil near foods with strong odors or flavors, as it can pick up the scents and result in an off-tasting product.

Where does it come from?

Most olive oil is imported from Mediterranean countries, especially Spain and Greece. About one hundred thousand metric tons of olive oil are im-

ported into the United States every year. Imports have tripled in the last decade—up from twenty thousand to thirty thousand metric tons during the 1970s and early 1980s. Olives can be grown in Australia and Florida but are most successful in southern and central California, as well as in southern European and Middle Eastern countries.

PALM OIL

Fast gaining popularity in the food industry, this inexpensive vegetable oil is made from the fruit and/or kernel of palm trees.

Palm oil was traditionally used for soap or was freshly pressed for food in Africa. It is orange to yellow in color in its natural state. When boiled, it has characteristics similar to butter.

Palm oil contains over 80 percent saturated fatty acids—very high for a vegetable oil—and 13 percent unsaturated fatty acids. For certain uses, such as snacks and confections, palm kernel oil is fractionated, a process that separates the unsaturated fatty

ADDITIVES

To retard spoilage or rancidity in shortening and liquid oils, some manufacturers add preservatives called antioxidants. Antioxidants slow down or stop oxygen from filling in some of the atoms in an unsaturated fat molecule. Unsaturated fats are mostly carbon and hydrogen, but there is room for more hydrogen (or oxygen).

When an unsaturated fat is hydrogenated, hydrogen gas is bubbled through it so that hydrogen atoms will saturate the fat molecule. This process extends the shelf life of oils.

The more common antioxidants used in fats and oils are:

BHA (butylated hydroxyanisole) and BHT (butylated hydroxytoluene)—These petroleum-derived chemicals have been used since the late 1940s, but they are claimed to be of minimal value in actually stopping oxidation. They can accumulate in body fat. At the present time they are on the U.S. Food and Drug Administration's GRAS (generally recognized as safe) list.

Citric acid (sodium citrate)—A naturally occurring substance found in citrus fruits and berries, this additive is considered safe. The chemical is made from by-products of fruits or by allowing a fungus to grow on beet molasses under controlled conditions.

Propyl gallate—This is often used with BHA and BHT for a synergistic effect, but it is also suspected of doing little in the way of antioxidizing fats. It is an ester of propyl alcohol and gallic acid. Propyl gallate breaks down into gallic acid during digestion and is secreted in the urine. It is on the GRAS list.

acids from the saturated fatty acids to make the oil nearly 100 percent saturated. This prevents candy coatings from melting at room temperature or in your fingers.

Palm oil is commonly used as the frying fat for potato chips and in margarine, gravies, and soups. Palm kernel oil is added to nondairy coffee whiteners, dressings, dips, whipped toppings, candies, and in cookies and waffles as filler fat.

The low cost of palm oil is due to the wages paid to workers who harvest the palms. Most palm oil is imported from Malaysia.

PEANUT OIL

What is it?

Peanuts were one of the first native North American sources of vegetable oil. They grow naturally in the southern region of the United States. Oil makes up about half of the peanut.

Peanut oil is frequently used in combination with other vegetable oils to make all-purpose cooking oil. Over three million metric tons of crude peanut oil are produced annually throughout the world. Most of it becomes cooking oil. It is usually extracted by the solvent method.

How do I use it?

Peanut oil is often used for popping popcorn, because its smoking point is 440 to 460°F. This allows popcorn kernels to be heated and popped before the oil starts smoking and breaking down. Pure peanut oil, or cooking oils that contain it, can also be used for frying. Peanut oil adds an extra nutty essence to cookies, muffins, or other foods that contain peanuts.

How nutritious is it?

Like most other vegetable fats, peanut oil contains a high percentage of unsaturated fats—it is about 45 percent polyunsaturated and 30 percent monounsaturated. The level of vitamin E is low compared to other oils, and there are only very small amounts of a few trace minerals present.

◆ Nutritive Value: Appendix, 122, 123.

How do I store it?

Refrigerate peanut oil to stave off rancidity. It may become cloudy or thicker from the cold temperature, but this does not affect the nutritional value or quality. The oil will liquefy again at room temperature. For maximum freshness, buy peanut oil in small quantities and at frequent intervals.

RAPESEED (CANOLA) OIL

An increasingly popular vegetable oil in the United States is made from the rape plant, a "four-letter word" in our society. The botanical version of the word is derived from *rapum,* the Latin word for turnip, a close relative of rape. Rapeseed oil is now more commonly referred to as canola oil, due to the successful production of this oil in Canada.

Rape is grown commercially in China, India, Canada, and northern European countries. Only a small amount of rapeseed oil is produced in the United States. Worldwide production is eight to nine million metric tons per year, making rapeseed oil one of the most highly used edible vegetable oils.

Rapeseeds are small, round, and usually black. They grow in long, slender pods similar to mustard, another relative of rape. The oil constitutes 40 to 45 percent of the seed. Rape foliage is used as a forage crop, and the meal that remains after oil is pressed out of the seeds becomes a protein-rich livestock food. It is thought that rapeseed protein will soon become an important ingredient in processed foods, such as baked goods and meat extenders.

One drawback of rapeseed oil is the presence of two antinutritional factors. One is a fatty acid called erucic acid; the other is glucosinolate. Erucic acid oxidizes at a slower rate than other fatty acids, which can cause undesirable accumulations of triglycerides. Glucosinolate has been known to promote goiter, the enlargement of the thyroid gland. Recent breeding experiments in Europe and Canada have, however, resulted in new varieties of rape that have little or no erucic acid or glucosinolate and higher levels of oleic acid.

Use canola oil as you would other vegetable oils.

SAFFLOWER OIL

Safflower oil is extracted from the seeds of the safflower, a plant in the thistle family that grows in semiarid regions, particularly in the southwestern United States.

Safflower oil is obtained from the seeds by expeller pressing, solvent extraction, or a combination of both. Each seed is about 40 percent oil.

Unrefined safflower oil is usually a deep amber-yellow color and has a mild, slightly nutty and earthy flavor. Refined safflower oil is typically a very pale yellow in color and has a bland taste.

Because it is fairly light in weight and color, safflower is a good all-purpose oil. Its smoking point (the temperature at which it will start to smoke) is high—440 to 480°F—which makes it suitable for deep-fat frying. Safflower oil is often used for sauteing and in baking. It is also used as an ingredient in salad dressings and mayonnaise.

Safflower oil has one of the lowest saturation levels of all commercial vegetable oils. It is 75 percent polyunsaturated and only 9 percent saturated. The remaining fatty acids are monounsaturated. Unrefined safflower oil is high in vitamin E.

Most of the safflower oil used in the United States is from plants that are grown in California and Arizona.

✦ Nutritive Value: Appendix, 124, 125.

SESAME OIL

What is it?

Pressed from the seeds of a tropical plant, sesame oil is one of the oldest vegetable oils used. It is also called *benne, ginglii,* or *teel oil.*

The sesame plant grows two to five feet high and produces long, oval, pointed leaves. The fruits are packed in four-celled capsules that hold many seeds.

Sesame seeds contain about 50 percent oil. They are one of the few sources of edible oil that can yield a commercially acceptable oil without being exposed to high heat or without being put through a high-pressure expeller process.

How do I use it?

Unrefined sesame oil is dark yellow to amber in color and has a pleasant, mild flavor. When refined, sesame oil is pale yellow and has a bland taste. Its smoking point is 465°F.

Sesame oil is good for sauteing vegetables, grains, and noodles, and for making salad dressings. It can also be used to make soap, shampoo, and skin lotions.

How nutritious is it?

Pure sesame oil contains about 42 percent polyunsaturated fatty acids and 14 percent saturated fatty acids. Vitamin E is also present.

✦ Nutritive Value: Appendix, 465.

Where does it come from?

Sesame seeds are grown in China, India, Africa, and Latin America; some are grown in Texas. A small amount of the total worldwide production is pressed into sesame oil. The United States imports about thirty-five thousand metric tons per year, up from the 1975 rate of about twenty-thousand metric tons. Italy and Japan are also large importers of sesame seeds.

SOYBEAN OIL

What is it?

Funny how something unheard of to most North Americans one hundred years ago can become our most widely used source of vegetable oil.

Soybeans are the number one cash crop of the United States, mainly because of their oil. With a 20 percent fat content, soybeans are higher in fat than most common beans. (Navy beans, for example, have 1.5 percent fat.) More than 90 percent of the soybeans used for human consumption is made into margarine, shortening, salad oil, and cooking oil.

Only 60 to 75 percent of the oil in soybeans can be extracted by the expeller or pressure process. Consequently, most soy oil is obtained by solvent extraction, which yields 95 percent of the oil.

Blends of soybean and cottonseed oils are marketed as salad and cooking oils by some companies. Check the label to know for sure what is in the oil.

How do I use it?

Natural (unrefined) soybean oil has a strong "beany" odor and is therefore more suitable for baking than as a salad oil. It can foam during frying, which may not be desirable in some dishes.

Refined soy oil—that which has been degummed, deodorized, and bleached—has one of the highest smoking points of all vegetable oils: 465 to 510°F. Thus, soybean oil is frequently used as a cooking oil as well as a salad oil.

Soybean oil contains about 3 percent phosphatides, often referred to as soybean lecithin. Lecithin acts as an antioxidant and emulsifier, making it especially suitable for baked goods. Refined oil that has gone through the degumming process has had the lecithin removed from it.

How nutritious is it?

Soybean oil is high in polyunsaturates and contains a good amount of vitamin E. The essential fatty acid linoleic acid is present and constitutes over 50 percent of the fatty acids in soybeans.

✦ Nutritive Value: Appendix, 126–129

How do I store it?

Store soybean oil in a clean, dark-colored jar, and refrigerate it to prevent rancidity. Avoid storing it near other foods with strong odors, as the scents may be picked up by the oil and may give it an off-flavor.

Where does it come from?

Soybeans originated in China about 1000 B.C. and were the staple food in East Asia for many years.

The bean became popular in the United States after scientists and agronomists researched it extensively and brought it over from the Orient in the 1920s. It gained wide recognition as an oil bean in the 1940s and 1950s, during which time margarine and vegetable shortening sales soared.

Today soybeans are grown in southwestern Minnesota, Iowa, and other midwestern states. Most of the soybean oil sold in the United States is manufactured by large food companies.

SUNFLOWER OIL

What is it?

Sunflower oil is extracted from the seeds of a flower in the daisy family. Sunflower seeds contain 35 to 50 percent oil.

Special varieties of sunflower seeds are grown for their high oil content. These varieties generally have smaller flower tops than those grown for birdseed or for the nut. Although 40 to 65 percent of the United States' sunflower crop consists of oil varieties, only 20 to 25 percent of this is used in domestic consumption—10 percent as vegetable oil and 15 percent as livestock feed. Many sunflower seeds are exported.

How do I use it?

Sunflower oil is good for baking and sauteing, and in salad dressings.

Unrefined sunflower oil is light amber in color and has a distinctive flavor. Refined sunflower oil is pale and bland tasting.

How nutritious is it?

Sunflower oil is quite low in saturated fats. It contains 44 to 66 percent polyunsaturated fatty acids and about 10 percent saturated fatty acids. The essential fatty acid called linoleic acid constitutes 68 percent of sunflower oil. It is also very high in vitamin E.

✦ Nutritive Value: Appendix, 130, 131.

Where does it come from?

Sunflower seeds were first grown by North American Indians and were introduced to Europe and Asia in the mid-1500s. They became quite popular there, especially in Russia, where the czars supposedly fed soldiers two pounds of sunflower seeds as a daily staple.

Sunflower oil is most popular in Canada and Russia. In the United States, the plants are widely grown in North Dakota, Minnesota, South Dakota, Texas, Colorado, and Kansas.

WHEAT GERM OIL

An extract of the heart of the wheat berry, wheat germ oil is generally consumed not as a cooking oil but as a dietary supplement. Wheat germ itself contains about 11 percent fat.

Consuming wheat germ oil between meals or when the stomach is empty will allow the nutrients to be better utilized and less affected by any rancid fats that may be present in the digestive tract.

The vitamin E content of wheat germ oil is extremely high, offering twice as much (or more) vitamin E as any other common vegetable oil. The level of unsaturated fats is also good—less than 20 percent of the fatty acids is saturated.

Refrigerate wheat germ oil to prevent rancidity.

FRUITS

What are they?

Sweet and succulent, sour and saucy—fruits are better described by taste than by words.

There are hundreds of kinds of fruits, from the everyday apples, bananas, and oranges to the exotic fiejoa, akee, and carambola.

Botanically, a fruit is the part of a flowering plant that contains or consists of one or more seeds. Grains, legumes, and nuts are called *simple dry fruits* because their shells or skins become dry and hard when mature. *Fleshy fruits* have soft or fleshy skins when mature; those foods that we generally consider to be fruits are all fleshy fruits. Certain vegetables such as cucumbers, peppers, tomatoes, and avocados are also fleshy fruits by this definition.

For consumer purposes, *fruits* are the fleshy fruits that grow on trees; generally taste sweet or are sweetened; are juicy; and are used mainly for eating raw, juicing into a beverage, cooking into preserves, or baking into desserts. Also, generally speaking, *berries* are small fleshy fruits that grow on plants and bushes rather than on trees.

In the past twenty years fruit consumption has increased steadily in the United States, from 85 pounds per person in 1975 to the current rate of about 100 pounds per person per year. Most fruit is consumed fresh; about 70 percent is noncitrus (apples, bananas, peaches, etc.), and 25 percent is citrus (oranges, grapefruit, etc.). The rest is either canned, sold as juice, frozen, or dried.

Buying tips

Most fruits should be purchased or picked when ripe, as indicated by color, texture, and sometimes odor. Their colors should be full and true to species or variety. They should appear healthy with no major bruises, moldy spots, or scars. Fruits vary in texture, from soft to firm and smooth to rough-skinned, so learn the individual traits of the various fruits.

A few fruits, such as muskmelons, will smell when ripe. Others will smell when they are over-ripe or rotten. Figs and pineapple, for example, can ferment and become sour or bitter smelling.

Although many fruits are grown domestically and are available most of the year, some types are imported, especially in winter and spring (see the chart on page 37 for dates of availability and peak season). Virtually all imported fruits are fumigated to deter insects during transit. A common fumigant is methyl bromide, a poisonous gas.

Fruit Beverages

Fruit beverages contain varying amounts of fruit juice and pulp. They are labeled as follows:

Nectar—Usually thick or syrupy, containing most or all of the fruit juice and pulp

Juice—The fruit liquid, with or without pulp, usually unsweetened

Juice concentrate—Juice that has had some of the water removed, so it can be reconstituted later

Juice drink or fruit drink—Typically a mixture of some fruit juice—usually 10 percent—and other liquid, either water or a combination of water and small amounts of different fruit juices and sweeteners

Ade (as in lemonade)—A small amount of fruit juice and pulp with a large quantity of water and sweetener

Powdered beverage mixes—Usually artificially flavored, colored, and sweetened crystals to which you add water to make a fruitlike beverage

AVAILABILITY AND STORAGE OF FRESH FRUITS

Fruit	Availability	Peak	Maximum Storage Time	Storage Temperature*
Apples	year-round	Sept.–Nov.	2 weeks or more	32–34°F
Apricots	June–Sept.	June–July	3 to 5 days	
Avocados	year-round	Oct.–Jan.	3 to 5 days	65–70°F (unripe)
Bananas	year-round	———	1 to 5 days	room temp.
Blackberries	July–Sept.	July–Aug.	1 or 2 days	
Blueberries	June–Aug.	July–Aug.	3 to 5 days	
Cherries	June–Aug.	June	1 or 2 days	
Cranberries	Sept.–Dec.	November	1 week	
Currants	June–Aug.	July	1 or 2 days	
Dates	year-round	November		
Figs (fresh)	July–Oct.	July–Oct.	1 or 2 days	
Gooseberries	May–Aug.	June–July	1 or 2 days	
Grapefruits	year-round	Jan.–Apr.	1 week	
Grapes	June–Mar.	summer	3 to 5 days	
Kiwifruit	year-round	June–Mar.	4 to 6 months	
Kumquats	May–Aug.	Nov.–Feb.	5 days	
Lemons	year-round	May–Aug.	5 days	
Limes	year-round	June–Sept.	5 days	
Mandarins	Nov.–May	Nov.–Jan.	5 days	
Mangos	Jan.–Aug.	June	3 to 5 days	room temp.
Melons				
Honeydew	June–Dec.	July–Oct.	3 to 5 days	
Muskmelon	May–Nov.	July–Oct.	3 to 5 days	
Watermelon	May–Oct.	June–Aug.	3 to 5 days	
Nectarines	May–Sept.	July–Aug.	3 to 5 days	
Oranges	year-round	Dec.–Mar.	5 days	
Papayas	May–June; Oct.–Dec.	May, Oct.	1 week	
Peaches	May–Sept.	July–Aug.	3 to 5 days	
Pears	July–Mar.	July–Mar.	3 to 5 days	
Persimmons	Apr.–Jan.	Sept.–Jan.	3 to 5 days	
Pineapples	year-round	Apr.–June	1 to 2 days	
Plums	May–Sept.	July–Aug.	3 to 5 days	
Pomegranates	Aug.–Dec.	October	1 week	
Raspberries	June–Sept.	July–Aug.	1 or 2 days	
Rhubarb	Apr.–June	Apr.–June	2 to 3 weeks	
Strawberries	year-round	Apr.–July	1 or 2 days	
Tangelos	Oct.–Apr.	Nov.–Jan.	5 days	
Tangerines	Oct.–Mar.	Nov.–Jan.	5 days	

*Refrigerate unless otherwise noted.

For the most food value and authentic taste, look for or make beverages that contain real fruit juice and a minimal amount of nonfruit sweeteners.

How do I use them?

Fruits are one of nature's convenience foods. Just wash the ripe foods, peel or cut off the skins in some cases, and eat. Fresh, raw fruits and juices are excellent thirst quenchers and sweet, quick-energy foods.

Fruits, especially berries, can be made into jellies, jams, or preserves. Pies, turnovers, and upside-down cakes combine fruits and grains for delicious desserts. Many fruits can be cooked into sauce or can be canned and frozen for long-term storage. The various methods and procedures for preserving, canning, and freezing fruits can be found in food storage books, such as *Putting Food By* by Hertzberg, et al. (Stephen Greene Press, Brattleboro, VT), and *Stocking Up* by Carol Stoner (Rodale Press, Emmaus, PA). Also consult your county, province, or state extension home economist or office, and publications by the United States or Canadian departments of agriculture.

How nutritious are they?

Fresh fruits, although mostly water, are excellent sources of natural sugar and provide food energy and carbohydrates. They are low in fat and generally contain little protein. Most provide bulk or fiber.

The minerals potassium, magnesium, calcium, phosphorus, and iron can be found in fruits, as can vitamins C, A, and traces of B-complex. Cooked, canned, and frozen fruits contain the same nutrients as fresh fruits, but in smaller quantities. Heating and prolonged storage generally decrease or eliminate vitamin C. Sweetened fruits are less nutritious because the extra sweetener displaces nutrients.

Dried fruits are very high in natural sugars but are low in water, so they are concentrated sources of food energy and fiber. The mineral content also increases in some fruits when they are dried.

✦ Nutritive Value: Appendix, 132–244, 466–475.

TREE FRUITS

The common tree fruits—apples, peaches, pears, plums, and cherries—are characterized by a seed core or pit in the center, surrounded by fleshy pulp.

There are hundreds, and in some cases thousands, of different varieties of fruits. For example, the United States Department of Agriculture has identified more than seven thousand varieties of apples. There are many varieties because when a new fruit tree grows from a seed, it will be of a different variety than that of the parent tree. This can be due to genetic mutation or cross-pollination.

Today, rather than planting fruit seeds, most fruit trees are propagated by grafting, a process of cutting part of an existing tree and fostering the growth of that part onto another growing tree. This

How do I store them?

Keep fresh, ripe fruits in a cool place or in your refrigerator. Not-quite-ripe fruits can usually be ripened at room temperature in a few days.

Store dried fruits in a dry, cool place, or refrigerate them in tightly sealed containers. If they dry out, steam them in a vegetable steamer for a minute or two until they are at the desired moisture level.

APPLES

What are they?

Apples are the most common fruit throughout the world. People in the United States eat about eighteen pounds of fresh apples per person every year, or about thirty pounds when canned, juiced, and dried apples are also considered.

There are over seven thousand varieties of apples, but only twenty varieties make up three-fourths of the United States' crop. The Red Delicious variety alone accounts for one-fourth of the total production.

thereby perpetuates and multiplies the particular variety from which the cutting came.

Although there are many different varieties of each fruit, only a few of them are produced commercially. Varieties of fruit that are disease resistant and are good shippers, or store well, are typically the varieties that are grown.

Most commercial fruit trees are subject to sprayings of soil fumigants, herbicides, fungicides, and growth regulators. This is done to obtain a marketable crop—that is, to satisfy consumers who want blemish-free and worm-free fruit. It is difficult to find growers who do not use some type of spray or chemical for their trees—even so-called organic orchardists. The growth regulators are for the growers' benefit, so they can have all the fruit ripen at the same time and thereby reduce or eliminate repeat pickings on the same trees. Most tree fruits are hand picked, although mechanized picking is becoming more common.

After picking, commercial packers may place unripe fruits in ethylene gas chambers to speed the ripening or, in some cases, cause the fruit skin to appear to be ripe. Ethylene gas occurs naturally in fruits and vegetables, but even the foods that give off ethylene gas are gassed prior to marketing. These include apples, bananas, peaches, pears, and tomatoes.

Buying tips

Apples are graded according to color and appearance, but not according to taste or quality of the fruit under the skin.

Extra Fancy is the grade for blemish-free, "perfect" apples. They also command the highest prices.

Fancy grade is for apples of good appearance; they are generally lower in price than Extra Fancy.

Windfalls (fruits that have fallen by the wind) or *seconds* are apples that may have blemishes and bruises. They are usually quite inexpensive and are sold only in areas where they grow rather than through supermarkets.

Most apples are sold by weight or individually. A bushel box will contain 96 to 144 apples and will provide 16 to 20 quarts of canned applesauce or slices.

To determine if apples are ripe, look for those that are bright red in color (unless they are of a green variety), are firm to the touch, and contain brown or black seeds. If possible, cut one open to judge its quality. Unripe apples taste very tart and have white seeds; overripe or old apples are mealy (caused by being left on the tree too long) or mushy (caused by prolonged storage). Avoid apples that are brown around the core, wormy, or excessively bruised. Waxed apples can cause indigestion and

Apple	Eating	Baking	Cooking	All-purpose
Red Delicious	x			
Golden Delicious	x	x	x	x
McIntosh	x	x	x	x
Rome Beauty		x	x	
Jonathan	x	x	x	x
Winesap	x	x	x	x
Greening/Pippin		x	x	

nausea in sensitive people, so avoid them unless you intend to peel the fruit.

The best time to buy apples is in the late summer and autumn, when harvesting occurs; apples available in early summer are generally mushy or of poor eating quality.

How do I use them?

Apple strudel, apple pie, apple butter . . . the list of recipes using apples is nearly endless.

Apples are generally classified as *eating, baking, cooking,* or *all-purpose.*

- *Eating* apples—those that are best consumed raw—are firm, crisp, juicy, and sweet to slightly tart.
- *Baking* types are large, fairly firm, and should have thick skins.
- *Cooking* or *pie apples* are often tart and juicy. They are used for pies, applesauce, and other desserts.
- *All-purpose* apples are good for eating, baking, cooking, juicing, or drying.

Some of the more common varieties of apples and their typical uses are listed on the previous page.

To make a 9-inch apple pie, use 2 pounds (4 to 6 apples). One apple provides approximately 1 cup of diced apple pieces.

When cutting apples for cooking or salads, sprinkle the pieces with lemon juice or dip them in a lemon juice and water mixture (¼ cup lemon juice to 1 cup water) to prevent them from turning brown.

Beverages containing apples are referred to as either cider or apple juice. Apple cider is made by crushing or pressing apples to extract the liquid. It is not pasteurized or filtered, so it must be refrigerated or used up in a short time to prevent fermentation. Country or hard cider is apple cider that has been allowed to partially ferment and contains some alcohol. Apple juice (sometimes called sweet cider) is cider that has been pasteurized and canned or bottled, or made from frozen concentrate.

Dried apples are wonderful for snacks or for adding to baked goods, pancakes, poultry stuffing, or cereal. You can also reconstitute them by soaking the pieces in warm water for a few hours until soft. These apple pieces can be made into applesauce.

How nutritious are they?

Apples are an excellent source of pectin and fiber. When eaten raw, they help clean the teeth and exercise the gums. They digest rapidly in the body— in ninety minutes if well-chewed.

Raw apples provide small amounts of many minerals, including potassium, magnesium, and calcium. Also present are vitamins A, B-complex, and C.

Canned (cooked) and dried apples offer the same nutrients as raw apples, although cooking destroys some vitamin C and drying eliminates vitamin A.

Apples contain negligible amounts of fat and protein.

✦ Nutritive Value: Appendix, 132–138, 466.

How do I store them?

For long-term storage of homegrown apples, pick them shortly before the fruit is fully ripe and refrigerate them at 32 to 34°F. Wrap each apple in newspaper to enhance keeping qualities.

Store-bought apples should also be refrigerated and will keep for two weeks or longer.

Dried apples are best kept in a cool, dry spot in a closed container. They will keep for about a year.

Where do they come from?

Originally from southwest Asia, apples are now found on every continent. They thrive in temperate climates—some varieties can withstand winters of –40°F.

In the United States, ten billion pounds of apples are produced commercially every year; more than 40 percent of them are grown in Washington state. New York, Michigan, California, and Pennsylvania also provide large quantities of apples. Some apples are imported from New Zealand, particularly during the Northern Hemisphere's spring and summer months (New Zealand's autumn and winter months).

APRICOTS, NECTARINES AND PEACHES

What are they?

These juicy golden fruits are botanically related and look quite similar to each other, but each has a luscious flavor of its own.

Like other tree fruits, propagation is by grafting rather than seed planting, to ensure that the same varieties will result. The trees begin to bear fruit at five years and continue to produce for thirty years—apricots for up to one hundred years.

Apricots, nectarines, and peaches are all roundish and have golden skins with red "cheeks." They have a slight groove, or seam, from the stem to the blossom end, which serves as a guideline for slicing them in half. These fruits contain almond-shaped, stonelike pits; they are related to almonds. Peaches and nectarines are sometimes referred to as *clingstone* (when the flesh of the fruit clings to the seed) or *freestone* (when the flesh is easily freed or removed from the seed).

Buying tips

Fresh apricots, nectarines, and peaches should be plump, fairly firm, have a slight give when touched at the seams, have a creamy golden color with red-blushed skins, and feel velvety. Avoid hard, green, dull, shriveled, bruised, and moldy fruits. Generally, nectarines and peaches will not become sweeter after picking, so they are best eaten when as close to being fully ripe as possible. They are highly perishable and should be handled carefully to prevent bruising. Green or firm apricots will ripen in about three days at room temperature, and ripe ones should be used as soon as possible. These fruits are in season from early spring to late summer.

Dried apricots and peaches should appear clean and be dry but pliable. Apricots are sometimes gassed with sulfur dioxide to retain their golden color and some of their moisture. Naturally dried fruits turn brown, which does not affect eating quality.

How do I use them?

Besides eating these fruits as fresh foods, you can slice them for fruit salads and cereal, blend them with yogurt for refreshing fruit shakes, or wedge them for garnishes on desserts.

There are few things as delicious as peach pie, but have you tried apricot ice cream? Or nectarine cobbler? For most recipes, these fruits are interchangeable.

Dried apricots and peaches are sweet, chewy morsels that can be cut up for trail mixes or granola or just eaten as snacks, a few at a time. Keep in mind that each piece of dried peach or apricot represents a part or a half of the fresh fruit, so eat only as many pieces of dried fruit as you would if they were fresh.

You can reconstitute dried apricots, nectarines, and peaches by soaking them in an equal amount of water for about 30 minutes. Use the swelled fruits for sauces, purees, as a spread, or cooked as you would frozen or canned fruits.

How nutritious are they?

Fresh apricots, nectarines, and peaches are high in vitamin A and contain several minerals. They provide carbohydrates and are low in fat. A small amount of protein is present.

Dried apricots, nectarines, and peaches are very high in vitamin A, as well as iron, magnesium, potassium, and calcium.

◆ Nutritive Value: Appendix, 139–146, 187, 197–206.

How do I store them?

Store fresh, ripe fruits in the refrigerator for three to five days until ready to eat. Unwashed peaches can keep for up to two weeks under refrigeration.

Dried apricots, nectarines, and peaches will remain usable for at least a year. They may dry out and become brittle. If this happens, lightly steam them in a vegetable steamer to add moisture and make them chewy.

Where do they come from?

Apricots, nectarines, and peaches all originated in China and eventually were planted in Europe, then in North and South America.

About 90 percent of both apricots and nectarines produced in the United Sates are from California. Some are from Idaho, Washington, Colorado, and Utah.

Although Georgia is reputed to be the peach state, California, South Carolina, and Pennsylvania produce more peaches.

These fruits are imported during the winter months from Chile, Argentina, Italy, and Iran.

Apricots

The name of this fruit is derived from the Latin word *praecoquum,* which translates as "early ripe." Indeed, the English called apricot *hastie peche,* because it is one of the first fresh fruits to appear in the summer.

Some of the more common apricot varieties are Royal, Tilton, Derby, and Moorpark. Fresh apricots constitute 21 percent of the total commercial crop of one hundred thousand tons annually. Canned apricots make up about 50 percent, dried apricots 17 percent, and frozen apricots 12 percent of the total production.

Nectarines

The Greek drink of the gods is *nekter,* hence the name of this refreshing fruit. Its use dates back to ancient times, although it is sometimes mistakenly referred to as a recent hybrid of peaches and plums, its cousins. However, a nectarine is not a fuzzless peach any more than a peach is a fuzzy nectarine.

About ten varieties of nectarines are grown commercially, including May Red and Red June (early varieties), Sun Grand (mid-summer), and September Grand (late season). Most nectarines are sold fresh or canned; some are dried.

Peaches

Sometimes called a Persian plum, this fruit is grown for commercial purposes in thirty-five states in the U.S. It is among the four most popular fruits for eating out of the hand, and it is also frequently canned, frozen, and dried.

The most popular variety of peach is Elberta—named after a woman, not after the province in Canada (Alberta) as may be believed. It is a freestone peach and accounts for about half of the peach harvest. It is usually sold fresh. Cling peaches are not a variety—the term refers to the clingstone (see page 41). Most cling peaches are canned or frozen.

Because the fuzz on peaches is often considered undesirable, defuzzing machines have been invented to brush the fruits.

AVOCADOS

What are they?

Alligator pears, ahuactl, vegetable butter, agovago pear . . . these are just a few of the other names for avocado.

Avocados are green, usually pear-shaped fruits of a subtropical tree in the laurel family. Unlike most tree fruits, which are sweet and juicy, avocados are

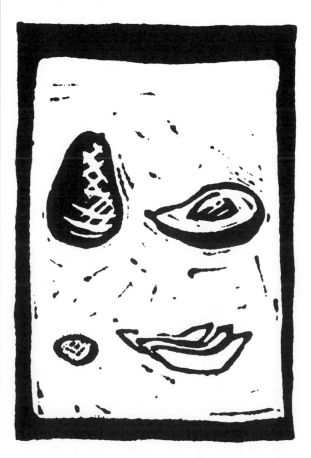

creamy and have a mild, nutty flavor. They are generally used as a vegetable.

Of the one hundred known varieties of avocados, fifty to seventy varieties are grown in the United States. Between 150 and 300 thousand metric tons of avocados are produced in the U.S. every year. The two main varieties grown for commercial purposes are:

- Hass—A dark green to purple-black rough-skinned avocado that has a higher oil content—and therefore more calories—than other varieties. Hass avocados originated in Guatemala and are grown in California. They are small to medium in size (eight ounces average) and are summer fruits, usually available from April to October.
- Fuerte—A medium-green, leathery-skinned fruit that ranges in size from eight to sixteen ounces. Fuerte avocados are of Guatemalan-Mexican origin and are also grown in California. They are available in fall and winter.

Approximately 85 percent of the domestically grown avocados are from California. The other 15 percent are from Florida. Of those grown in Florida, the summer types are bright green and smooth-skinned; they are originally from the West Indies. Florida's fall and winter avocados have bright green but rougher and thicker skins; they are of Guatemalan origin or are West Indian-Guatemalan hybrids.

Florida avocados are usually larger than those grown in California and can grow to five pounds. Florida avocados also contain less fat and consequently fewer calories than California avocados.

Avocados become mature on the trees but will not ripen or soften until they are picked. To avoid bruising, most avocados are hand-picked and hand-packed.

Buying tips

Avocados should be fairly heavy for their size and free of bruises, dark sunken spots, cracks, or other irregularities. Ripe, ready-to-eat avocados will feel soft when you press them between the palms of your hands. Firm ones can be ripened at room temperature in a few days by placing them in a paper bag or in a fruit basket. The skins darken as the fruits become ripe.

How do I use them?

To prepare an avocado, first wash it off and cut it in half, being careful not to sever the large seed pit. Twist the halves to separate them, then pick out or lift the pit with the knife. (Save the pit to grow a houseplant if you'd like.) Scoop out the flesh or peel off the skins. You can now slice, dice, mash, or scoop little balls out of the avocado. This fruit is normally eaten raw, but you can heat it gently. Prolonged heat, however, will cause it to become bitter.

Guacamole, for which avocados are most popular, is a dip made by mashing the ripe fruit and adding lemon juice, garlic, salt, Worcestershire sauce, tomatoes, and other ingredients as you wish. It is eaten with corn chips, crackers, or raw vegetables.

Avocados are also good in sandwiches and salads. Try making appetizers by stuffing avocado halves with fish or fruit pieces. Have you ever eaten avocado ice cream? Try it sometime!

How nutritious are they?

Although they are nearly 75 percent water, avocados contain more solids than many other fruits or vegetables. Avocados are 5 to 22 percent fat—most of which is monounsaturated fatty acids. There is no cholesterol in avocados.

Avocados also provide some carbohydrates, protein, and fiber. Vitamins A, B-complex, and C are present, as well as potassium, magnesium, iron, calcium, and phosphorus.

✦ Nutritive Value: Appendix, 147, 148.

How do I store them?

Firm, unripe avocados should be stored at room temperature. Colder temperatures—below 55°F—can injure the fruit. Soft, ripened fruit should be refrigerated until ready to use.

The flesh of halved or otherwise prepared avocados will turn brown due to oxygen in the air. This can be prevented by adding lemon juice or lime juice to the surface of the halves or by mixing the juice with pureed avocado. Keep the avocado pit in any unused half and tightly wrap it with plastic film to prevent flesh discoloration.

For convenience, you can freeze pureed avocados or guacamole. Whole or sliced avocados should not be frozen however, as the flesh will become mushy.

BANANAS

What are they?

Bananas—the long, slender fruits of a tropical plant—have been in the human diet as least as long as life has been recorded. They are actually berries and are unique in that the inedible peels are easily removed, making them a nutritious, naturally packaged, and easy-to-eat treat for children or adults.

There are about thirty different varieties of bananas. The most common ones are Cavendish (also called Vallery), which have blunt ends; Gros Michel, which have tapered ends; and plantains, which are large and starchy, and are typically used as a vegetable (see page 167).

Bananas grow on tall, treelike plants in bunches with clusters of hands that have ten to fifteen fingers. Only one big bunch grows per plant, and it can weigh from 60 to 100 pounds and contain nine to sixteen hands. The fingers (individual bananas) grow pointed ends up. It takes about a year for fruits to develop. After harvesting, the plant is removed and is replaced with a new planting.

Bananas are picked while green and are either allowed to ripen slowly or are ripened quickly in rooms of ethylene gas. There is reportedly no difference in taste between slowly ripened and artificially ripened bananas. Tree-ripened bananas are said to be not as sweet as those picked while green and ripened off the plant. They would also split open and be subject to insect infestation if left on the tree too long.

Buying tips

When shopping for bananas, look for solid, well-developed bunches with no signs of bruises or cuts. Flat or thin bananas have been picked too early and will not ripen completely. Three medium-sized bananas equal approximately 1 pound.

Most retail stores receive bananas at the "green tip" stage—when the body is yellow and the ends green. Green bananas can be ripened at home, and they will ripen faster in a paper bag. The bag will keep the naturally occurring ethylene gas around the fruit. Avoid green bananas that have been refrigerated, indicated by dull or smoky skins. Cool temperatures cause the flesh of bananas to remain starchy or to never fully ripen. They ripen best at 60 to 70°F and are usually ready to eat in two or three days.

How do I use them?

Bananas are, of course, delicious by themselves, but you can also blend them with yogurt and other fruits or fruit juices for a refreshing smoothie. Add them sliced to fruit salads and cream pies, or roll them in a bowl of chopped nuts or coconut flakes for a textured treat. Try baking bananas as you would apples.

You can also dry banana slices, halves, or thin chips for a munchy snack. Use ripe, but not mushy, bananas.

Overripe bananas need not be thrown out. Mash them for banana bread or cookies; 2 or 3 bananas make 1 cup of mashed fruit.

For the sweetest and fullest flavor, eat bananas that have completely yellow skins. Those with brown speckled skins are sweeter than bananas with barely yellow peels.

How nutritious are they?

Bananas are rich in potassium, magnesium, and many other minerals. They contain vitamins A and B-complex and have twice as much vitamin C as apples. They are high in carbohydrates but low in fat and protein.

✦ Nutritive Value: Appendix, 149, 150.

How do I store them?

As mentioned above, ripen green bananas at home at room temperature. Bananas can be refrigerated once the brown spots appear. The skin will turn completely brown but the inside will remain yellow and quite edible. You can also freeze peeled whole or mashed bananas; use them within a month.

Where do they come from?

Bananas originated in Southeast Asia and were one of the first cultivated fruits. The U.S. consumes 60 percent of the bananas produced in the world. The Central American countries from which bananas come (Panama, Honduras, Costa Rica) are sometimes referred to as banana republics.

BERRIES

What are they?

Berries are usually small, sweet, and juicy fruits that grow on plants and bushes. There are hundreds of kinds of berries—both edible and poisonous—and they are often found growing wild in woods, fields, and marshes. The more common edible kinds are strawberries, blueberries, cranberries, blackberries, raspberries, gooseberries, and currants.

When picking your own berries, try to handle them as little as possible, and place them in shallow trays rather than in deep bowls to prevent them from squishing. To retain flavor and juice, do not wash or soak them in water. Try dry-washing them in a piece of cheesecloth: Roll them by holding the ends of the cloth and swinging your arms back and forth like a seesaw for a few minutes.

Buying tips

Because of their fragility, most berries are packaged in pint- or quart-size baskets. To get more from less, some retailers "dink" the basket by emptying the contents then loosely refilling more baskets than what they originally had.

Look for fully rounded baskets of ripe, plump berries. Avoid those that have become soft, mushy, or moldy, or berries that are green (unripe) and hard. Except for strawberries, berries should have the stems removed to prevent them from being poked and bruised.

✦ Nutritive Value: Appendix, 151–154, 157, 158, 233–235, 237–239, 468, 469, 471.

Blackberries and Raspberries

Blackberries and raspberries are close relatives. Both are members of the rose family, grow on thorny brambles or canes, and have distinct fruit shapes. A single berry is actually a group of drupelets—tiny fruits clustered together. Each drupelet contains one seed.

The main differences between blackberries and raspberries are that green (unripe) blackberries are red in color and the stem core stays inside the berries, whereas ripe raspberries have a hole where the stem core once was. Also, blackberries prefer a warmer climate, while raspberries grow well in northern areas. The flavor of each is distinct.

Although blackberries are black (dark purple), raspberries can be both red and black—the red varieties being more common. Black raspberries are sometimes called *black caps* and are usually found in their wild state in early summer. Blackberries look quite similar to black raspberries but they are larger, juicier, and bear later in the summer.

Two other bramble berries are closely related to blackberries and raspberries. The *loganberry,* either a blackberry and raspberry cross or a hybrid blackberry, originated in the California garden of James Logan. It is dark red and very long in comparison to the other two berries. *Boysenberry,* a cross between black raspberry and loganberry named after Rudolph Boysen, is another large, elongated and dark red berry.

Blackberries and the other bramble berries make fine fruit pies, jams, and juices. Add them to pancakes or blend them with other fruits for tangy beverages. A dish of yogurt and berries is quite colorful and appetizing, as commercial yogurt makers have found. You can cook the berries or just eat them raw, right off the cane.

Blackberries and raspberries provide vitamins A and C, small amounts of B-complex, and some minerals. Raspberries are also high in pectin, which helps to thicken homemade jam.

Blueberries

This berry has several names—*whortleberry, bilberry, hurtleberry*—and cousins—*saskatoons* and *huckleberry.* There are several types of blueberry plants as well: low-bush, rabbit-eye, and high-bush.

Low-bush blueberries grow wild in the northern United States and Canada, and they are usually small but very flavorful. Rabbit-eye blueberry bushes grow to heights of thirty feet, requiring ladders for picking. These berries grow in the southern United States and are generally processed rather than marketed fresh. The plants of high-bush blueberries grow to heights of ten feet and produce large, firm, light blueberries—the type most often found in grocery stores.

It has only been in the last 60 years that blueberries have gone from being a wild delicacy to an important cultivated crop. During the 1960s commercial production of this second most popular berry increased 500 percent. Blueberries are grown in Michigan, Maine, Washington, Oregon, and Canada.

Ripe, fresh blueberries should be plump, full of color, and have a powdery bloom on the skins. They are highly perishable, lasting only about seven days after picking, so avoid shriveled, green, or dark, soft, and shiny berries, as well as those in stained or leaky containers. Blueberries are available from May through September and are at their peak in July and August.

Use blueberries in muffins, pancakes, cereals, salads, pies, and fruit shakes. Keep them refrigerated until ready to use, or freeze them, with or without additional sweetener. To freeze, just dry-wash them and place in tightly sealed containers.

Cranberries

Another cousin of the blueberry, although red or pink in color and larger in size, is the cranberry. The name was chosen because the plant's blossom grows downward and looks like the head of a crane. Cranes also like to eat cranberries, which often grow in one of the birds' favorite habitats: sandy peat bogs.

Cranberries are harvested in the fall and are at peak season in November, hence their traditional association with Thanksgiving feasts.

Most of the cranberries sold in the United States are marketed by Ocean Spray, an eight hundred-grower/member cooperative. Cranberries grow in Massachusetts, New Jersey, Oregon, Washington, and Wisconsin.

During the preparation for marketing, cranberries are sorted and graded by a bouncing test, which allows the berries to bounce over four- to seven-inch barriers. Those that can't bounce are too soft and therefore unmarketable, so most of the cranberries that reach the consumer have passed the hurdles test. About a pound of cranberries is eaten per person in the United States every year.

Look for firm, plump, bright-colored cranberries. Avoid shriveled, crushed, or soft ones.

Cranberries are rather tart and generally need sweetening. They add a zesty zing to salads, breads, and relishes. Try them in pies, waffles, or stuffing. Dried cranberries perk up trail mixes and granola. They can also be reconstituted for sauce.

To prolong storage, do not wash cranberries until ready to use. Better yet, freeze them raw and have cranberries for mid-winter and early spring delights.

Strawberries

By far the most popular berry is the strawberry. The origin of its name is unknown, although it may be due to straw being used as a mulch around strawberry plants. The small, wild strawberry of Europe and North America was crossbred with a walnut-sized strawberry of Chile in 1835 to produce the commercial fruits we know and consume.

Although strawberries contain many seeds, most plants are propagated not with seeds but by shoots—runners that grow from an existing plant. They are easy to grow and are one of the first fruits to be eaten in spring. The strawberries known as June berries bear once, in June, while everbearing berries begin to bear in early summer and continue to produce through mid-summer.

The best-tasting and most nutritious strawberries are those that have been sun-ripened on the plants. The amount of vitamin C in strawberries increases the longer the berries remain in the sun, unpicked.

They should be fully red, slightly soft, and fragrant, with stems intact. To retain the sweet juice, do not remove the green caps until the berries have been rinsed in cold water, drained (stem side down), and allowed to dry on an absorbent surface.

Strawberries are wonderful for eating out of the hand, in fruit salads, and blended with rhubarb for pies. Strawberry jams and preserves can be made with honey, but use only as much honey as you need to sweeten them, as the flavor of honey may overpower the delicious taste of the berries.

Always keep fresh **strawberries** refrigerated, uncovered. For longer storage, strawberries can be dried or frozen. To dry strawberries, slice thinly and place on drying trays (see Dried Fruits, page 57). To freeze them, just add a little sweetener to strawberry pieces or halves, then pop them into the freezer.

Fresh strawberries provide vitamins A, C, and small amounts of the B-complex, as well as some minerals. Cooking, freezing, and drying them greatly reduce the vitamin C content.

Gooseberries and Currants

Two bush berries that grow wild in certain unrestricted areas of North America are gooseberries and currants. Because they are carriers of a blister-rust fungus that causes white pine trees to die, many of these fruit bushes are eradicated rather than allowed to bear fruits. Plants that survive in the wild or that are cultivated in unforested areas provide delicious, slightly tart, round berries.

Gooseberries can grow to about the size of marbles. They are so named because it is thought that they were traditionally served with cooked goose.

Currants grow like grapes in clusters and are fairly small. So-called dried currants are actually a type of miniature raisin from the Corinth grape.

Both gooseberries and currants come in red and white (yellowish-green) varieties. Black currants grow in Europe.

Use raw gooseberries and currants for simple desserts or snacks, or cook them into pies, jellies, sauces, and jams. They are available from late spring through August.

CHERRIES

What are they?

Cherries are small, soft fruits related to peaches and plums. Cherry trees grow in moderate to temperate climates and are beautiful in early spring when blossoms appear. The fruits hang from long, thin stems and bear large seeds (or pits) surrounded by juicy flesh and thin skins.

The two main types of cherries available are sweet and sour. *Sweet cherries* are large, heart-shaped, usually dark-colored (maroon to nearly black), and have smooth skins. The more popular varieties are Bing, Lambert, Chapman, and Royal Ann (Napoleon). The latter variety is yellow and is typically canned, dyed red, and bottled as maraschino cherries.

Sour or *tart cherries* are smaller, round, and usually red or pinkish. Most sour cherries are marketed canned or frozen for sauce or pie filling rather than fresh.

Less common types of this fruit are:

• Chokecherries—Small, red, very tart cherries often eaten by birds before any fruit can be harvested for human consumption
• Sand cherries—Wild fruits growing in the Rocky Mountains
• Ground cherries—Actually related to tomatoes, they grow on short, sprawling plants. The fruits of ground cherries are found inside papery husks (similar to Chinese lanterns), and are round, yellow or green, and marble-sized

Buying tips

Cherries are rarely picked before they are fully ripe. Ripe, sweet cherries are dark or full-colored, plump, soft but not mushy, and have glossy or fresh-looking stems. Avoid bruised, shriveled, moldy, and dull-skinned cherries. Those with dry, brittle stems are overripe.

Sweet cherries are available from May to July. Sour cherries ripen too fast for fresh marketing purposes.

How do I use them?

Besides eating cherries as fresh fruits, use them in fruit salads, desserts, baked goods, and for canning or freezing. Be sure to wash them, but do not soak in water.

One drawback to cherries is removing the pits. You can cut them in half and take out the pits by hand, which is rather tedious, especially if a large quantity is involved. A mechanical cherry pitter works well and makes canning, freezing, and drying preparations much easier. Reportedly, poking a clean hairpin or an artist's pen point (in a clean holder) into the stem end will also remove the pit.

To make dried cherries, pit them and cut in half. Place pieces in single layers on drying trays and dry them for a day or so at 110 to 120°F. (The sweeter the fruit, the longer the drying time.) Use dried cherries in baked goods, granola, trail mixes, pancakes, or waffles.

Consult a food storage or preservation cookbook for details on canning, freezing, and making jelly from cherries.

How nutritious are they?

Cherries are a good source of carbohydrates and contain little fat and protein. The minerals phosphorus, potassium, and calcium are present, as well as vitamin A, a minimal amount of B-complex vitamins, and vitamin C. Sour, raw cherries are exceptionally high in vitamin A (although not necessarily edible without sweetener added). Canned cherries lose some vitamin C and are generally sweetened, which increases the calories and displaces some nutrients.

✦ Nutritive Value: Appendix, 155–156.

How do I store them?

Keep fresh, sweet cherries refrigerated until ready to eat, and use within a week if soft fleshed, two to three weeks if firm fleshed.

Dried cherries should last up to a year if stored in a dry, cool area.

Where do they come from?

Cherries were found growing all over the world, successfully propagated by birds which, after eating, flew to another area and disposed of the pits.

The cultivated varieties are of European origin. Probably the most popular sweet cherry variety, Bing, was named after a Chinese worker.

In the United States today, most of the cherries come from Washington, Oregon, California, Michigan, New York, and Utah.

CITRUS FRUITS

What are they?

Citrus fruits—oranges, grapefruits, lemons, limes—are semitropical fruits that originated in Southeast Asia. Botanically, they are considered berries. Their seeds are found throughout the fleshy fruit, although the skins are not usually eaten.

Trees of citrus fruits are evergreens that grow to varying heights, seemingly reflecting the size of their fruits. Lime trees grow to about fifteen feet, whereas grapefruit trees grow to fifty feet.

As the name implies, citrus fruits contain citric acid, which gives the fruits their tartness. Most citrus fruits have both sour (tart) and sweet varieties. Sweet oranges, sour lemons, and sour limes are usually preferred for consumption.

Buying tips

All citrus fruits are tree ripened and ready to eat when they appear in the marketplace. Some may have green patches on the skins, which could be because of the variety, but they are ripe and will not change color. Only dark brown (noticeably bruised) or fuzzy green (moldy) fruits should be avoided, as well as those with soft spots and a puffy appearance (except for mandarin oranges, which are often puffy). Fruits that have begun to deteriorate are weak and mushy, sometimes brown and wrinkly at the stem ends.

Citrus fruits that contain a lot of juice are generally heavy and have smooth, thin skins. Lightweight fruits are usually old and dried up. Very rough skins indicate thick skins and therefore less juice and less fruit inside.

How do I use them?

Citrus fruits are excellent for juicing to provide thirst-quenching beverages for breakfast or any other time of day. Citrus juices, especially lemon juice, add a pleasant essence to steamed vegetables, dressings, desserts, or fish and poultry dishes. When squeezing your own, roll the fruit with your palm on a hard surface before cutting. This breaks the juice capsules and results in more juice.

Lemonade and limeade are made from the fruit juice and pulp, water, and a sweetener. Pink lemonade is artificially colored for appearance only.

A tangy fruit salad can be made with pieces of all the common citrus fruits or mixed with strawberries, bananas, and apples. They blend well with jelled desserts and are attractive as garnishes, sliced thinly across the center as coins.

Lemon and orange peel are fine flavorings for cookies, breads, and salads. Grate them with a small-holed grater or chop them very, very fine. If possible, use fruits that have not been waxed or sprayed with pesticides. Orange peels from Florida and Texas fruits are often dyed, solely to compete with the bright orange-colored California fruits—which are sometime preferred by consumers because they *look* orange. Dyed oranges will have "color added" stamped on the skins. But russeted, light orange, spotted, or otherwise imperfect skins generally do not reflect the quality of the citrus fruit inside. And the off-colored skins are fine for grating. About 3 oranges or 5 to 6 lemons will provide $1/2$ cup grated peel.

How nutritious are they?

Citrus fruits are known for their high vitamin C content, the highest amount of which is in the juice. Orange juice made into frozen concentrate loses only a trace of vitamin C.

Another nutrient in citrus fruits, especially in the white insides of the skins and the membranes, is called bioflavinoid. Sometimes referred to as vitamin P, bioflavinoids are needed by the body to absorb vitamin C. (See pages 223–224.)

Citrus fruits also contain potassium, calcium, and magnesium. Grapefruits and oranges provide a good amount of vitamin A as well.

✦ Nutritive Value: Appendix, 164–170, 177–183, 188–195, 240–242.

How do I store them?

To keep citrus fruits fresh and juicy, store them in your refrigerator or in a very cool place. Do not keep them in plastic bags or film-covered trays, as they may become moldy because the plastic causes moisture to collect and drop onto the fruits. Citrus fruits are best stored loose and should last one to two weeks.

Don't worry about grapefruits with skins that have become dark and sunken from prolonged refrigeration. The fruit inside will be unaffected.

Orange juice should be kept refrigerated and stored in a nonmetallic container to preserve vitamin C. Avoid fizzy orange juice, as it has begun to ferment.

Grapefruits

Grapefruits are so called because they grow in clusters like grapes. They are found mainly in the Caribbean Sea region, especially in Florida. The fruit was thought to have evolved from pomelo, and it used to be called *shaddock,* after a sea captain who brought it to the West Indies. This formerly bitter citrus may have crossed with a sweet orange to become the sour-sweet grapefruit we know.

Both white (yellow) and pink grapefruit are grown. *White grapefruits* are usually smaller in size and quite tart. *Pink grapefruits* are naturally colored; the ruby red type was discovered growing in the Rio Grande Valley of Texas in 1929—a quirk of nature. They are fairly large and are distinguished by a red blush on their yellow skin. Both white and pink grapefruits have thin, slightly pebbly skins; some are seedless.

Most grapefruits are from Florida, where 70 percent of the world's supply grows. Most of the pink (ruby red) grapefruits are grown in Texas. Equal amounts of the total grapefruit crop are used for fresh markets and for canning as juice and segments. The season lasts all year, although it peaks in mid-winter and drops off in summer.

Uglifruit

This is a citrus fruit that resembles grapefruit in size but has brownish wrinkly skin and red flesh. It tastes like a grapefruit-orange cross and is fairly sweet and juicy. The fruit is grown in the West Indies, particularly Jamaica. It is generally considered a specialty item in the United States.

Lemons

This bright yellow, roundish or egg-shaped citrus fruit is full of tartness and zing. The *sour lemon* is grown commercially, but the *sweet lemon*—also edible—is grown as an ornamental tree. The main varieties of sour lemons are Lisbon, a smooth-skinned winter fruit with a long nipple stem end; and Eureka, which has a flat nipple and only a few seeds. Eurekas are available most of the year, with the season peaking in summer. Lemons with greenish tints on the skins are more acidic. Rough or pebbly skins are a sign of lower juice content.

Citron

Citron is a fairly large, lemonlike fruit with thick skin but not much flesh or juice. The rind is candied for fruitcakes or is pressed to obtain oil. This oil is quite fragrant and is used in the manufacture of medicines, liqueurs, and perfumes. This should not be confused with citronella oil, which is distilled from a tropical grass of southern Asia and is sometimes used as an insect repellent.

Limes

Limes are green, usually small fruits resembling lemons in shape and taste. Several varieties are grown: Bearss, a seedless lime from California; Persian, a very acidic fruit from Florida usually made into juice;

and Key Lime, a round acidic Mexican fruit also grown in Florida. The skins of limes are usually pebbly and should be green. Yellow skins indicate storage in sunlight, which causes them to deteriorate and be less acidic. Those with brown surface spots or russeting are fine, however. You can purchase limes year-round. Peak season is June to September.

Kumquat

A small (one- to two-inch) oblong or roundish fruit that looks like a miniature orange, kumquats have edible skins and are sold with the leaves still attached. They should be squeezed before eating to break and blend the juicy pulp. You can also pickle, preserve, or candy them.

Mandarins

Although consumers in the United States often consider mandarins to be oranges that come in cans, this species covers the citrus fruits of *tangerines, temple oranges,* and *tangelos.* The skins are generally pebbly and dark orangish red, and they separate easily from the flesh of the fruit. Most are quite seedy and slightly tart, but juicy. They are available from November to May.

- Tangerine—This term is often mistakenly used to describe mandarins. The name is from Tangiers, a seaport of Morocco, where the fruit is popular. Several varieties of tangerines are available, such as Satsuma, a sweet and nearly seedless Japanese tangerine; Kinnow, a thin-skinned, yellowish, harder to peel fruit; and Clementine, a larger, deep orange, bumpy-skinned tangerine.
- Temple—An orange and tangerine hybrid, the temple orange is fairly large and tangy in taste. This fruit is available from December to April.
- Tangelo—A cross between *tange*rine and grape-fruit (pom*elo*), this fruit is quite seedy and often has a nipplelike stem end. The main tangelo varieties are Minneola, Seminole, and Orlando. They taste similar to tangerines and oranges, but they are not much like grapefruits in taste or appearance.

Oranges

Oranges, the second most popular fresh fruit, are available most of the year for eating, juicing, or making marmalade. The word orange is derived from *nagarunga,* a Sanskrit term meaning "fruit favored by the elephants." An estimated 80 percent of the commercial oranges in the United States become bottled juice or frozen concentrate. An increasing amount of bottled juice and frozen concentrates are from oranges grown in Brazil and other Latin American countries.

The main types of oranges are:

- Navel—These oranges have a bellybuttonlike spot at the blossom end and are seedless, usually large, and sweet. They are favored for eating out of the hand. If the skins are bumpy, they are also likely to be thick and thus contain less flesh. This type of orange is not a recent hybrid; it has been known of since the 1600s. About 10 percent of the annual United States orange crop is Navels.
- Valencia—This is a juice orange that ranges in size from small to nearly grapefruit size. It usually has numerous seeds within its sweet, juicy, pulp. The skin is smooth and thin. About 50 percent of the oranges grown in the United States are Valencias, and they are available throughout most of the year.
- Seville—This is a sour orange, usually imported from Spain and used for candied peel, marmalade, and curaçao liqueur. The leaves and flowers are used in cosmetics for fragrance.

DATES

What are they?

Dates are the sweet, chewy fruits of certain palm trees. They have been referred to as "candy that grows on trees."

The date palm is a desert plant that grows to one hundred feet in height and has a straight, shaggy-barked trunk. The trees are dioecious, which means there are both male and female trees. To pollinate the female trees that produce the fruit, a male flower sprig is tied to female flowering branches. One male tree will pollinate forty to one hundred female trees. Each female tree produces up to six hundred pounds of dates which grow in five to one hundred bundles that weigh up to forty pounds each. One bundle holds one thousand or more dates.

Although there are about one hundred varieties of dates, only six are of commercial importance in the United States:

- Deglet Noor—This variety constitutes 85 percent of the date production. The fruits are medium to large in size and amber in color. When dried, Deglet Noor dates are medium to deep brown and quite sweet. Different grades of Deglet Noors are available—from Fancy to Choice to Standard—judged according to size and softness. Bread dates are Deglet Noors that have been dried to a lower moisture content and are hard, dry, and chewy but not sticky.
- Medjool—These large, meaty dates can grow four to five times as large as Deglet Noors if they are thinned heavily.

Both of the above varieties are of African origin; Deglet Noors are from Algeria, and Medjools are from Morocco.

- Khadrawi—A soft, sticky, chewy date that contains invert sugar, Khadrawis can crystallize or become sugary, but this will not affect the eating quality. This dark-skinned date is one of the earliest dates to ripen.
- Halawi—This date looks very much like Deglet Noor but it has its own distinct, sweet flavor. It is light amber in color.
- Barhi—A very soft, very sweet fruit.
- Zahidi—Not quite so sweet as other dates and small to medium in size. They are golden colored and of different flavor than most dates.

These last four varieties originated in Iran.

Buying tips

Fresh: Shop for plump, well-colored dates with glossy, smooth skins. If they are dull and shriveled, they were stored too long.

Dried: Well-shaped, whole dates are best. Avoid broken, wormy, or fermenting dates. If your source has sample dates, feel and taste them to know if they will suit your needs. Packaged dried dates are often pitted and pasteurized to prevent mold growth, or they have corn syrup added to keep them moist and chewy.

How do I use them?

Dates are excellent, quick-energy snacks—they are 75 to 80 percent all-natural sugars. Add pitted and chopped dates to breads, puddings, or cookies. They are great in fruitcake, muffins, trail mixes, and granola.

You can substitute date sugar for other sweeteners. To make a cup of date sugar, remove the pits from and slice 36 dates. Spread the slices on an ungreased baking pan, without allowing them to touch. Place the pan in a warm (250°F) oven for 12 to 15 hours. Occasionally open the oven door to release moisture and to check on the drying progress. Dry the date pieces until they are hard and completely free of moisture; they should feel like rocks. After cooling, grind them in a food grinder or add them slowly to a blender until they become sugarlike and powdery.

How nutritious are they?

Dates are high in carbohydrates and food energy. They contain some potassium, calcium, and magnesium, as well as small amounts of B-complex and vitamins A and C. They are very low in fat and contain some protein.

✦ Nutritive Value: Appendix, 159, 160.

How do I store them?

Keep fresh dates refrigerated in a tightly closed container to maintain freshness and prevent absorption of other food odors. Soft dates are best stored in a cool, dry place and should be used within six months to a year. Bread dates will keep indefinitely.

Where do they come from?

Dates have been grown in the Middle East and African deserts since 3500 B.C. About half the dates sold in the United States are grown in the Coachella Valley of California, where commercial date pro-

duction began in 1890. The remaining half are dates imported from Iran, Iraq, Egypt, and their bordering countries.

FIGS

What are they?

Known as the most nutritious of fruits, figs have been cultivated for centuries and cherished for just as long. The sweet, rich taste of figs is alluring and nearly addictive.

Fig trees grow in warm, semiarid climates to about twenty feet in height and bear fruit within one to three years after planting. Botanically, figs are only receptacles for the fruits inside—the small, crunchy, so-called seeds. Figs grow stem down, and the tiny openings at the other end, that face the sun, are for pollinating. No blossoms ever form on

---

CAPRIFICATION

Calimyrna figs set fruit by an unusual process known as *caprification.* A tiny insect called the *Blastophaga* wasp grows inside an inedible male fruit (caprifig). During the process of crawling out of the caprifig's top opening, the female wasp picks up pollen on her wings and body parts. Her goal is to lay eggs inside another male caprifig. But unfortunately for the wasp, she ends up in one of the more numerous female Calimyrna figs, and her attempts to lay eggs inside it are to no avail—the structure of the female fig will not allow it. However, her crawling around inside the female fig causes the pollen of the male caprifig to be deposited, thus resulting in the pollination of the (edible) female fig.

Only one *Blastophaga* wasp out of thousands ever finds a male caprifig—enough to provide a new generation of female wasps to repeat the process.

the fig trees; the flowers grow inside the receptacles.

There are hundreds of varieties of figs. The four most common ones grown in the United States are:

- Calimyrna (California Smyrna)—A large, "white," tan-skinned variety with sweet flesh, this variety is referred to as a *caprifig* because of caprification (see page 52).
- Adriatic—A prolific bearer, the Adriatic fig is similar in appearance to Calimyrna but smaller and not as sweet. It is good as a fresh fruit but is also dried.
- Mission—A black or dark purple-skinned fig of medium to large size and pleasantly sweet taste. It is sold fresh and dried.
- Kadota—A small, white, thick-skinned fig generally canned or sold fresh. It has only a few small seeds.

Calimyrna, Adriatic, and Mission figs each constitute about 30 percent of the dried fig sales. Kadotas make up the other 10 percent.

Buying tips

Most figs are sold dried or canned, although they are available fresh where grown. Fresh figs should be soft and plump. Avoid mushy, sour-smelling fruits or those with broken skins—they are overripe. Shriveled or partially dry figs are okay. Peak season for fresh figs is July through October. Dried figs are sold year-round.

Dried figs should be slightly moist and sweet-smelling. Dried out, moldy, or fermenting (sour smelling) figs should be avoided. Occasionally, dried figs will have potassium sorbate added to inhibit mold growth and to keep them moist. It takes three pounds of fresh figs to make one pound of dried figs. They are available throughout the year.

How do I use them?

Figs are a very versatile fruit, even though they are mostly eaten as snacks. You can stew them for breakfast, chop them for baked goods, or stuff them for desserts.

Fig newton cookies have long been favorites of both children and adults. To make your own, grind figs into a paste and spread on half a layer of thinly rolled out cookie dough. Fold the other half of dough over the layer with the fig paste, cut into strips, seal edges, and bake until brown.

Have you ever tried pickling figs? How about making fig preserves? You can substitute figs in any recipe calling for apricots.

How nutritious are they?

Figs are loaded with natural food energy (55 percent sugars) and provide carbohydrates and fiber. They contain a small amount of fat and a fair amount of protein.

The minerals calcium, magnesium, phosphorus, and potassium are found in abundant levels in figs. Also present are vitamins A and B-complex.

✦ Nutritive Value: Appendix, 161, 470.

How do I store them?

Fresh figs are highly perishable, so keep them refrigerated and use them within a few days. Dried figs are best stored in a cool, fairly dry place (below 45°F). If they develop surface sugar, simply dip them in lukewarm water.

Where do they come from?

Figs originated in western Asia and the Mediterranean sea region. Spanish missionaries established a fig orchard during the mid-1700s in San Diego, California, where the Mission fig was developed.

Most of the figs produced in the United States are from California. Fresno, California, is known as the fig capital of the world. Figs are also grown in Texas and other parts of the southern United States.

Figs and fig paste are imported to North America from Greece, Turkey, Italy, Portugal, and Spain.

GRAPES

What are they?

Grapes—those luscious, juicy little fruits on the vine—are grown and eaten all over the world. In fact, they constitute the largest fruit industry on the globe. They are sold as a fresh fruit, dried into raisins, crushed for juice and wine, and preserved or canned for jelly and fruit cocktail.

The grape plant is a series of twining, narrow vines that climb—if supported by a trellis or by tall plants—to six feet or higher. The fruits bear in bunches, with five to fifty grapes per bunch, depending on the variety. A typical vine will produce fifty bunches in a season and will last fifty to sixty years.

Grapes are classified as table or wine varieties, as well as by continent of origin (European, Asiatic, American). Some of the more popular grape varieties are:

- Concord—Flavorful, dark purple grapes that are savored as table grapes and favored for jelly, juice, and wine. This variety is native to North America.
- Thompson Seedless—This variety alone makes up half of the California grape acreage. Fresh Thompsons are light green, medium to large, and in season from June to November. Dried Thompsons make up 95 percent of all the raisins produced (see below).
- Ribier—Large, purple-black, mildly sweet grapes available from July through February.
- Emperor—A later variety (September through March) with large red berries and a cherrylike flavor.

These last three varieties are European types.

Buying tips

Fresh table grapes should be plump and well formed, have a bloom (a powdery look) on their skins, and have green, firm stems. Shiny grapes were overhandled; brown, dry stems (except on Emperors) indicate overaged and less flavorful grapes.

How do I use them?

Table grapes are refreshing summer snacks. They perk up fruit salads and desserts. Grapes and cheese have long been paired in European cuisine.

For an interesting twist, add fresh grapes (halved and seeded) to fruitcake. Try grapes in casseroles, sauces, curries, or stuffing. A small cluster of grapes makes an excellent garnish to hors d'oeuvre trays or main dishes.

Grape juice, usually made from Concord grapes, is a fine beverage for meals or over ice. Blend it with apple cider or other fruit juices, or with milk to make a "purple cow."

How nutritious are they?

Grapes provide potassium, magnesium, phosphorus, and calcium. They also contain vitamins A, B-complex, and C. Although mostly water, grapes have natural sugars and thus supply carbohydrates and food energy (calories). Small amounts of protein and fat are present.

✦ Nutritive Value: Appendix, 171–175.

How do I store them?

Grapes do not ripen after being picked from the vine, so they will shrivel and dry up or ferment if they are not refrigerated. They will keep for a week or two under refrigeration.

Where do they come from?

Grapes were one of the earliest foods cultivated. They are thought to have originated in Asia, although grapes were growing in North America when early Viking explorers came over from Norway. They called the country Vinland.

About 90 percent of the table grapes marketed in the United States are grown in California; over half of these become raisins. New York, Washington, and several other states also produce grapes in significant amounts. Out of all the grapes grown in the United States, 65 percent are used for wine, juice, and brandy.

Raisins

What are they?

Raisins are dried grapes. They are also the most popular dried fruit in North America.

Nearly all of the raisins produced are of the Thompson Seedless grape variety. Most of these are dried naturally in the sun and become dark purple or black. A small percentage of Thompson raisins are artificially dried with sulfur dioxide gas to retain the light color. These are called *golden seedless* raisins.

Three other regular-sized raisins are produced,

although in very limited quantities. They are:

- Muscat—A wine grape that is dried and often used in fruitcake
- Monukka—A large, dark, robust-flavored raisin
- Sultana—What Europeans call Thompson Seedless raisins

Miniature raisins, often referred to as Zante currants, are produced from the black Corinth grape variety and are dried for the confectionary market. They are mistakenly called "currants" because of their resemblance to the bush berries and the mispronounced name (Corinth sounds like currant).

Buying tips

When shopping for raisins, look for clean, well-developed fruits. They should not be mashed, dried out, sugary, or wormy.

Packaged raisins are often sealed in containers that do not allow you to see the contents. Look on the package for a "sell by" date, or write to the company to find out the product code that tells when they were packed and possibly when they should be taken from the shelves.

How do I use them?

Raisins are quite versatile and can be used for many different dishes, such as cookies, candy, granola, and breads. They add color and sweetness to garden salads, custard pies, and rice pudding.

For a simple sauce or dessert, stew raisins by simmering a cup of them in a cup of water or fruit juice. Then drain, saving the liquid for baking or cooking. You can, of course, eat them alone or with yogurt and cinnamon, other dried fruits, and nuts.

Raisin paste, made by grinding raisins in a food grinder until crushed and sticky, is a fine substitute or replacement for other sweeteners in baked goods and candies. Try mixing it with sesame tahini, sunflower seeds, and a bit of honey, and roll into bite-sized balls.

Ever had "ants on a log?" Take a stalk of celery, fill the hollow space with peanut butter, and dot it with raisins. This is a fun and nutritious snack that youngsters can make and eat.

How nutritious are they?

Raisins are a storehouse of minerals: potassium, phosphorus, magnesium, iron, and calcium are in abundant supply.

Also present in raisins are vitamins A and B-complex, and a small amount of vitamin C. They are high in carbohydrates and food energy, and they contain some protein but little fat.

✦ Nutritive Value: Appendix, 231, 232.

How do I store them?

Raisins should be stored in a tightly closed container in a cool place. They will last up to one year.

Where do they come from?

Raisins have been around as long as grapes have been grown—since early human history.

California is the source of almost all raisins marketed in the United States. Over half of the table grapes grown in that state are dried into raisins. A two thousand grower/member marketing cooperative, Sun-Maid, produces over 40 percent of these raisins.

GUAVA

Guava is a small, fragrant, tropical fruit originally from Mexico and now grown also in Florida, California, Hawaii, and South America.

Guava trees are short and bushlike. The fruits are one to four inches long, roundish, and have yellow or green skins with white, pinkish, or red flesh. A number of small seeds are found in the middle.

Ripe guavas are fairly firm but slightly soft to the touch. You can ripen hard ones at room temperature in a few days. To eat, cut them in quarters, then slice off the skin and seeds. Guavas are fine as raw fruits or cooked like apples in pies, jelly, casseroles, or puddings. Sweet potatoes and guavas are traditionally served together in Mexico.

Guavas are a good source of vitamins A and C and potassium. Store them in your refrigerator until ready to use.

✦ Nutritive Value: Appendix, 472.

KIWIFRUIT

Named after the New Zealand national bird, kiwi (pronounced **kee-***wee*) is also called *Chinese gooseberry* and tastes similar to the American gooseberry.

The fruit is distinctive: egg-shaped with brown, furry skins, about two inches in diameter and three inches long, with bright green, syrupy flesh and rays that shoot out from the center. Tiny edible black seeds surround the creamy yellow center.

Kiwifruit grows on vines and is heavily trellised to support the fruits. In New Zealand, blossoms appear in December, and the fruit is usually picked in early spring. In California, kiwifruit is harvested from late October through January.

Ripe kiwifruit is firm but should give when it is squeezed between your hands. To speed ripening, put firm kiwifruit in a plastic bag for a few days to keep the ethylene gas (a natural ripening agent) with the fruit. It is available year-round.

To use kiwifruit, slice it in half and eat it with a spoon. Add kiwifruit to salads, desserts, or cheese sandwiches. Do not cook the fruit, however, as the flavor would dissipate from the heat. Kiwifruit can tenderize meat, so rub the fruit over steaks or other cuts of meat.

Kiwifruit is reportedly high in vitamin C and contains other vitamins and minerals. There are about 66 calories in an average kiwifruit.

Store kiwifruit in your refrigerator, where it will keep for up to six months.

✦ Nutritive Value: Appendix, 176.

MANGO

A multishaped tropical fruit related to cashews, mango is a luscious, juicy, orange-fleshed fruit with both rainbow-colored and yellow skins. It can be round, kidneylike, or avocado-shaped—as well as long and narrow—and range from egg size to five pounds. Mangos are native to India and are now grown in Mexico, Haiti, and southern Florida. Over one thousand varieties are known.

Green mango skins indicate the fruit will not fully ripen, while black-spotted skins indicate over-ripe fruit. A ripe mango will yield to pressure between your palms; firm ones will ripen in a few days at room temperature. Mangos are in season from January to August and peak in June.

Because mango skins can be irritating to skin and mouth, they need to be removed. A potato peeler works well (unless the mango is extremely soft). You can also peel the fruit by cutting it in half, removing the large seed inside, and then cutting the skin twice to form a wide strip across the middle, down to (but not through) the flesh. Peel off the strip, then remove the ends. You can now slice or wedge the mango, puree it, or juice it. Mangos that are not quite ripe are fine for cooking and baking.

This fruit is extremely high in vitamin A and has vitamin C, magnesium, calcium, and potassium. Store mangos at room temperature and eat them as soon as they are ripe.

✦ Nutritive Value: Appendix, 184.

MELONS

What are they?

There is nothing like biting into a fresh, ripe, juicy slice of melon on a hot summer afternoon to satisfy a sweet thirst.

Melons come in all sizes—from the round muskmelon to the oval honeydew to the huge, cucumber-shaped, striped watermelon. Each type has a particular taste and aroma. They grow on sprawling vines with large, fuzzy leaves, and they are related to squash and cucumbers.

The melon family includes:

- Cantaloupe and Muskmelon—Often referred to as the same melon, the true cantaloupe is grown only in Europe. It has a pebbly rind, as does the nutmeg muskmelon, but it does not have the netting marks. Muskmelons have deep-grooved rinds—almost as indicators for cutting—and have netted rinds, a light crisscross pattern over the tannish green skin. They have orange flesh and a mass of seeds in the center. *Musk* refers to fragrance—ripe muskmelons will have a pleasant smell on the stem end.

- Watermelon—Several varieties of watermelon are sold. The Charleston Gray watermelon is oblong; its skin is green/gray-striped and its flesh is bright red. Some grow to forty pounds or larger. Peacock (medium to large) and Sugar Baby or Midget (small) watermelons have solid green rinds and are round in shape. Some may have yellow or orangish flesh. Sugar Baby contains many small, black seeds but is very sweet and juicy. One sign of ripeness is a brown, dry stem. Another sign is to hold a watermelon in one hand and thump it with the fingers of your other hand. It should sound hollow, with a slight ring. When purchasing a sliced half or portion of watermelon, look for dark brown seeds. White or streaked seeds indicate immature, less sweet fruit.

- Honeydew—These smooth, whitish-skinned melons have lime-green skin and very sweet flesh. A light, patched netting over the skin indicates a very sweet melon; a velvety bloom (a powdery look on the skin) with slight stickiness indicates a ripe honeydew. Avoid those that feel like billiard balls, as they were picked too soon.

Other melons sold in the United States include:

- Casaba—A large, pumpkin-shaped fruit with yellow or light green skin and sweet, juicy white flesh. It should have a slightly soft blossom end but will not have an aroma. Casabas are available from late summer through autumn.

- Cranshaw—A hefty muskmelon hybrid with salmon-orange flesh and mild flavor. It can weigh up to 9 pounds. The skins are rough and thick and may be golden yellow or dark green. Look for those with a soft blossom end and those that have a noticeable melon aroma. Cranshaws with a sunken spots have begun to rot, so avoid them. Cranshaws are available from mid-summer to mid-autumn.

- Persian—A honeydew-size melon that looks similar to cantaloupe, with netting and green rinds. The orange flesh is thick and full flavored. It is available from early summer to early autumn.

- Santa Claus—Oval, light green melons with mild, sweet flesh. They are so named because of their availability in December.

- Spanish—A large fruit with dark green corrugated skin. It tastes similar to Cranshaw and is available from mid-summer to mid-autumn.

DRIED FRUITS

Dried fruits, such as raisins and prunes, are made from fresh, ripe fruits that have had the water evaporated off, either by sun drying or artificial heat. Dried fruits are chewy, concentrated, sweet snacks and make fine additions to granola, pancakes, trail mixes, party appetizers, and baked goods. They can also be reconstituted and used like fresh or canned fruits. Eat only as many dried fruits as you would if they were fresh. (Two pear halves equal one fresh pear, for example.)

To dry fruits at home, buy or build a food dehydrator, use a cool oven, or place fruit pieces on a high shelf by a wood stove.

Fruits for drying should be ripe and at full flavor. Wash and allow fruit to drain. Then cut in slices or pieces as desired. Arrange the pieces on trays, being careful not to have any pieces touching each other. Trays can be of framed netting, screens, or cheesecloth-covered pans. In general, the fruits should be dried at a low temperature, 100 to 150°F. Unless the dehydrator or oven has air vents, periodically check and assist in the drying process by opening the door to release moisture.

FRUIT PROCESSING TERMS

Honey-dipped—Dried fruit sprayed or dipped with a honey and water solution to prevent mold growth and retain moisture. Honey acts as a preservative. "Honey-dipped" pineapple (and possibly other fruits) is actually dipped in a sugar and water solution—see page 62.

Potassium sorbate (also called sorbic acid)—An additive to some figs and prunes to keep them moist and prevent mold growth. It breaks down in the body as fat would, providing food energy. It is on the Generally Recognized As Safe (GRAS) list of the United States Food and Drug Administration (FDA).

Sulfur dioxide (sulfite)—A gas applied to some dried apples, apricots, golden seedless raisins, and other fruits to retain their light color. (Naturally dried fruits will turn brown due to oxidation.) Sulfur also helps retain vitamin C and carotene. Sulfites form naturally in the body and are converted to sulfate, which passes through the body. An excessive amount of sulfur dioxide on dried fruits (more than .05 percent) would be noticeable because of its distinctive rotten-egg smell. Sulfur has been used for thousands of years as a preservative and is considered safe, though not always necessary. Sulfur dioxide is on the GRAS list of the FDA.

Fruit leather is made by pureeing fruit pulp in a blender or food mill then pouring or spreading the mixture into shallow trays. The trays are then placed in a food dehydrator until enough water evaporates to leave a pliable, chewy wafer.

Buying tips

Look for melons with even-colored rinds, good symmetry, and pleasant fragrance. Avoid those that are off-colored, lopsided, or flattened; that have cracks or soft spots; and that sound sloshy when shaken.

The sweetest melons are those that have been fully ripened on the vine. With the exception of honeydews, they do not become sweeter after picking but merely dry up or ferment and rot. Melons are available from May through December, depending on the type.

How do I use them?

Simply cut open a melon, remove the seeds, and eat a portion as a breakfast wake-me-up or before-meal appetizer. Fantastic fruit salads can be made using melon wedges with oranges, bananas, apples, strawberries, and blueberries. For parties, float melon balls in a punch bowl of fruit juices.

Have you ever tried drying melons? Just remove the rind and seeds, slice into $1/4$-inch pieces (watermelon in $1/2$-inch pieces) and dry on trays in single layers for 12 to 18 hours at 110 to 120°F. They will be leathery and very sweet. You can reconstitute the pieces by soaking a cup of them in a cup of water for about an hour. To reduce the sweetness, add a small amount of lemon juice or grapefruit juice.

You can make watermelon pickles from watermelon rinds. They are a unique accompaniment to meals.

How nutritious are they?

Melons are over 90 percent water, but they contain natural sugars to provide carbohydrates and food energy (calories).

Muskmelons and watermelons are very high in vitamin A and contain some B-complex and C. They are excellent sources of potassium and also supply calcium, phosphorus, and other trace minerals.

✦ Nutritive Value: Appendix, 185, 186, 243, 244.

How do I store them?

For fullest flavor, keep melons at room temperature away from direct sunlight. Refrigerate after cutting. They will last for about a week.

Where do they come from?

Muskmelons originated in Persia (Iran). Watermelons come from the central part of Africa.

Today, melons grow in home gardens in almost all climates. Domestic commercial production is in Florida, Texas, Georgia, and California. Melons are imported from Mexico in winter and spring.

Carambola
(Star Fruit)

Carambola is a tree melon that originated in Malaysia and is now grown throughout Asia. The tree grows to about thirty feet and is an evergreen, producing three crops a year.

The fruit is about five inches long and has pointed ridges similar to an acorn squash. If you cut it crosswise, the slices resemble a star.

Use fresh carambola as you would melons. You can also juice it, make jams from it, and dry it. Dried star fruit is available in some natural food stores.

✦ Nutritive Value: Appendix, 467.

PAPAYA

A large, pear-shaped fruit, papaya is sometimes called the melon that grows on trees. It originated in the American tropics and grows in Florida, Mexico, and Puerto Rico. Most papayas now come from Hawaii.

Some papayas grow to eighteen inches long, but the most common length is about six inches. The smooth skin turns from green to yellow when ripe. The ripest papaya has nearly all yellow or orangish skin and feels slightly soft to the touch. Ripen green ones at room temperature for a few days out of direct sunlight, then refrigerate them for up to a week.

Papaya flesh is similar to muskmelon, but it sometimes has an almost peppery taste. In the center lie shiny, black, peppercorn-size seeds, which should be discarded. Eat papaya as you would melon, or puree it, or serve it with citrus fruits.

Dried papaya—long orange strips of the fruit's sweet flesh—is a great snack for hiking trips. Cut them into chunks for cookies, fruitcakes, and granola.

Papaya is low in calories but high in vitamin A. Some minerals are also present. Papain, an enzyme found in the green skin and leaves, is used as a meat tenderizer and aids in digestion of protein. Papaya is available year-round; its peak season is from April through October.

✦ Nutritive Value: Appendix, 196.

PASSION FRUIT

Passion fruit is a brownish yellow or purplish skinned, egg-shaped fruit with a punchy flavor. It is full of small black seeds surrounded by golden orange flesh.

The name is derived from an interesting interpretation of the fruit's flowers. The various parts are said to represent certain aspects of the Passion (crucifixion) of Christ. Passion fruit is also called *granadilla*.

Several types of passion fruit are grown: purple, sweet, and giant. The purple and sweet passion fruits are three to six inches in length and are more commonly available than the giant passion fruit, which is not so flavorful. Ripe passion fruit yields to gentle pressure and can be eaten like a melon—spooned or sliced. You can puree it for fruit juice or make jelly and desserts from it.

Passion fruit is grown in Hawaii, Florida, southern California, and South American countries.

✦ Nutritive Value: Appendix, 473.

PEARS

What are they?

Pears are probably the easiest fruit to identify by the shape: the small stem end gradually broadens

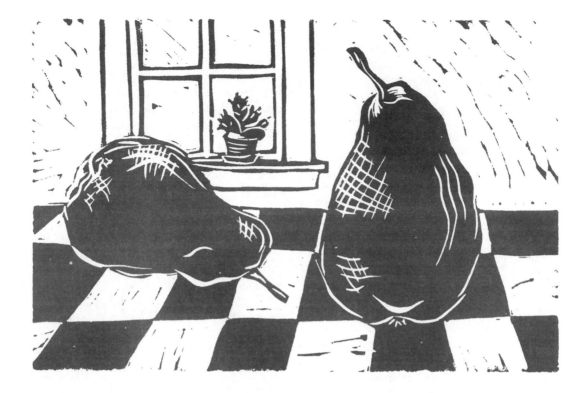

to a plump blossom end, like a bell. They are related to apples and have a similar seed core.

Pear trees are especially long-lived. They can bear fruit for seventy-five to one hundred years. Several thousand varieties of pears are known, but like other fruits only a small number of them are grown on a commercial scale. The more popular varieties are:

- Bartlett—Usually large, golden yellow summer pears popular for eating out of hand and for canning. They were growing wild in England in the late 1700s, and today they are the most common variety grown—over 65 percent of pear production. Bartletts are available from mid-July to early November.

- Bosc—Medium-sized, dark yellow, brown-russeting skins with long, narrow necks. They are popular for desserts and are available from October through May.

- Anjou—Another winter variety, Anjous are yellowish green, rounded, and have a thick, barely noticeable neck. They are spicy-sweet and juicy, medium to large in size.

- Comice—Similar in size and color to Anjou and favored for cooking and desserts. A red blush distinguishes this variety from Anjou.

- Winter Nelis—A fooler: these pears are ripe when the skins are green, with light brown russet spots. They are used mostly for dessert and are sold from October to May.

Buying tips

Firm to slightly soft pears are best. Pears are picked while green and develop their sweetness after harvest, but green (unripe) pears can be ripened at room temperature in a few days. Green-skinned varieties, however, stay firm and hard, even when ripe. Avoid bruised, mushy fruits. If you are going to cook them, they do not need to be completely ripe.

How do I use them?

Pears are as versatile as apples. Add them to baked goods, salads, desserts, and beverages.

Try baking pear halves with a spread of mayonnaise and a generous sprinkling of Parmesan cheese for an interesting side dish. Mash ripe pears and add to a pumpkin or fruit-pie filling for a pleasantly sweet extender.

To dry pears at home, wash and core them, then cut into 1/4-inch slices or rings. Spread in single layers on drying trays and dry at 110 to 120°F for 10 to 14 hours. Pear halves will dry in a day or so. They should be chewy and bendable but not brittle.

How nutritious are they?

Fresh pears are over 80 percent water. They provide carbohydrates, fiber, and small amounts of vitamins and minerals.

Dried pears are about 25 percent water and thus provide more nutrients by weight. They are rich in potassium and magnesium, have a good supply of iron and phosphorus, and provide small amounts of vitamins A and C and protein.

✦ Nutritive Value: Appendix, 207–213.

Where do they come from?

Pears are thought to have originated in both Europe and Asia. Those grown in North America are of European descent.

Commercial U.S. production of pears is mainly on the West Coast—California, Washington, Oregon, and Colorado—although some are grown in New York and Michigan. About 40 percent of the commercial pears are marketed fresh, with the remaining 60 percent canned. Less than 1 percent are dried.

How do I store them?

Keep fresh, ripe pears in your refrigerator, but allow them to sit at room temperature before eating for full flavor.

Dried pears store well in a cool, dry area in a tightly closed container.

Other "Pears"

Prickly pear—Not related to pears, this thorny, elongated, egg-shaped fruit is actually a type of cactus.

It is also called *Opuntia* (botanical name) and *Indian fig*. The skin turns from green to yellow to red, and the flesh is sweet but seedy.

Quince—A pearlike fruit with a distinct smell. It is yellow when ripe but not edible when raw. Quince is cooked and sweetened for marmalade and jams, or it is added to pear and apple dishes.

PERSIMMON

Without a second glance, you might think a persimmon is a tomato. Its bright orange-red skin and flesh, with a green cap stem, make persimmon an interesting fruit.

This "apple of the Orient" was found both in Southeast Asia and, in smaller form, in the southern United States. The Oriental persimmon (Japanese *kaki*) is fairly large, sometimes acorn shaped, and seedless. It must be fully ripe before eating—that is, soft and slightly shriveled; as the tannic acid in unripe persimmons causes the fruit to be very astringent (bitter and mouth puckering). The American type contains one to eight large seeds and has sweet, edible flesh even before being fully ripe—that is, brownish red and soft.

Persimmons that are sold in stores are usually the larger Oriental type and are from California. They are in season from September to January.

Persimmons are fine raw, cut into wedges, or spooned like pudding. Use them as you would pears and apples for pies, cookies, and cakes. One-half teaspoon of baking soda to a cup of persimmon pulp will reduce astringency in baked goods, as heat tends to increase the fruit's bitterness.

Keep ripe persimmons refrigerated and handle them gently, as they will easily break or become mushy. Persimmons that are not quite ripe will ripen at room temperature in a few days. To speed the ripening process, put them in a plastic bag with ripe apples.

The wood of persimmon trees (of the ebony family) was used to make golf clubs. Persimmon is the national fruit of Japan.

✦ Nutritive Value: Appendix, 474.

PINEAPPLE

What is it?

Pineapple is neither a pine nor an apple. Its resemblance to a pine cone prompted Spanish explorers who saw it growing in the West Indies to call it *piña de Indias* (pine of the Indies). "Apple" was added by English-speaking Europeans. But native West Indians called it *na-na,* from which its botanical name *(Ananas comosus)* comes.

The main varieties of pineapple are Smooth Cayenne, the most popular for fresh and canned pineapple; Sugar Loaf, a large, heavy type; and Red Spanish, squarish and thick-skinned.

Dried Pineapple

The dried pineapple available in North America is usually imported from Taiwan, although some is from other tropical areas. The typical procedure for drying the fruit is to slice off the shell, cut out the core, and slice the fruit into $1/4$-inch to $1/2$-inch rings. Once the rings are spread on drying pans, a sugar and water solution is poured over them. They are partially dried, then soaked again with sugar and water. This is repeated until the rings are about 80 percent sugar. This type of dried pineapple is erroneously called *honey-dipped.* A less common practice is to use pineapple juice concentrate rather than sugar and water. This kind of dried pineapple is referred to as *unsweetened* or *natural.*

Buying tips

Ripe, juicy pineapple has golden-orange skin and glossy pips (circular spots or eyes of the shell), and it feels heavy. It should have a dull-sounding thump when tapped with a finger. If it sounds hollow, it is not ripe. An easily removed spike from the pineapple crown is usually an indication of ripeness.

Reportedly, pineapple does not ripen or become sweeter after being picked, so those for the fresh market are allowed to mature as much as possible before being shipped by airplane.

Overmature pineapple becomes mushy or soft, and then it ferments or becomes rotten. Shriveled, dull-colored, or greenish fruit should be avoided. Buy a large pineapple to get the most flesh for your money. Pineapples are available all year, with peak supplies available from April to June.

How do I use it?

Pineapple is a wonderful dessert by itself, in pies and sherbets, or mixed into fruit salads and baked goods. Its juice is lively and refreshing.

Fresh, whole pineapple can be cut in several ways. One is to remove the crown by twisting it off, then cutting the base and the sides from top to bottom. Use a sharp knife and try to leave as much fruit as you can. The eyes can be removed by cutting diagonal grooves, or by using a sharp vegetable peeler as you would for removing potato eyes. Then cut the fruit across into slices or vertically for wedges or spears, and remove the core.

Another cutting method is to cut the pineapple in half from the base to the crown, then quarter it. Remove the core, then take a long, curved grapefruit knife to remove the skin. Cut the quarter pieces into wedges or cubes.

Dried pineapple is great for snacking and adding to trail mixes. It can be reconstituted by soaking a cup of rings in a cup of water or pineapple juice for 1 or 2 hours. Use it as you would use canned pineapple.

How nutritious is it?

Fresh raw pineapple is 85 percent water. It is high in carbohydrates and contains negligible amounts of fat and protein. It is a fairly good source of potassium. Small amounts of other minerals and vitamins A, B-complex, and C are also present.

Canned pineapple with heavy syrup is heavily sweetened with sugar and has more calories but less vitamin C than fresh pineapple. No data for dried pineapple was listed in the sources used.

Pineapple has an enzyme called bromeline that can aid in digestion. However, this enzyme also causes fruit salad that contains fresh pineapple to become soggy after half an hour or so.

✦ Nutritive Value: Appendix, 214–219

222

How do I store it?

Although fresh pineapple is only at peak perfection for about a day, you can refrigerate it for three to five days. If it is cut, place it in a sealed plastic bag to prevent dehydration.

Dried pineapple will keep for a year or longer if it is stored in a dry, cool place. It can ferment in a warm area.

Where does it come from?

Pineapple is native to tropical Central and South America and the islands of the Caribbean Sea. It was brought to Hawaii and other countries in the Pacific, where it also thrives.

Much of the pineapple sold in North America is from Hawaii, Honduras, Mexico, the Dominican Republic, and Costa Rica. An increasing amount is being shipped from the Philippines. Most is canned as sliced, crushed, or juiced pineapple. The people in the United States consume more pineapple than the people in any other country.

PLUMS

What are they?

Plums, like their cousins peaches and cherries, are soft, roundish tree fruits with hard seed pits or "stones" in the center. They have been eaten since the Stone Age.

Thousands of plum varieties exist, but only about twenty varieties are grown commercially. Commercial plums are usually classified as *European*—purple or blue skins, small, firm; or *Japanese*—red to yellow, large, juicy. The queen of plums, the Santa Rosa plum, accounts for 35 percent of the California harvest. Other popular varieties are El Dorado, Laroda, Nubiana, and Casselman. Native North American plums usually grow wild. One of the more popular of these varieties, Sloes, is used to make sloe gin.

Buying tips

Fresh plums should be plump, full color, firm to slightly soft, and have a bloom (a powdery look) on the skins. Avoid hard, shriveled, split, bruised, and soft plums. You can ripen firm plums at room temperature a few days before eating. Plums are in season from early May through September.

How do I use them?

Fresh plums are excellent summer snacks—good for picnics or lunches. Add them, quartered and pitted, to fruit salads or desserts. You can also cook them for puddings, sauces, preserves, pies, and cakes. Don't cook them too long, though, or they will become mushy. Keep fresh plums refrigerated for up to five days.

How nutritious are they?

Plums provide carbohydrates and some minerals and vitamins. When dried into prunes, they are excellent sources of vitamin A, iron, potassium, calcium, and magnesium.

✦ Nutritive Value: Appendix, 222–227.

Where do they come from?

Plums were originally from Asia and China, but they now grow all over the world. California produces about 75 percent of the world's supply, as well as 90 percent of the fresh plums sold in the United States.

Although Little Jack Horner was said to use his thumb to pull out a plum from his Christmas pie, the legend behind this nursery rhyme is that a steward named Thomas Horner was sent by an abbot to King Henry VIII. With him was a "pie" of deeds, which were to transfer Church properties over to the King. En route, Horner pulled out a "plum" for himself—one of the deeds—and said, "What a good boy am I!"

POMEGRANATE

This "seedy apple" is unique in that its hard, reddish brown shell-skin contains a multitude of seeds, each surrounded by bright red, juicy pulp and sectioned by a spongy membrane.

Pomegranates originated in the area called Persia (now Iran), although they were also found growing

---

UMEBOSHI PLUM

A type of plum reputed to have medicinal value is the umeboshi or salt plum.

Umeboshi plums are pickled in crocks for two years, using a special acid bacterial process. They are often packed with an herb called chiso. Umeboshi plums are used in Japan and other countries of East Asia, and figure prominently as a condiment in the macrobiotic diet.

Use umeboshi as a vinegar substitute in mayonnaise, dressings, and sauces. Be forewarned: umeboshi plums are very salty and should not be eaten alone.

---

most common variety used is the California French prune.

After harvesting and washing, ripe plums are dried for 15 to 24 hours under controlled conditions of temperature and humidity, then they are stored until they are packed for the markets. Right before packing, the prunes are again washed and then moisturized via a hot water bath. Some prunes are honey-dipped or have potassium sorbate added to keep them moist and chewy. Three pounds of fresh plums are needed to make a pound of prunes.

Buying tips

Prunes should be plump, firm, and of good color. Those with glossy skins and very soft texture are usually moisturized with potassium sorbate or are honey-dipped. Avoid extra hard or nearly dried up prunes unless you plan to cook them. Wormy or fermented prunes should never be eaten.

How do I use them?

Prunes can be eaten as is, a few at a time. Cooked, pitted prunes are fine for a breakfast sauce or pureed for a fruit spread on breads.

To plump or cook prunes, pour $1/2$ cup each of cold and boiling water or fruit juice over a cup of prunes, and let them sit overnight in a covered container. Another method is to place 1 cup each of prunes and water in a pan and bring to a boil. Cover, then allow them to simmer (not boil) for 10 minutes. Never boil prunes, as this will cause the skins to split and the flavor to be lost.

Prunes are best kept in a cool, dry area in a closed container and should be refrigerated for extended storage.

Prunes and prune juice are popular remedies for constipation, as they provide bulk to aid in the elimination of wastes from the intestine.

✦ Nutritive Value: Appendix, 228–230.

in California and Georgia. Today, most of the pomegranates sold in the United States are from California. Peak season is in October; supplies are available from September to December.

There are several ways to eat a pomegranate. One is to just cut it open, scoop out the pulp, and eat it. The white seeds are edible, although they are usually discarded. Another method is to roll the whole fruit on a hard surface to break the pulp pockets, then poke a hole in the shell and drink the liquid with a straw or suck out the juice.

The sweet juice of pomegranate is sometimes used in fruit juices, jelled desserts, and sauces. Grenadine liqueur is made from pomegranate.

Keep pomegranates in the refrigerator for up to a week, or freeze the pulpy seeds for longer storage.

✦ Nutritive Value: Appendix, 475.

PRUNES

What are they?

Prunes—what the French call plums and from which the botanical name is derived—are dried plums. Only certain plum varieties, usually the purple plums, can be successfully dried into prunes. The

RHUBARB

This plant is not really a fruit. It is a relative of dock, a common weed. Rhubarb can grow in temperate to moderate climates to heights of three to five feet.

The plants have wide, curly leaves and sleek stalks one to three inches thick.

The leaves and roots of rhubarb are toxic—they contain a high level of oxalic acid, a substance that can interfere with calcium absorption. Rhubarb stalks, however, are quite edible, although they are tart and in need of sweetening to be palatable. They are green to red or red-streaked, and can be eaten from early spring to early summer. In summer and fall the stalks are needed by the plant to foster growth of the next year's shoots.

To cook rhubarb for sauce, wash the stalks and cut off the bottoms and top part near the leaves. Then dice them into 1-inch cubes. Cook the cubes in a small amount of water and some sweetener to taste. When the fibrous stalk has become stringy and mushy, it is done. Rhubarb sauce can be preserved like jam or just eaten for a simple dessert or side dish.

You can also use rhubarb for baking. It is sometimes called *pie plant,* so make a rhubarb pie that lives up to its nickname. Use uncooked pieces or sauce mixed with a sweetener or blended with strawberries. Also try rhubarb crisp—like apple crisp—topped with yogurt.

Nutritionally, rhubarb offers vitamins A and C, is a good source of calcium, and has some potassium.

Fresh rhubarb stalks will wilt if kept at room temperature, but they will remain fresh for several weeks in your refrigerator. Diced raw or cooked rhubarb can be frozen.

✦ Nutritive Value: Appendix, 236.

GRAINS

Whole grains and grain products have been staple foods in almost all cultures for thousands of years. It was the cultivation of grains that led to agricultural development, which in turn resulted in commerce and industry.

In the modern human diet, grains are still a common source of carbohydrates and the cheapest source of calories, protein, and other nutrients. Numerous types of grains are cultivated, and each culture, country, and climate favors certain types. Among the cultivated grains are rice, wheat, rye, millet, corn, oats, barley, and buckwheat.

In North America our experience with grains is mostly with wheat flour products. It may be hard to imagine the link between a sweet roll and the kernels of wheat growing in a farmer's field until you understand the process of growing, processing, and manufacturing the grain.

What are grains?
Basically, a grain is a seed made up of three parts. The *bran (or hull)* is the tough outer layers of the kernel that protect the grain. The *germ* is the "heart" or life-giving part of the seed, which would germinate it by providing the nutrients needed to create the first tiny leaves and rootlets. The *endosperm* is the starchy bulk or center of grain, which would nourish the seedling during its early growth before leaves have begun photosynthesis.

Grains and grain products on the market are referred to as *whole* or *refined*. A grain is *whole* when it contains all of its three parts. Grains are *refined* to varying degrees by removal of the bran (called *hulling* or *polishing*) and/or the germ *(degerminating)*. The more grain is refined—that is, the more bran and germ are removed—the lower its nutritional value will be. Many of today's commercially produced grain products—such as breakfast cereals, white flour, white bread, white rice, and degerminated cornmeal—are extremely refined, having most or all of the bran and germ removed.

How do I use them?
Whole grains are not difficult to use. They do not require much attention during cooking, and best of all, they taste great!

There are three basic ways to prepare grains for eating: cooking, soaking, and sprouting.

Cooking
Regular method—Rinse the grain in a colander or sieve, or put it in a pot of water and swirl with your hands to loosen any hulls or particles that may float to the surface. Drain the grain through a strainer, then panfry it—with or without oil—in a heavy skillet until golden brown. Add about twice as much water or other liquid as you have grain (see Cooking Chart, page 67). Bring water to a boil, then cover the skillet, reduce the heat, and let the grain simmer until tender or fluffy.

Pressure cooking—This method requires less water and is faster than regular cooking, so energy and preparation time can be saved. Refer to pressure cooker manufacturer's instructions for proper use of your pressure cooker. Adding a small amount of oil to the cooking water will prevent a clogged vent. (See Cooking Chart on page 67 for measurements and cooking times.)

Baking—Another form of cooking grains is by baking them in an oven. Use flours or cracked grain products to make breads, cookies, and other pastries.

Soaking

Semiprocessed grains, such as bulgur and buckwheat grits, can be reconstituted by soaking them overnight or by pouring boiling water over them and allowing them to fluff up. Some instant grain products, such as instant oatmeal, just need hot tap water to be ready to eat.

Sprouting

Wash grains, remove any broken pieces, then measure about 2 tablespoons of seeds into a quart-size glass jar. Now follow the directions for sprouting seeds on page 145. You can sprout wheat, barley, buckwheat, rice, rye, millet, flax, and triticale seeds.

How nutritious are they?

In general, whole grains are valuable sources of carbohydrates, protein, B-complex vitamins, vitamin E, iron, zinc, magnesium, and dietary fiber.

Refined grains, by contrast, are less nutritious—most of the B-complex vitamins, vitamin E, unsaturated fatty acids, and some protein are removed. If a refined grain product is enriched, only three or four of the B-complex vitamins and iron are replaced. The remaining B-complex vitamins, several minerals, and protein that are lost during the refinement process are not replaced by enrichment.

♦ Nutritive Value: Appendix, 245–276, 476–483.

How do I store them?

Store grains in airtight and bug-proof containers in a cool, dry place. Flours and cracked grain products should be refrigerated to prevent rancidity. You can also freeze grains and grain products.

Sprouted grains should be refrigerated and will keep for about a week. Store them in a glass container rather than a plastic bag to prolong freshness.

AMARANTH

What is it?

While poets may imagine amaranth as a flower that never dies, horticulturists are bringing new awareness about the life of the plant once honored by pre-Columbian Aztecs.

Amaranth is a tall, bushy plant with broad leaves and a showy flower or seed head. A relative of pigweed (a common garden weed), amaranth is grown for the leaves as a vegetable and for the seeds as a grain. The seed head resembles corn tassels, al-

COOKING CHART

1 Cup	Regular		Pressure*	
	Water (cups)	Time	Water (cups)	Time
Rolled oats, Rolled wheat	2–2½	20 min.		
Bulgur wheat	1½–2	20 min.	1	10 min.
Barley, pearled	2	25–30 min.	1½	10 min.
Millet	2	30–45 min.		
Cracked wheat, Cracked rye	2–2½	25–30 min.		
Buckwheat	2–2½	25–30 min.		
Brown rice—				
short	2½	35–45 min.	1½	15–20 min.
medium	2	35–45 min.	1	15–20 min.
long	1½	35–45 min.	¾	15–20 min.
Steel-cut oats	3	60 min.		
Barley, hulled	2½–3	1½ hours	2–2½	15–20 min
Whole wheat, Oats, Rye, Triticale	2	1–2 hours	1½	15–20 min.

*At full pressure

though it is somewhat bushier, and it yields hundreds of round, dark seeds.

How do I use it?

Amaranth has a mild, sweet, nutty flavor that lends itself well to cookies, breads, and other baked goods. Use 1 part amaranth flour with 3 or 4 parts wheat flour or other grain flours. Amaranth flour is also good in homemade pasta and is used in some commercial crackers.

Amaranth seeds can be cooked for hot cereal. It becomes rather gelatinous when it is boiled. The seeds are also good puffed like popcorn, or sprouted by spreading the seeds on moistened paper towels in a flat pan and covering the pan with aluminum foil. The sprouts are ready in 4 to 6 days. Eat the sprouts in salads or vegetable entrees.

How nutritious is it?

Amaranth is a high-protein grain, showing a whopping 15 to 18 percent protein that is high in the amino acids lysine and methionine. It is a high-fiber grain with notable levels of calcium and iron. Unlike most grains, amaranth is high in vitamin C and also contains vitamin A. It has a fairly high amount of fat, about 7 percent.

How do I store it?

Amaranth is best stored in a cool, dark place in a tightly covered container. Amaranth flour should be refrigerated to prevent rancidity and should be used within three to six months. Amaranth sprouts will keep for about a week under refrigeration.

Where does it come from?

Amaranth was originally grown by Aztecs in what is now Mexico, where it was used as a basic food as well as in religious ceremonies. When the Spaniards conquered Montezuma and his people in 1519, they banned the Aztecs' religious ceremonies and the growing of amaranth. Consequently the plant was reduced to relative obscurity and was used only in specific areas of Mexico, primarily for confections.

Since 1975 amaranth has been gaining avid support in the United States and is now readily available in many natural food stores and directly from growers in Colorado, Illinois, Nebraska, and other states.

BARLEY

What is it?

Barley, a deliciously chewy grain, is most often consumed in the form of beer. Of the barley grown in the United States, one-third is malted to make beer, and less than one-tenth is used for direct human consumption—most of that as pearled barley. The rest is used for animal feed.

The barley kernel has a spikelet (two outer husks), endosperm (starchy middle part), and a germ (embryo). Pearling is a scouring or abrasive process that removes the outer layers of the barley kernel. *Scotch* or *pot barley* is what remains after three pearlings. *Pearled barley* has undergone six pearlings and has many nutrients removed—almost all of the fiber is gone, along with over half the protein, fat, and minerals. *Hulled barley* is the whole grain with only the inedible spikelet removed. *Hull-less barley* is a special variety that has a softer, easily removable hull. *Malted barley* is made from whole barley that has been sprouted and toasted.

How do I use it?

Barley has a good texture and a mild grain taste. It is especially tasty in soups, and it is a pleasing addition to stews and casseroles. You can serve it alone as you would rice.

Hulled barley takes about $1^{1}/_{2}$ hours to cook and uses $2^{1}/_{2}$ to 3 cups of water per cup of barley. If you have a pressure cooker, use 2 to $2^{1}/_{2}$ cups of water per cup of grain and cook 15 to 20 minutes after full pressure is reached.

Hull-less barley cooks a bit more quickly than the hulled variety. Use the same proportions of water to grain.

Pearled barley takes 25 to 30 minutes to cook and requires 2 cups of water per cup of grain. For soups, just add the barley to the soup stock one-half hour before serving.

Try sprouting barley as you would other seeds. (See directions on page 145). If you want malted barley, take the sprouted seeds when they are $1/4$-inch long and spread them on a cooking sheet or pan. Toast them in the oven at 250 to 300°F for about 20 minutes—until the smell of malt fills the air. Then grind the seeds in a food grinder or blender and sift away the fibrous hull. Malted barley can be added to milkshakes or other beverages, or to baked goods such as homemade grape nuts and crackers.

A syrup made from sprouted and malted barley is called *malt syrup*. It is high in maltose sugar. Malt syrup is used in beer making, commercial milkshakes, and other sweets. (See page 134 for more details.)

Barley flour (finely ground barley) can be added to breads to produce a cakelike product with delightful sweetness. It will enhance the growth of yeast cells in leavened breads, as the maltose in barley provides additional nourishment for the yeast.

You can also use barley to make a nutritious, hot grain coffee. Spread it on baking pans about $1/2$-inch deep, then toast it in the oven at 400°F for $1^1/2$ hours or until it is richly brown. Be sure to stir it every 20 minutes or so, so it roasts evenly. When done, grind it in a blender or food grinder to the consistency desired. Use as you would regular coffee—experiment with quantities until the desired strength or flavor is achieved.

How nutritious is it?

The endosperm of barley is surrounded by aleurone cells, which contain most of the barley's nutrients. As stated above, pearling removes these cells, and with it most of the fiber, much of the minerals, and the protein. Hulled barley contains about as much protein as the average cereal grain, and it is especially high in niacin, thiamine, and many minerals.

✦ Nutritive Value: Appendix, 245.

Where does it come from?

The cultivation of barley dates far back into human history. It is a staple grain in the Far East and was frequently mentioned in the Bible and Chinese sacred books, giving evidence of its use in the East four thousand years ago.

Barley was commonly used during the Middle Ages in Europe. It was brought to the New World by Dutch and British colonists primarily to make beer. *Barleycorn* was a term used for beer in England, since both barley and corn can be used for beer-making, but also because *corn* was the common term for any grain. The "spirit" of John Barleycorn was popularized and personified during this time.

BUCKWHEAT

What is it?

You wouldn't know it by looking at them, but buckwheat "grains" are actually the seeds of an herb. The name was derived from the word *bockweit,* a Dutch term for beech wheat, because of buckwheat's resemblance to beechnuts and its nutritional similarities to wheat.

The buckwheat plant is bushlike and grows to about three feet in height. The leaves of the plant are heart shaped, and the stems grow clusters of very fragrant flowers, often pollinated by bees, who produce dark buckwheat honey.

Buckwheat seeds are called *groats.* Coarsely ground groats are called *grits,* and finely ground groats become *buckwheat flour.*

Buckwheat groats are difficult to hull because the seeds are three cornered, thus they require special hulling machines. Two major buckwheat mills in the United States are Pen Argyl in Pen Argyl, Pennsylvania, and the Birkett Mills in Penn Yan, New York.

How do I use it?

Buckwheat groats can be cooked for a breakfast cereal. Heat a small amount of oil in a deep pan and saute groats until all the grains are coated. Add 2 to $2^1/2$ times as much boiling water as you have grains, then cover and simmer about 20 minutes. Save any liquid for soup stock or cooking purposes.

Groats may also be toasted and eaten as a crunchy snack by themselves or in combination with other nuts and seeds. Kasha, a traditional grain dish of eastern European countries, is easy to make and is good to add to soups and casseroles or as a substitute for potatoes or rice. To make kasha, simply roast 1 cup of groats in a heavy pan. Stir in 1 egg and cook until dry. Add 2 cups water or soup stock and salt to taste, cover tightly, reduce heat, and simmer gently for 20 to 30 minutes. Add butter before serving, if desired.

Buckwheat grits cook much more quickly and are often cheaper than groats. Use 2 parts water to 1 part grits and cook 10 to 15 minutes. Grits have traditionally been used as a filler in Polish sausage.

The most common use of buckwheat, however, is in pancakes. Buckwheat flour adds a hearty flavor to waffles, dumplings, and other breads.

How nutritious is it?

The nutritional value of buckwheat is, as mentioned above, quite similar to that of wheat. The notable vitamins present are thiamin and riboflavin (B-complex vitamins), and notable minerals are calcium and phosphorus.

Dark buckwheat flour contains more of the hull than light buckwheat flour. The amino acid lysine is present in the hull, so dark buckwheat flour is a slightly better protein source than other flours.

✦ Nutritive Value: Appendix, 251, 476, 477.

Where does it come from?

A relative of rhubarb, dock, and other plants in the Polygonaceae family, buckwheat probably grew wild in Asia. Prehistoric Chinese people cultivated it, and it was eventually carried into eastern Europe by migrating tribes.

Ancient Phoenicians used buckwheat to make *far* (refined flour). Later, it became a staple food of people in the Mediterranean, who called it *farinha*. Today, however, most farina is made from wheat.

CORN (MAIZE)

What is it?

Corn (or maize) is a grain that is considerably larger than most other cereals. It grows on stalks, and the corn ears are eight to twelve inches long and two to three inches in diameter. About one thousand kernels form on each ear (or cob). These are the edible parts of the corn, usually yellow to white in color.

Cornmeal or flour is generally made from *dent corn,* so called because the seeds indent after drying. Dent corn is harder and starchier than the sweet corn eaten as a fresh vegetable.

Other types of corn are *popcorn* (see page 73–74); *pod corn,* a relatively uncommon type that has a separate husk for every kernel; and *flint corn (Indian corn),* which has multicolored kernels. *Blue corn,* popular in the southwestern United States, is now being used by corn chip and tortilla manufacturers to make uniquely colored products with a rich corn flavor. Blue corn has about 20 percent more protein and higher levels of lysine and minerals than yellow corn.

How do I use it?

Dried corn—If you buy or dry your own dent corn, just soak it in water to reconstitute it, then add it to soups, casseroles, or other dishes. It may also be ground into meal or flour.

Cornmeal—This is coarsely ground whole kernels, which may or may not have been hulled and degerminated. Use cornmeal for muffins, pancakes, and breads, or as breading for fish and poultry. It can also be cooked by itself for cornmeal mush (corn pone).

Corn flour—Finely ground corn, frequently used to make tortillas or other flat breads and added to baked goods, such as cookies and bread. Corn flour can be made from either whole kernels or hulled, degerminated corn. It is sometimes sold as *masa harina.*

How nutritious is it?

Corn is the only common grain that contains vitamin A. Yellow cornmeal is higher in vitamin A than white cornmeal.

Corn also has notable quantities of the B-complex vitamins. Degerminated cornmeal is usually enriched with artificial B-complex vitamins and iron. The niacin (vitamin B_3) in corn is largely in a bound form, which makes it unavailable to the human body. Due to this unavailability, a niacin-deficiency disease known as pellagra is found in some cultures in which corn is a main food. The traditional Native American cultures, however, treat corn with alkaline substances that release the bound niacin and make it usable by the body. Some examples are lime (from limestone) used in tortillas and wood ashes used in hominy.

The amount of protein in corn is fairly high. It is best complemented with beans, nuts, or dairy products to form a complete protein (See Protein Complementarity below).

Corn provides the minerals calcium, magnesium, phosphorus, potassium, iron, and zinc. Commercial pancake and muffin mixes may be high in sodium.

✦ Nutritive Value: Appendix, 246, 247, 253–256.

How do I store it?

Whole corn may be left on the cob and shelled as needed or stored in an airtight container. Dried whole-kernel corn keeps far longer than ground cornmeal or flour because the hull protects it.

Store corn flour and cornmeal in covered containers in a cool, dry place, and refrigerate them if used infrequently. Cornmeal and flour can become rancid due to the high oil content in the germ, which is exposed to air after grinding. This is why it is often degerminated.

Where does it come from?

Maize originated in Central and South America. It is thought to have grown wild in southern Mexico about nine thousand years ago. The Incas of Peru hybridized corn and used vast irrigation systems to feed themselves. This grain is still the staple food of native Central and South Americans.

Today, corn is grown all over the world. About 90 percent of the dent corn produced is fed to livestock or poultry. The remainder is used for human consumption and for industrial by-products such as alcohol, ether, and varnishes.

PROTEIN COMPLEMENTARITY

Protein is made up of twenty-two different substances called *amino acids*. The human body can produce fourteen of these amino acids on its own, but the other eight—called *essential amino acids*—must be obtained from the food we eat.

In order for our bodies to make use of the protein we consume, these essential amino acids must be present in the digestive system simultaneously and in specific proportions. When they are, our bodies create *complete proteins*. Some foods, such as legumes and grains, however, contain all eight essential amino acids but not in the correct proportions. These foods are called *incomplete proteins*.

You can create a complete-protein meal by combining foods that are deficient in certain amino acids with foods that are strong in those same substances. This is called *protein complementarity*. Grains, for example, are deficient in two amino acids that are found in legumes, and vice versa. The two food groups fit together like pieces in a jigsaw puzzle, with nutritious—and delicious—results. The traditional cuisine of many nations illustrates this simple rule of nutrition: bean and pea dishes are served with bread, tortillas, rice, or other grains at mealtime.

MILLET

What is it?

Millet is one of the oldest foods known to humans. It is the chief source of carbohydrates for the northern Chinese as well as many people in Africa and India. It is cultivated mostly in the Eastern Hemisphere, particularly in countries with primitive agricultural practices and high population densities. It grows well on poorly fertilized and dry soils.

In North America, millet is grown mainly for bird seed and cattle feed. A small part of the total crop is processed for human consumption. Millet is related to sorghum, a grain that is cooked into a sweet, molasseslike syrup (see pages 137–138). Foxtail, a wild millet, grows freely in roadside ditches and some farm fields, where it is considered a weed.

How do I use it?

Millet can be cooked in the same way as rice, using 2 parts water or stock to 1 part grain. It cooks in 30 to 45 minutes. You can presoak millet to shorten the cooking time 5 to 10 minutes, or pressure cook it with 1 1/2 times as much water as you have grain for 10 minutes once full pressure is reached.

Cooked millet is good in casseroles, breads, stews, soufflés, and stuffing. Use it as a side dish as you would rice, or serve it under sauteed vegetables or with beans. When millet is cooked, a mucilaginous substance rises to the surface upon cooling, which can result in an interesting texture, especially when millet is added to soups or bean dishes.

You can also sprout millet and use it as a breakfast cereal. Harvest the sprouts when the shoots are the same size as the grains. (See page 145 for directions on sprouting.)

Millet flour can be used in breads and pastries to add variety in taste. It does not contain gluten, however, so it will not rise unless it is mixed with wheat flour.

How nutritious is it?

Millet is high in B-complex vitamins and protein. It contains lecithin as well as the minerals calcium, iron, magnesium phosphorus, and potassium.

Millet is considered to be one of the least allergenic and most easily digestible of all grains.

✦ Nutritive Value: Appendix, 478.

Where does it come from?

Millet has been used for centuries in Egypt, northern China, and other Eastern and Middle Eastern countries. In the United States, millet was first grown and used like corn by white colonists. It constitutes a minor agricultural crop now. Most of it is grown in the Midwest.

OATS

What are they?

Oats are one of the few whole grains commonly eaten by North Americans. Almost everyone likes oatmeal for breakfast!

PARCHED CORN

Parched corn, also called corn nuts and corn nuggets, is a snack food made from whole corn kernels. These crunchy morsels are made by soaking the corn in water or brine (salted water) until they swell. They are then deep-fat fried or baked at 350°F or hotter until golden brown. Salt is usually added after this.

Besides eating them as snacks, try them in cookies, casseroles, or breads as you would real nuts.

Parched corn contains mostly carbohydrates and thus provides lots of calories. It has about 10 percent protein and about 5 percent fat—higher if deep-fat fried. Salted parched corn is high in sodium.

Keep these snacks in an airtight container away from insects and rodents.

Oat groats are hulled, whole kernels. They are cleaned, dried, and toasted to make the hulls brittle, then the two outer layers of the hull are removed. After hulling, the inner part of the grain is scoured to remove some of its outer skin. During the hulling process, the oats are exposed to a temperature of 200°F, which deactivates the enzyme lipase. Lipase causes a soapy taste when it is combined with certain fats. The heating process also gives the oats a slightly roasted flavor.

A hulled oat groat is softer than a wheat berry. It can be pounded with a wooden mallet or rolled on a flat surface with a rolling pin so it will cook more quickly than it would in its original form. Oat groats may be used as a hot cereal; they taste more like cooked wheat or rice than oatmeal, however. Allow 1 to 2 hours for cooking, using 2 parts water to 1 part oats. Groats can also be sprinkled into soup, soaked overnight and added to bread dough, or cooked like buckwheat for kasha.

Steel-cut oats are oat groats that have been thinly sliced lengthwise with sharp blades. They are available in coarse and fine grinds. The finer the slicing of the oat, the quicker it cooks. Steel-cut oats are usually cooked for hot cereal, although they may be added to breads and cookies or used as a supplement in vegetable or meat dishes. Use 3 cups water to 1 cup grain and cook for about 1 hour.

Old-fashioned rolled oats are oat groats that have been heated until soft and pressed flat with steel rollers. They will cook more rapidly than oat groats or steel-cut oats—in 20 minutes, using 2 to 3 cups water per 1 cup oats.

Quick-cooking rolled oats are oat groats that have been thinly sliced into 3 or 4 small pieces, then heated and prepared in the same way as old-fashioned rolled oats. They cook faster because the pieces are smaller—in about 5 minutes.

Instant oatmeal is made by precooking oat groats in water, drying them, and rolling them extremely thin. Instant oatmeal is ready to eat with the addition of boiling water.

All three forms of rolled oats have the same nutritional value, although instant oatmeal is usually packaged with flavorings and sugar.

Oat flour (also called *flaked oats*) is produced by grinding oat groats until fine. It gives a moist sweetness to breads, pancakes, biscuits, and other pastry products. Oats are low in gluten, so be sure to use oat flour with wheat flour when making leavened bread—about 1 cup of oat flour to 4 cups of wheat flour.

Oat bran is the outer layer of oat groats. Oat bran has been cited as an effective agent in lowering blood cholesterol because it has a higher percentage of water-soluble fiber than other cereal grain brans, and this is thought to be beneficial in removing substances that contribute to high cholesterol levels. Oat bran can be added to breakfast cereals, muffins, or any other foods for which you would use wheat bran. (See page 82 for more information on wheat bran.)

How nutritious are they?

Oats are a good source of carbohydrates and provide protein, B-complex vitamins, and the minerals calcium, iron, magnesium, phosphorus, and potassium. Oats cooked with salt will, of course, contain sodium.

Oats are very good for digestion and can act as a mild laxative. Rolled, flaked, or crushed oats are the most easily digestible of all the forms of oats.

✦ Nutritive Value. Appendix, 248–250.

Where do they come from?

Oats were found growing wild in barley fields in parts of Russia, northern Africa, and the Near East about 2500 B.C. They were taken to Europe where they thrived in the cooler climates of Scotland, Ireland, and England.

Oats were planted in Massachusetts during the 1600s and used for the colonists' porridge. Most of the oats grown in North America today are used as animal feed.

POPCORN

What is it?

Popcorn is a type of maize that looks similar to other types of corn, except the ears and kernels are smaller. The kernels have a hard hull and a higher percentage of endosperm than other corn.

When popcorn pops, the moisture inside the kernels turns into steam and creates pressure of up to 250 pounds per square inch at 400°F. This pressure forces the kernel to burst—the endosperm explodes through the hull.

Yellow popcorn is from a variety that produces kernels that are yellow to orange in color; it pops into large pieces. *White popcorn* is from a variety that produces pale kernels, and it generally pops into small pieces. *Red popcorn,* a relatively uncommon variety, has red to violet-colored kernels and pops into small or medium-size pieces.

How do I use it?

To make popcorn on the stove, heat oil or fat in a pan, add kernels, cover the pan, and shake the pan occasionally. When the popping subsides, remove pan from heat and pour popped corn into a bowl. Use about 1 tablespoon of oil per ¹/₄ cup (2 ounces) of popcorn kernels; this will yield about 2 quarts of popped corn. For best results, use peanut oil or coconut oil, as they have a high smoking point. Do not use unrefined corn oil, as it will foam and smoke.

If all of the kernels don't pop, they may be too dry. This can be prevented by adding a little water with the oil before heating, or by placing a damp paper towel in the storage container.

Most people eat popcorn as a snack, with or without melted butter and salt. For variety in taste, sprinkle tamari on the popped corn, or try adding herbs such as marjoram, thyme, or rosemary, either dry or mixed with melted butter. You can also shake nutritional yeast or grated Parmesan cheese onto the popcorn for a zesty taste.

A traditional use of popcorn is to make popcorn balls. For a healthier version, mix peanut butter and maple syrup or sorghum together, then add it to popped corn and shape into balls or candy clusters. Throw in some peanuts to make a healthy Cracker Jacks-like snack.

How nutritious is it?

Contrary to some beliefs, popcorn is not fattening. One cup of plain popcorn has only 30 calories. Adding butter, however, does increase the calories.

Popcorn is high in fiber and contains some B-complex vitamins, calcium, phosphorus, potassium, and zinc. It contains protein but is generally not considered a protein food.

✦ Nutritive Value: Appendix, 262–264.

How do I store it?

Like all grains, popcorn should be kept in a cool, dry place in an airtight container. It can be refrigerated. Popped popcorn will stay fresh for only a short time, unless it is tightly sealed in a plastic bag.

Where does it come from?

Popcorn is believed to have originated in Mexico. Archeologists have found ears of corn in Bat Cave, New Mexico, that are estimated to be 5,600 years old.

Aztecs and West Indians were using popcorn when the white European explorers arrived. The Iroquois people popped corn in pottery vessels placed in heated sand, and made popcorn soups and other foods when French explorers visited the Great Lakes region in the early 1600s. Popcorn was also brought to the first Thanksgiving dinner in 1620. Today, most popcorn is grown in the Corn Belt of the Midwest, especially in Iowa. An estimated 46 quarts of popcorn are eaten per person per year in the United States.

QUINOA

What is it?

Quinoa (pronounced **keen**-*wah*) is a plant that originated in the Andes region of South America. This herb, a relative of the common North American garden weed lambsquarters, grows from three to six feet in height and produces a bushy head of colorful seeds. These round, usually pale yellow seeds resemble millet, although they are flat and have a band around the center.

Quinoa seeds are covered with a resinous, bitter substance called saponin. To rid the seeds of this they must be washed in alkaline water before they are marketed and eaten.

Because of its uniqueness and limited production in the United States, the price of quinoa seems fairly high when compared to that of other cereal grains (except wild rice). But it quadruples in size upon cooking, so you get more per pound.

How do I use it?

Quinoa is very easy to cook. Just rinse the seeds under the tap, strain off the water, and then cook them using 1 part quinoa to 2 parts water for 15 to 20 minutes. The cooked seeds have an interesting sproutlike appearance and a light but flavorful taste.

Cooked quinoa is great with vegetables, in soufflés and casseroles, and as an accompaniment to seafood. The uncooked seeds can be added to soups as you would barley or rice.

Quinoa flour, made by grinding the seeds, is also versatile. Use it in pancakes, muffins, crackers, cookies, and pastries. Cook it for baby food: boil 1 cup water, stir in ¼ cup quinoa flour, and cook 20 minutes over low heat.

Sprouting quinoa seeds is also easy. Soak about ⅓ cup seeds in a jar for 2 to 4 hours. Drain, then remember to rinse the seeds twice a day. In 2 to 4 days, the sprouts will be about an inch long. Put them near a window to allow them to turn green, then eat them in salads, sandwiches, or as a garnish. (See page 145 for more information on sprouting.)

How nutritious is it?

Here quinoa shines, with 16 to 20 percent protein. It is high in the essential amino acids cystine, lysine, and methionine—amino acids typically low in other grains.

Quinoa also has good amounts of iron, calcium, and phosphorus. It is higher in fat (6 to 7 percent) than other grains, which may be why it seems to melt in your mouth. B-complex vitamins and vitamin E are also present.

How do I store it?

Quinoa seeds are best kept in a cool, dry place in a covered container. Use them within a year.

Quinoa flour, because of the high oil content, should be refrigerated to prevent rancidity. Use it within three to six months.

Fresh quinoa sprouts should also be refrigerated. Use them within a week.

Where does it come from?

The Incas of what is now Peru, Ecuador, and Bolivia once relied on quinoa as a staple food, but after the Spanish conquests of the 1500s quinoa became a minor crop, grown only by peasants in remote areas for local consumption.

The availability of quinoa in the United States has been spurred by the cultivation of it in Colorado since the early 1980s by two entrepreneurs who learned of the food from a Bolivian. They began test plots in high arid fields in the central Rockies and began test marketing in 1985. It has since become more widely available in natural food stores throughout North America.

RICE

What is it?

A staple food for over half the earth's people, rice is one of the main grains grown for human consumption. About four hundred pounds of rice per person per year are consumed in the Far East, compared to 17 pounds in the United States.

Brown rice is whole rice with only the hull removed. It is available as *short-, medium-,* and *long-grain rice.* The shorter grain contains more of the starchy substance called glutin (not to be confused with gluten), so the main difference between short- and long-grain rice, besides size, is that short rice cooks up sticky and long rice comes out fluffy.

Converted (parboiled) rice is processed by steeping and steaming the grain in water before milling. Vitamins and minerals from the hull, bran, and germ are infused into the starchy part of the grain. The rice is then milled in the same way as ordinary white rice.

White rice has the hull, bran, and germ removed. White pigments, such as chalk or talc, and preservatives may be added to white rice.

Sweet rice is a short-grain, waxy variety that cooks into a very sticky mass. It is often used in desserts,

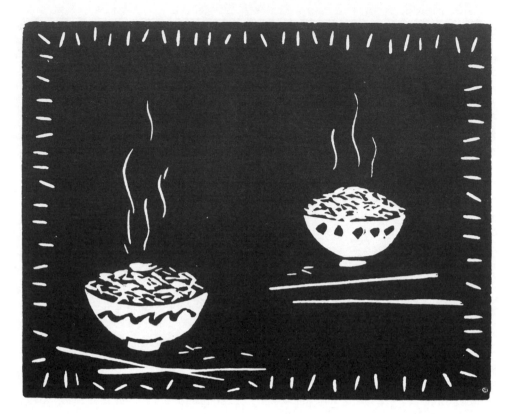

in gravies, and for baby food cereal. Mochi, a Japanese dish, is made from cooked sweet rice that is pounded in a mortar until it becomes a heavy paste. The paste is then cut into cakes and baked or deep-fried.

Basmati rice, a special long-grain rice imported from India or Pakistan, has a distinct aroma and flavor. *Trimati* (also called *Texmati*) rice is a cross between domestic long-grain and basmati rice. It is grown in Texas and may be erroneously labeled as basmati rice.

Rice flour is finely ground rice. It has a tiny crystalline appearance and is excellent for pie crusts, batter breads, and crackers, adding a pleasant sweetness.

How do I use it?

Rice is generally cooked by simmering. First, clean it by picking out specks, small stems, or spoiled grains. If you are in the habit of washing or rinsing rice prior to cooking, you may like to know that up to 10 percent of the thiamine in brown rice (25 percent in white rice) is lost by washing it.

Place the rice in a clean pot or skillet and add water in the following proportions:

1 cup short grain + 2½ cups water
1 cup medium grain + 2 cups water
1 cup long grain + 1½ cups water
1 cup basmati + 2 cups water

Bring the rice to a boil, cover it, and turn heat to lowest setting. Allow it to simmer gently until the water is absorbed. Do not stir the rice, because as it cooks little passageways form to allow it to cook evenly. Disturbing this network will result in a gummy, sticky texture. Brown rice—all lengths—takes 35 to 45 minutes to cook. Converted rice takes about 15 minutes. White rice takes 30 minutes.

For variety, add spices, onions, mushrooms, tamari, or other flavorings to the rice before cooking.

How nutritious is it?

Brown rice is higher in fiber, vitamins, and minerals than white rice. Converted rice contains similar levels of protein, vitamins, and minerals as brown rice. It is usually enriched with thiamine and iron. White rice has less protein and half the vitamins and minerals of brown rice. It is sometimes enriched with B-complex vitamins.

✦ Nutritive Value: Appendix, 265–270.

Where does it come from?

Rice probably first grew as a wild grass in Southeast Asia. It has been cultivated for over five thousand years.

Today, about 350 million metric tons of rice are grown every year, most of it in Asia. The United States grows about 1 percent of the world's crop.

Wild Rice

What is it?

Wild rice is a grass that grows in lakes. It has rounded, hollow stems and flat, pointed leaves. The hooked roots secure the plant to the bottom of the lake. It grows best in lakes and rivers with fresh water, cool temperatures, muddy bottoms, and uniform depth. Tiny flowers with pale, yellow-green blossoms form during July, and the seeds (rice) appear two to three weeks later. Wild rice is harvested in August and September.

Although wild rice looks similar to other rice, the plants are not in the same botanical family.

Traditionally, wild rice is harvested by canoeing out to where it grows, bending the ripened seed head stems into the boat, and beating them to remove the seeds. When the craft is full of rice, the harvesters return to shore where they may partake in a ceremonial hulling of the grain. Two to 3 pounds of unhulled seeds yield 1 pound of edible wild rice.

Much of the wild rice available to consumers today is actually domesticated. Paddy wild rice is carefully seeded and cultivated, then mechanically harvested, just as in other commercial grain farming operations. Commercial production and harvesting of paddy wild rice started in the 1960s when machines were developed especially for this purpose.

How do I use it?

Prepare wild rice as you would other rice, using $2^{1}/_{2}$ to 3 cups of water per cup of wild rice. It should be rinsed carefully to remove any dust or foreign particles.

Wild rice triples in volume when it is cooked, so you will need less raw wild rice per serving than you would regular rice.

Wild rice is commonly used as a side dish with meats and as a Thanksgiving entree in stuffings or casseroles. It has a unique flavor, so you may want to mix it with other rice until you are used to the hearty, wild taste.

Another way to eat wild rice is to pop it like popcorn. The kernels will double in size—not nearly so much as popcorn. It is a crunchy, robust snack.

Try grinding wild rice into flour and using it in baked goods, pancakes, waffles, or muffins. Use leftover cooked wild rice in homemade bread.

How nutritious is it?

Wild rice contains twice as much protein as white rice. The amino acids lysine and methionine are more prevalent in wild rice than in most other cereals.

Wild rice is low in fat and high in B-complex vitamins. Notable amounts of magnesium, potassium, phosphorus, and zinc are present in higher proportions than in white rice.

✦ Nutritive Value: Appendix, 483.

How do I store it?

Wild rice will keep indefinitely when stored in a tightly covered container in a cool, dry place. Cooked wild rice should be refrigerated and used within a week, or frozen.

Where does it come from?

Wild rice is the only grain native to North America. It was a staple food for the Sioux and Chippewa Indians. Native legends say it was discovered when a young brave, during a ritual of survival, resorted to eating the plant's seeds for lack of other edible foodstuffs.

Two-thirds of the wild rice harvest is from northern Minnesota. The remainder comes from Wisconsin, Michigan, New Brunswick, and the Rocky Mountain region.

RYE

What is it?

Rye is a cereal grass that is second only to wheat in world popularity for bread baking. It has a strong, hearty flavor in bread and as a cereal.

Rye is the most popular grain for bread flour in Scandinavia and Eastern Europe. In the United States, however, one of the main uses for rye is rye whiskey.

How do I use it?

Rye berries are whole kernels with the husks removed. They can be cooked alone or with rice (1 part rye to 2 parts rice) for 1 to 2 hours, using about twice as much water as grains.

Dark rye or *whole rye flour* is made from whole rye berries that have been ground in a flour mill. *Light rye flour* is made from rye that has had the bran and/or germ removed. It may also have been bleached.

Rye flour makes delicious, robust bread. It does not, however, respond favorably to commercial yeasts, so you must add some wheat flour to your dough to enable the yeast to develop. As little as 1 part wheat flour to 3 parts rye flour will improve the rising capabilities of the dough without diluting the rye flavor.

Many commercial rye breads look very dark, but they are often made mostly of wheat flour and have artificial coloring added. Read the label: If rye flour is listed before wheat flour, there will be more of it present.

Cracked rye or *rye cereal* is rye berries that have been broken or ground into small pieces. It can be cooked for a hot breakfast cereal and can be combined with cracked wheat or rolled oats for variety. Bring rye cereal to a boil using twice as much water as grain, and simmer, covered, for 10 to 15

minutes. Add powdered or whole milk for a smoother cereal.

Rolled rye or *rye flakes* are made by heating rye berries until soft, then pressing them flat with steel rollers. Add rye flakes to soups and stews, cereal, meat loaf, casseroles, or granola. Make cream of rye by simmering 1 part grain and 4 parts water over low heat for 15 minutes.

Rye sprouts can be made like any other sprouts. They are good in salads and breads. Just soak rye berries overnight, drain off the water, cover the jar with a screen, rinse the seeds twice a day, and wait two or three days until the sprout is as long as the seed. Then eat! (See page 145 for more information on sprouting.)

How nutritious is it?

Rye contains B-complex vitamins, protein, calcium, iron, magnesium, phosphorus, and potassium. Dark rye flour contains significantly more protein, calcium, iron, phosphorus, and potassium than light rye flour.

✦ Nutritive Value: Appendix, 479, 480.

Where does it come from?

Rye may have originated in southwest Asia, although recorded history first mentions it as a grass found in northern Europe. It was considered a weed in early Greece but became popular during the days of the Roman Empire. During the Middle Ages rye spread throughout Europe and became a basic grain for bread.

Dutch immigrants brought rye to the United States and used the grain for both flour and rye whiskey. The countries of the former Soviet Union produce more than half the world's rye crop. The United States grows about 1 percent of the world's crop.

TEFF

What is it?

Abyssinian love grass, also known by its scientific classification *Eragrostis abyssinica,* is simply called teff by Ethiopians. This Amharic word translates as "lost" in English, perhaps due to the tiny grains that roll all over the place. About 150 teff seeds stuck together would be the same size as one kernel of wheat.

Teff has been a staple grain in Ethiopia and the eastern highland regions of Africa (ancient Abyssinia) for several thousand years. Teff seeds were found in a pyramid that is thought to date back to 3359 B.C. Brown, red, and ivory (white) teff is grown as a food grain as well as an annual hay grass. Teff straw is sometimes mixed with mud to make thatch huts. Teff grows to a height of four feet and has been used as an ornamental grass in North American gardens. Commercial production of teff in North America is almost exclusively by Wayne Carlson of Caldwell, Idaho, who worked in Ethiopia in the 1970s, took a liking to that country's cuisine, and has since grown and marketed teff first to Ethiopians living in North America and now to natural food outlets.

How do I use it?

Teff has long been used in Ethiopian cuisine, particularly for making *injera,* the national bread. A spongy flatbread, injera either serves as a wrapper for food, or it is torn and eaten like buns or chapati. The teff seeds are pounded or ground into flour, mixed with water, and allowed to ferment with natural airborne yeasts at room temperature for 2 or 3 days. When the batter is sour and bubbly, it is poured onto a griddle and baked like a pancake.

Teff flour is also great in Western-style baked goods such as muffins, cookies, cakes, and waffles. Teff has no gluten so is recommended for people who have allergies to other grains.

Teff seeds are used to make hot porridge and can also be added to confections, soups, and stews. Cooked teff has a slightly robust, nutty flavor and is somewhat mucilaginous, which makes it good for puddings or as a thickener in gravies. Mix cooked teff with herbs, garlic, and onions to make grain burgers or fillets. You can substitute teff seeds for sesame seeds (1 part teff to 2 parts sesame seeds). Teff seeds can also be sprouted.

A fortified product called faffa is distributed by the Ethiopian government and is a mixture of teff flour, chick-pea flour, skim milk powder, sugar, salt, and vitamins. Faffa is cooked as a porridge for infants, mixed with the false banana (a traditional Ethiopian food), and used in making both leavened and unleavened breads.

How nutritious is it?

Teff is amazingly high in iron. Brown teff in particular is very iron-rich: one two-ounce serving supplies 25 percent of the U.S. Recommended Daily Allowance of iron. Teff also provides thiamine (vitamin B$_1$), calcium, and protein. The lysine content of the protein is low, however, so it is best to serve with beans, peas, or other high-lysine foods for protein complementarity. Teff is a good source of dietary fiber.

✦ Nutritive Value: Appendix, 508.

How do I store it?

Keep teff seeds and flour in a cool, dry place away from insects and rodents. Leftover cooked teff can be refrigerated but should be used within a few days.

TRITICALE

What is it?

Triticale (pronounced *tri-ti-**kay**-lee*) is the world's first human-made grain. It was developed by cross-breeding several different species of wheat (botanical name: *triticum*) and rye *(secale).* When ripe, triticale is similar to wheat except the grain head is about twice as large.

The developers of triticale considered it science's gift to the world, an aid to the "underdeveloped" nations where, ironically, whole grains have been eaten for thousands of years.

Triticale has been promoted as a more nutritious and higher yielding crop than either wheat or rye alone. However, tests and experimental research in several midwestern states have shown this to be not always true.

How do I use it?

Triticale tastes like both rye and wheat. Use triticale berries as you would wheat or rye berries by cooking them whole or grinding them into small pieces or flour.

To cook whole triticale berries, bring 2 cups of

water to a boil. Add about 1 cup of berries, then cover and simmer for 1 to 2 hours.

Use triticale flour with wheat flours or other grain flours, or as a direct substitute for bread and other baked goods. However, because triticale has less gluten than wheat, bread dough with only triticale flour requires gentler kneading and only a single rising.

Try making triticale pancakes, pie crusts, or chapatis—anything you would normally make with wheat or rye flours.

How nutritious is it?

Triticale is higher in protein than either rye or wheat, and it contains a greater percentage of some of the amino acids. Also present are B-complex vitamins and minerals.

Where does it come from?

Research on triticale was published as early as 1876, but only in the last fifty years has much attention been given to it. The grain was developed in Sweden. Serious research was conducted at the University of Manitoba in Canada, and at the Jenkins Foundation for Research, founded in California in 1968. This research center conducts tests in thirty states and forty-eight countries around the world.

Triticale is grown commercially in the Grain Belt states of North and South Dakota, Nebraska, and Minnesota.

WHEAT

What is it?

Wheat is by far the most popular grain in North America. We eat about 130 pounds of it per year, mostly as bread and baked goods. Wheat ranks with meat and dairy products as a main source of nourishment in North America.

There are three common types of wheat grown today:

- Hard winter or Spring—Usually red but sometimes white wheats, grown for their high protein content. These wheats are generally ground into flour.
- Soft red winter—Lower in protein and generally

SEITAN—"WHEAT MEAT"

Meat eaters may chide vegetarians for wanting imitation meat products, but everyone may be intrigued to discover seitan (pronounced **say**-tan), a unique food made from gluten, the protein in wheat.

Gluten is obtained by mixing approximately 7 parts whole wheat or unbleached wheat flour (*not* pastry flour) with 3 parts water. This becomes a stiff dough that is formed into a ball and covered with cold water for 20 minutes to 4 hours. The dough is then gently kneaded under the water until the starch, bran, and germ separate and the gluten forms a mass. The water is poured or strained off, then fresh cold water is added and the kneading and rinsing process is repeated until the water becomes clear, in 10 to 15 minutes. After this, the glu-

---

milled into pastry flour for crackers, pie crusts, cakes, and cookies.

- Durum—Planted in spring, this wheat is typically used for pasta products. (See page 86.)

The wheat seed, or berry, consists of three main parts: the bran, or outer layers; the germ, or embryo of the seed, which would cause it to germinate; and the endosperm, or starchy middle part, of which most wheat flour consists. See the following pages for more information on bran, wheat germ, and wheat flour.

Most of the wheat sold in the marketplace is the product of modern milling methods that separate and sift wheat berries into its three parts. Bran and wheat germ are commonly used in animal feeds, while the endosperm is used for human consumption. Those who eat white bread or other white flour products may want to add bran and wheat germ to their diets to make up for the big nutritional difference between white flour and whole wheat—or they may choose to eat more whole grain products.

How do I use it?

Wheat can also be eaten in the following forms:

Wheat berries—You can cook wheat berries in 1

ten can be made into cutlets, steaks, hamburger substitutes, or poultry analogs.

Several health-food companies and members of the Seventh Day Adventist Church have been selling and using gluten products since the 1940s. In Japan, seitan has been used for many years. It is thought to have originated there in the diets of vegetarian Buddhists. Gluten products are frequently sold in Asian food markets. A derivative of gluten, *monosodium glutamate,* has also been used in East Asian countries for centuries to add a meatlike flavor to vegetable dishes.

Seitan, monosodium glutamate, and other gluten products should be avoided by people who are sensitive to gluten.

to 2 hours, using 1 cup berries to 2 cups water. They are good in casseroles, soups, or as a side dish.

Cracked wheat—Cracked wheat has a nutty flavor and texture and can be cooked in about 30 minutes, using 1 cup cracked wheat and 2 to 2½ cups water. Add it to bread or cook it as a breakfast cereal.

Couscous—The endosperm of durum wheat is cracked or pelletized to make couscous. Couscous cooks in about 10 minutes, using 2½ cups water per 1 cup couscous. It has a uniquely enticing flavor.

Bulgur—Bulgur is precooked wheat that is cracked and dried. See page 84.

Rolled wheat (sometimes called *wheat flakes*)— Rolled wheat is made in the same way as rolled oats: by steaming the berries until soft, then pressing them between steel rollers. Add them to cookies, granola, or other foods just as you would rolled oats, or cook them for a hot cereal. Rolled wheat takes about 20 minutes to cook, using the same proportions of grain and water as cracked wheat.

Farina—Farina is made from the endosperm only and looks like little white pellets. Cook it for hot cereal using 1 cup farina and 2 to 3 cups water (depending on how dry you like it). It cooks in 3 minutes or less.

Wheat sprouts—Soak wheat berries overnight in a jar, drain, then cover the jar with a screen. Rinse them 2 times a day, and harvest when the sprouts are about as long as the seeds. Use wheat sprouts in salads and breads. (See page 145 for more information on sprouting.)

Wheat grass—If you sprout the berries in a flat tray with soil and allow them to grow to about 6 inches, you can harvest the grass and extract the juice with a special wheat-grass juicer. The green, nutrient-rich liquid has a strong taste, which can be made palatable by diluting it with other liquids.

How nutritious is it?
Whole wheat contains protein, B-complex vitamins, iron, calcium, phosphorus, and potassium. The endosperm contains most of the protein and carbohydrate, as well as some of the B-complex vitamins in wheat. Bran stores most of the fiber, niacin, pyridoxine, and pantothenic acid. Wheat germ contains most of the thiamine, vitamin E, and many trace minerals.

Cracked, rolled, and cooked wheat products have slightly less nutritional value than whole wheat. Wheat sprouts and wheat grass contain vitamin C.

✦ Nutritive Value: Appendix, 252, 272–276, 481, 482.

How do I store it?
Keep wheat products in airtight containers away from rodents and insects. Refrigerate wheat germ and cracked, rolled, or ground raw wheat products to prevent the oil in the germ from becoming rancid. Wheat sprouts and wheat grass should also be refrigerated.

Where does it come from?
Wheat is thought to have originated in the Middle East, in the areas now called Egypt, Iran, and Turkey. It dates back to prehistoric times. The Chinese were using wheat in about 2800 B.C. It was the chief grain of the Roman Empire.

Wheat is presently grown on more acres in the world than any other grain—about five hundred million acres of wheat is cultivated yearly. In the United States, wheat is grown mainly in Kansas,

North Dakota, Montana, Minnesota, South Dakota, Idaho, and Washington state. Total worldwide production is about 350 million metric tons per year. In Canada wheat is grown in Alberta, Saskatchewan, and Manitoba.

BRAN

Bran is the name for the outside layers of grain that protect it until the kernel is planted. Almost all grains have bran or a hull, but most of the bran on the market is from wheat. It is high in fiber, stores many of the grains' minerals and vitamins, and accounts for 13 percent of the wheat berry.

Bran is typically used in breakfast cereals, casseroles, or in baked goods such as cookies and muffins. You can stir-fry bran with butter until browned to make a nutlike topping for salads and desserts. Make a quick snack by mixing bran with ample syrup or honey, dried fruits, and nuts, then pressing the mixture into a candy bar. Bran can also be added to beverages.

Bran contains dietary fiber, a necessary element for eliminating waste products from the intestines. Lack of fiber in the diet has been linked to bowel problems, cancer, diverticulosis, appendicitis, hernias, and varicose veins.

The outer layers of bran are coarse and have little food value, but the inner layers contain protein and other nutrients. They make up 93 percent fiber, 50 percent of the B-complex vitamins, and a large portion of the trace minerals in wheat.

Bran also contains phytic acid, a substance of concern to some nutritionists. Phytic acid can combine with certain minerals—such as calcium, zinc, and iron—to form indigestible compounds, thereby limiting the body's intake of these minerals and possibly leading to deficiency. Apparently, some people's bodies produce an enzyme that combats this effect. The phytic acid in bran and other whole grains can be deactivated by sprouting or by long, slow cooking (at least 100°F for 2 hours). The long rising and baking times in bread making are perfect for this. It is best to avoid eating large quantities of raw or slightly cooked bran or whole grains.

✦ Nutritive Value: Appendix, 481.

WHEAT GERM

What is it?

Wheat germ is the center of the whole wheat berry. It would germinate the plant and provide nutrients to help it grow. Although wheat germ comprises only about 2 to 3 percent of the total wheat berry, this "heart of the wheat" contains twenty-three nutrients.

How do I use it?

Wheat germ can be eaten alone as a breakfast cereal, combined with other grains and flours, or used in a wide variety of recipes. It can also supplement just about any food you like.

For instance, you can substitute wheat germ for part of the flour in home-prepared foods. If a recipe calls for 1 cup wheat flour, use $^3/_4$ cup wheat flour and $^1/_4$ cup wheat germ. For breading on fish, poultry, or meat use 1 part wheat germ to 1 part wheat flour. You can also extend meat loaf and meatballs with wheat germ.

The delicate, nutty flavor of wheat germ enhances the taste of cakes, cookies, and pie crusts. When your recipe calls for bread crumbs, try wheat germ instead. Sprinkle it on cooked green beans, peas, tomatoes, or other vegetables right before serving. Mix it into yogurt, omelettes, or casseroles. Use it as a coating for candy balls as you would coconut or sesame seeds.

How nutritious is it?

Wheat germ contains more protein for its volume than whole wheat, although it is weaker in certain amino acids. For complete protein utilization, eat wheat germ with nuts, seeds, dairy products, or green vegetables. (See Protein Complementarity, pages 71, 112.)

Wheat germ also contains major amounts of B-complex vitamins and vitamin E. These vitamins are partially destroyed by toasting, although commercially toasted wheat germ may be enriched and also contain vitamin A.

Important minerals such as calcium, iron, magnesium, phosphorus, potassium, selenium, and zinc are present in raw wheat germ. Toasted wheat germ loses the magnesium and selenium.

✦ Nutritive Value: Appendix, 482.

How do I store it?

The oil in wheat germ can become rancid quickly—within a week—so raw wheat germ should always be refrigerated in an airtight container. But it in small quantities to ensure a fresh supply, or freeze it if you want to keep it for long periods.

Toasted wheat germ may be kept on a shelf until it is opened. Thereafter it should be refrigerated.

WHEAT FLOUR

What is it?

Wheat flour is finely ground wheat berries. There are different types of wheat flour, named according to the amount of refining or processing it has had.

Whole wheat flour is made from hard-wheat berries. Generally, most of the bran and wheat germ are present in the flour, as well as the endosperm. Hard wheat contains a high amount of gluten (a form of protein); this flour is therefore good for bread making because gluten causes bread dough to rise.

Whole wheat pastry flour is made from soft-wheat berries, which contain less gluten than hard wheat. This flour is best suited for pastry, cookies, and pie crusts. It can also be mixed with hard-wheat flour for bread.

White wheat flour is made from wheat that has had the bran and germ removed during the milling process, leaving only the starchy middle part (the endosperm). White flour is usually enriched with three B-complex vitamins (thiamine, riboflavin, and niacin) and iron to make up for the loss of nutrients due to the removal of the bran and germ. White flour may also be bleached—treated with such agents as chlorine dioxide, benzoyl peroxide, or acetone peroxide—to make the flour whiter. This process destroys any vitamin E and B-complex vitamins that may have survived the milling process. After bleaching, white flour often has dough conditioners added that reduce the need to knead dough. Such flour is referred to as *bromated* or *phosphated* flour.

Unbleached wheat flour (also called unbleached white or noncommercial white) is white wheat flour that may have some of the bran and germ present. It is sometimes available in food cooperatives and natural foods stores.

Gluten flour is a mixture of wheat flour and gluten, the proteins of wheat that remain after the starch, bran, and germ are washed from the flour. Gluten flour is used to enhance the leavening of breads and may be found in commercial wheat bread, other baked goods, and flour blends. It has a protein content of about 40 percent.

Note: Any flour or product that lists wheat flour as an ingredient may contain anything from white flour to whole wheat flour. Some commercial whole wheat flours have had the germ removed to prolong storage. Read the label: If it doesn't say "100 percent whole wheat flour," parts of the wheat may have been removed.

How do I use it?

If you've ever done any baking, you know that wheat flour is the most common ingredient for bread, cake, and cookie recipes.

Bread made from whole wheat flour is generally more substantial in weight than bread made from white flour. It requires a little extra kneading in order for the gluten to develop and rise. For lighter but still more nutritious and tasty bread, use about $1/3$ part white flour to $2/3$ part whole wheat flour—or experiment with other types of flour, such as rice flour, millet flour, cornmeal or corn flour, and oat flour. The more varied the flours, the more flavorful and wholesome the bread.

Pie crusts and other pastries can be made with any type of flour, but for a lighter and flakier texture you should use pastry flour or a blend of flours.

Pancakes and waffles made with whole wheat flours should have a leavening agent added, such as baking powder, baking soda, or beaten egg whites, to ensure uniform baking and to reduce the heaviness that may result if you use only whole wheat flour.

Wheat flour can also be used in gravies and sauces to thicken them. Use about 2 tablespoons flour per quart of liquid.

How nutritious is it?

Nearly all the nutrients found in wheat are also found in whole wheat flour. Some nutrients may be destroyed in the milling process if the flour becomes too hot. A whole wheat flour that is *stone ground* will be subjected to less heat because the milling process involves rubbing stone against stone at fairly low speeds, rather than metal against metal (steel roller mills), which creates more heat. Consequently, more nutrients are likely to be retained in stone ground flour.

Whole wheat flour is high in B-complex vitamins, vitamin E, essential fatty acids, and important trace minerals such as calcium, iron, magnesium, phosphorus, potassium, selenium, and zinc.

White flour lacks fiber (bran), most of the B-complex vitamins, vitamin E, and some of the minerals. Enriched flour contains only some of the nutrients that were removed or destroyed in the milling process—namely, thiamine, riboflavin, and niacin.

✦ Nutritive Value: Appendix, 272–276.

How do I store it?

Always keep whole wheat flour in an airtight container such as a glass jar, durable plastic carton, or metal canister. Keep it refrigerated to prevent rancidity.

White flour that does not contain wheat germ should also be kept in an airtight container in a cool place. It has a longer shelf life than whole wheat flour and does not need to be refrigerated.

BULGUR

What is it?

Bulgur is a form of wheat that is quick to prepare, nutritious, and has an appealing, nutty flavor. It is made by boiling wheat kernels, drying them, removing some of the bran, and finally cracking the kernels.

One of the oldest processed foods, bulgur is believed to have originated in Syria thousands of years ago. It has since been a staple food in the diets of people in the Middle East.

Most bulgur is produced from hard red winter wheat grown in Kansas, Nebraska, and Texas. Although it can be prepared at home, most bulgur is processed by modern technological methods.

How do I use it?

Bulgur is a versatile food. It can be mixed with salads, fruits, vegetables, meats, poultry, and fish, or just eaten by itself. You can boil, bake, fry, or roast it, or just soak it in water for a few hours. Bulgur cooks more quickly than rice.

To cook bulgur, heat a small amount of oil in a deep pan and saute the grain until all the pieces are coated. Add $1^{1}/_{2}$ to 2 times as much boiling water as you have grain. Cover and simmer about 10 minutes. Do not wash the grain before or after cooking, and avoid lifting the lid or stirring it during the cooking process. Add more liquid if necessary to prevent scorching, and save any excess liquid for soup stock. Use cooked bulgur as a breakfast cereal or side dish as you would rice.

Bulgur can be reconstituted rather than cooked: Spread it in a shallow pan to about 1 inch deep and pour enough boiling water over it to leave about $^{1}/_{2}$-inch of standing water. When the water is absorbed, stir the grain with a fork until it is cool.

For camping or for special recipes, prepare bulgur by soaking it in tap water for several hours. Soaked bulgur will keep up to a week if it is covered and refrigerated.

In bread recipes, use 1 cup soaked bulgur with 5 cups of wheat flour. It is not recommended for use in cakes and cookies, as the bulgur would become dry and hard.

You can also add bulgur as a dry ingredient to soups, chili, casseroles, stews, meat loaf, or goulash.

How nutritious is it?

Bulgur has the same nutrients as whole wheat but in slightly smaller quantities. It is rich in protein and in the B-complex vitamins. There are about 85 calories per half cup of cooked bulgur.

✦ Nutritive Value: Appendix, 252.

How do I store it?

Dry bulgur can be kept for several months in an airtight container in a cool, dry place. Cooked or reconstituted bulgur should be used within a few days.

MAKE YOUR OWN BULGUR

Boil 4 cups water. Add 2 cups wheat berries. Cook them for 45 minutes or until the wheat is tender. Drain off water; save it for soup stock.

Spread berries on baking pans and roast them in a 250°F oven for 1 hour or until dry. Now grind them coarsely in a food grinder.

Store for future use in airtight containers.

WHEAT COUSINS

Kamut

Kamut (pronounced *kah-moot*) is an ancient Egyptian word for wheat. It is also a registered trademark for products made with kamut.

This cereal has, in a sense, been resurrected from the dead. Apparently abandoned two thousand years ago, after Romans and Greeks brought higher-yielding strains of wheat to Egypt, kamut is now rising from obscurity to become an important grain in both special-diet and natural-food markets.

The modern-day legend of this durum-like grain goes like this: In 1949, while stationed with the U.S. Air Force on the Iberian Peninsula, a Fort Benton, Montana, farm boy named Earl Dedman was given three dozen giant seeds by a fellow airman who had gone to Egypt on leave. The inch-long kernels were allegedly from either King Tut's excavated tomb or another ancient tomb near Dahshur, Egypt. Dedman sent the seeds to his wheat-farming father, who planted them back home. All but four sprouted, and the seeds produced by the thirty-two successful plants were saved and sown the next year. After six years, fifteen hundred or fifteen thousand bushels of grain, nicknamed "King Tut's wheat," were harvested. The big seeds would show up at Chouteau County fairs; most was fed to hogs. Some also wound up in North Dakota, where it

gained a reputation as "junk wheat"—found to be highly susceptible to wheat rust and a contaminant of durum wheat. In 1986, after planting the grain as a garden novelty for several years, Mack and Bob Quinn of Big Sandy, Montana, decided to grow the big wheat organically for whole-grain bakeries. Their acreage expanded from one and one-half acres the first year to several hundred acres in the 1990s. This father and son team is probably the only commercial farming operation in the world now producing kamut. They received a Variety Protection Certificate from the United States Department of Agriculture in 1990.

Kamut is favored for pasta and is considered superior to durum pastas by at least one manufacturer. It can also be milled into flour for baking purposes, cooked for tabouli salad, or sprouted. Commercially, the grain is rolled or shaped and sold as dry cereal flakes and "ohs." Green kamut plants are also pressed and blended with wheat-grass juice for a potent, energy-rich drink.

The flavor of kamut has been described as buttery, although some find it has a slightly biting aftertaste. Even though kamut is a distant relative of wheat, it does not produce the same allergic reactions in people who are sensitive to gluten.

Nutritionally, kamut ranks higher than other types of wheat in crude protein, magnesium, zinc, lipids, and most amino acids. It also provides B-complex vitamins, calcium, phosphorus, potassium, and copper.

Spelt

Long, long ago, a plant that peasants depended on for their sustenance grew in the hills of central Europe. This plant, an ancient type of wheat called spelt, provided the grain from which bread and pilaf were made. For hundreds of years, the Egyptians, Romans, and Greeks, as well as uplanders of central and southern Europe, grew and ate spelt. It is mentioned in the Bible (Ezekiel 4:9 and Exodus 9:31, 32). St. Hildegard of Bingen of the twelfth century, credited with curing the sick, was spurred by a vision that instructed her to feed spelt to the people.

Some people refer to spelt as German wheat; the

Germans call it *Dinkel* and the French call it *epeautre*. As other varieties of wheat became popular, this hearty, coarse grain fell out of use and by 1900 was relatively rare. With its small brown kernels that cling to the chaff (hull), spelt was not a favored grain for processing and milling, although it grows well in marginal soils.

Spelt is currently undergoing a quiet renaissance, with kernels, flour, and breads showing up in natural-foods and specialty markets throughout North America. Its robust flavor and chewy texture are quite a contrast to bland, highly refined white flour products, which is exactly why some people like it.

Spelt can be ground into flour like other wheat and used for biscuits, breads, crackers, muffins, pancakes, pastas, pie crusts, and tortillas. The hearty flavor tells you it's a substantial food to be taken seriously. Try it as a hot breakfast cereal or cook it as you would rice. Spelt is also popular in soups, particularly in the Provence region of France. Spelt grits and flour are mixed with rye to make a delicious dark German *Brot* (bread).

The nutritive value of spelt is reportedly similar to soft wheat, although it may provide more protein and B-complex vitamins than its cousin. Spelt contains gluten but is apparently more easily digested than common wheat, so it is acceptable for people with wheat allergies.

In the United States, spelt is currently being researched and grown in Ohio.

Pasta

What is it?

Pasta, also known in North America as noodles, is a food made from a paste of flour and water. This mixture is cut or formed into many different shapes and sizes, each shape and size having a particular name—lasagne, spaghetti, rigatoni, fettucini, ziti, and so forth.

While North Americans are familiar with only about ten types of Italian-style pasta, Italians have literally hundreds of shapes and sizes from which to choose, and they customarily eat some type of pasta every day. Asian and eastern European cuisines also make use of noodles—wonton, ramen, chow mein noodles, ribbons, and egg noodles.

Durum wheat is the most common variety of wheat used for commercial pasta because of its high protein content (14 to 15 percent). The more protein present in the pasta, the more it will expand during cooking. Pasta will generally expand four to seven times its original dry size during the cooking process.

Most pasta sold in North America is white, from refined wheat flour. But whole wheat, corn, buckwheat, spinach, soy, and egg pastas are becoming increasingly popular. Besides flour and water, other ingredients used in pasta include soy flour, wheat germ, eggs, and artichoke flour. Disodium phosphate may be added to shorten the cooking time. This additive is considered safe and by U.S. law must be listed on the label. White pastas are usually enriched with synthetic B-complex vitamins, food yeast or wheat germ, and iron.

How is it made?

Wheat meal *(semolina),* wheat flour, and other ingredients are mixed with just enough boiling water to make a workable dough. Manufacturers use large kneading machines that make the dough tough and smooth. This dough is then put into a cylinder and squeezed out by a screwpress through a perforated plate called a trafila. Macaroni, for example, is pressed through a trafila that has a steel pin in each hole, which forms the hollow tube. A trafila with a narrow slit is used to make flat noodles.

Automated knives rotate beneath the trafila to cut the pasta as it comes out of the holes. Long types, such as spaghetti, can be cut by hand to the proper length.

Once the pasta is cut into a shape and size, it is dried in large, heated rooms with continuously circulated and filtered air. Then the dried products are inspected, packed, and weighed according to size.

Buying tips

When shopping for pasta, observe the color, resilience, and breaking texture to determine quality. White pastas should be slightly golden and translucent—not grayish or cloudy. A test for spaghetti is

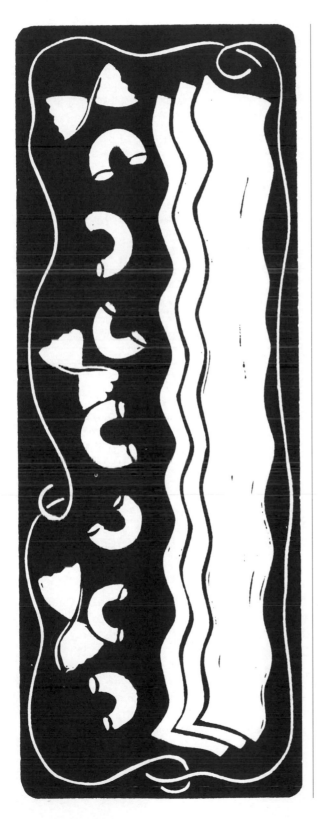

to grab a bunch in your hands: it should have the springiness of fresh twigs. Try breaking a flat noodle or strip of lasagne—if it is a good-quality pasta, the fracture will be jagged and not look starchy.

For the most authentic pasta and noodle products, locate Italian, Asian, or Polish grocery stores or manufacturers.

How do I use it?

Each type or shape of pasta has its own traditional use. Typically, spaghetti and lasagne are eaten in dishes of the same names. Others, such as macaroni, shells, and flat noodles, are added to soups, salads, and casseroles or are cooked and served as entrees with sauce and cheese.

The chart on page 88 shows the various kinds of pasta, their uses, and how long to cook them.

Cooking

The traditional method of cooking pasta is to bring a large saucepan of water to a rapid boil. Approximately 1 quart of water per $1/4$ pound (4 ounces) of pasta is best. Add salt if desired, using 1 teaspoon per quart of water. If possible, use salt that does not contain calcium chloride, as this would make the water hard, and pasta cooks best in "sweet" or soft water.

Now add the pasta gradually, so the water keeps boiling. Keep spaghetti, lasagne, or other large noodles whole rather than breaking them. Fan out these types and ease them into the pan until they are covered with water. Do not cover the pan, as this would cause the water to foam and boil over.

To prevent pasta from sticking, add a tablespoon of oil or a dot of butter to the cooking water, stir the pasta with a long fork while cooking, and make sure the water continues to boil for the full time as specified on the chart or package.

An energy- and nutrient-saving technique is to cook the pasta as stated above, but cook it for only 2 minutes if it is a fine pasta and 3 minutes if it is a thick pasta. Stir well, turn off the heat or take the pan off the burner, then wrap the sides of the pan with a cloth or towel and put the lid on. Now start timing it for the length of cooking according to directions. After the time is up, remove the cloth and lid. As you will see by looking at the cooking water, it will be clearer rather than cloudy (as in traditional pasta cooking)—an indication that vitamins and minerals have been retained in the pasta.

The test for doneness is a matter of taste. It is generally recommended that pasta should be cooked *al dente,* which means "to the bite"; the pasta should be slightly resistant and elastic instead of soggy. If it tastes raw or starchy or is hard to bite, resume cooking until it is done. A zanier test is to pick out a piece of pasta and throw it at a wall. If it sticks, it's done.

At this point, drain off the water by pouring it through a colander. If you'd like, save the water for soup stock by putting a bowl underneath the colander. Serve the pasta immediately, or return it to the cooking vessel until you are ready to eat.

Do not rinse pasta under cold water if it is to be eaten for the immediate meal, as this causes the pasta to lose its resilience and makes for a less delectable serving. Who wants to eat spaghetti if it's cold? However, if you plan to serve it at a later time that day, precook the pasta until not quite done, drain it (save the water), rinse it in cold water, and cook it again in the same water for about 30 seconds before serving.

PASTA INGREDIENTS

Dough is made of durum or high protein wheat flour, semolina, and water. Mixtures sometimes include farina, gluten flour, wheat germ, soy flour, artichoke flour, or vegetable puree (spinach, beets, tomatoes).

Name	Amount Per Pound	Cooking Time	Used For
Alphabets	3 cups	7–12 minutes	Soups
Bows (butterflies)	3–4 cups	12 minutes	Casseroles, soups
Macaroni (elbows)	3–4 cups	9 minutes	Salads, casseroles, macaroni and cheese
Lasagne	10 2-foot-long strips	8–12 minutes	Lasagne (main dish)
Mostaccioli (curlicues, spirals)	5–6 cups	8 minutes	Casseroles, soups
Rigatoni	4–5 cups	10–15 minutes	Main dishes
Rings	3–4 cups	7–12 minutes	Soups, salads
Shells	3–4 cups	7–12 minutes	Casseroles, salads, soups
Spaghetti	1½-inch diameter, 1-foot-long bundle	8–12 minutes	Spaghetti (main dish)

NOODLE INGREDIENTS

Dough is the same as that used for pasta, except eggs are added. The type of wheat may be of lower protein value. Noodles are more fragile than pasta and less salt is needed in the cooking water.

Name	Amount Per Pound	Cooking Time	Used For
Chow mein	7–8 cups	—	Chow mein, casseroles, confections, snacks
Flat (ribbons)	6–7 cups	5 minutes	Main dishes, soups
Ramen	6–7 cups	3–5 minutes	Casseroles, soups, main dishes
Wonton skins	—	varies	Egg rolls, soups

Use leftover pasta within a day or two, preferably in a baked dish or with a spicy or sweet sauce.

How nutritious is it?

Pasta is high in carbohydrates but low in fat. Cooked white pasta contains about 5 percent protein, which is best complemented with cheese or seafood to get a balanced protein. (See Protein Complementarity, pages 71, 112).

Pasta also contains calcium, phosphorus, iron, and B-complex vitamins. Pasta made with spinach, beets, or other vegetables will also contain vitamins A and C. Whole grain pasta products have a higher fiber content and are superior in certain nutrients and trace elements.

✦ Nutritive Value: Appendix, 257–261.

How do I store it?

White pasta without eggs can be stored up to two years without detriment, provided it is kept in a closed container in a cool, dry cupboard away from insects. Reportedly, pasta that has been stored a month or longer has better cooking qualities than freshly prepared pasta.

Pasta that contains eggs can spoil quite rapidly, so be sure to buy only what you need for a meal or two and then replenish your stock.

Soy pastas are also more susceptible to spoilage than white pasta, so refrigerate them until ready to use.

Cooked pasta can be refrigerated for up to two days without spoiling. It can be frozen and used later for a baked hot dish.

Where does it come from?

The making and eating of pasta dates back to 3000 B.C., when a Chinese cookbook, the *Hon Zo,* listed instructions for preparing macaroni. But Italians are generally given the credit for discovering pasta (*pasta* means "paste" in Italian). They have certainly popularized it! Pontedassio, Italy, features what is probably the world's only museum devoted to noodles, the Museo Storico degli Spaghetti (Historical Museum of Spaghetti). The small village is near the Ligurian Sea about two hours from Genoa, and the museum is open only by appointment.

The Japanese may have been using noodles in their cooking even before the Chinese or Italians, although they have traditionally used rice or buckwheat instead of wheat as the flour grain.

SERVING TIPS

1 pound of pasta serves:
   4 people for a main dish entree
   6 people for a first-course dish
   8 people for a side dish
Serving with sauce: Allow ½ cup sauce per person

LEGUMES

What are they?

Legumes—dried beans and peas—have been in the human diet for thousands of years. In some Western cultures they are traditionally known as "poor people's meat," but in the Far East they have been among the most highly valued foods since ancient times.

Beans and peas are grown all over the world, some being more adaptable to certain climates than others. The plants reach heights of about two feet as a bush; some grow on vines and spread on the ground. Pods form after the plants blossom. These pods contain the seeds, or beans.

The more popular edible dry beans grown in North America are lentils, lima beans, kidney beans, pintos, split peas, navy beans, and soybeans. There are hundreds of other beans available throughout the world, in all different shapes, sizes, and colors. In the markets of Mexico, India, and Africa you'll see many unique seeds that the people of these countries eat as a regular part of their diet.

Buying tips

When shopping for beans, look for ones of uniform size. They will cook evenly, since large beans generally take longer to cook than small ones. Avoid those that are cracked or that have pinholes (insect damage). Dull-colored beans are less fresh (have been stored longer) than bright-colored beans. Freshness does not affect the nutritional value of beans, but the cooking time will be longer because they will be drier and thus require more water than freshly harvested dry beans.

How do I use them?

Dry legumes can be cooked whole, flaked, or rolled like grains. Some can be roasted and eaten as a snack, sprouted to become a fresh vegetable, or ground into flour and used in baking.

Cooking

As a general guideline, 1 cup of dry beans will yield $2^1/_2$ cups of cooked beans, enough for 4 average servings.

Before cooking, dry legumes should be rinsed and sorted to remove any stones, dirt, or foreign objects. Cover them with 3 or 4 times their volume of warm water, then do one of the following: Soak overnight or longer (in the refrigerator after 8 hours, so they won't ferment or turn sour); *or* place the beans and water in a large pot, bring to a boil, and simmer for 5 to 10 minutes. Remove from heat and cover tightly to let them soak for 2 to 3 hours. The longer the soaking period, the shorter the cooking time.

Adding a dash of baking soda to the soaking water shortens the amount of time necessary for the soaking process. It also softens the bean skins so beans will not burst and become mushy during pressure cooking. Baking soda can destroy B-complex vitamins, but if the soaking water is discarded, no soda will remain for the cooking process, hence no vitamins will be destroyed.

After soaking, bring beans and water to a boil. Some sources recommend pouring off the soaking water and cooking with fresh liquid to help prevent flatulence. Another source says the soaking water should be saved, as it contains water-soluble nutrients.

Once the beans start boiling, lower the heat and simmer, partially covered, according to the times indicated on the cooking chart. Add more water if necessary to prevent scorching or sticking.

Pressure Cooking

Beans and peas can be pressure cooked, which saves much time and energy. Use just enough water to cover the beans, and cook at full pressure until tender (see Cooking Chart, page 92). Some beans, especially soybeans and split peas, tend to foam and can clog the pressure cooker vent. To avoid this, add a tablespoon of oil to the water before cooking.

Unsoaked beans can also be pressure cooked, which is handy when you want beans but forgot to soak them the night before. Bring water to a boil, using 3 to 4 times as much water as you have beans. Add the beans, bring to full pressure, and cook 10 to 15 minutes longer than you would had the beans been soaked.

Roasting

Cooked beans can be roasted to make nutlike snacks. Soybeans and chickpeas are good for this: Cook the beans to a firm consistency, then spread them on a lightly oiled baking sheet. Sprinkle with salt or tamari, if desired, and bake at 200°F for about 1 hour, or until the beans are well browned. You can also roast beans in a lightly oiled frying pan over medium heat on top of the stove. Be sure to stir them constantly to avoid burning and to assure consistent roasting.

Sprouting

To make bean sprouts, soak about $1/3$ cup dry beans in water overnight in a quart jar. Then follow the directions for sprouting seeds on page 145. Mung beans, chickpeas, whole dried peas, lentils, and soybeans are especially suited for sprouting. Be careful with soybeans, however, as the sprouts can mold

easily and should be cooked before eating to destroy trypsin inhibitors (see page 102).

How nutritious are they?

Legumes are excellent sources of protein, carbohydrates, several B-complex vitamins, and minerals. When sprouted, they also provide vitamin C.

Legumes contain about the same amount of iron and B-complex vitamins as beef, but they are very low in fat and contain little saturated fat and no cholesterol.

✦ Nutritive Value: Appendix, 279–288, 296, 302, 310, 318–320, 346–352, 357, 358, 417, 418, 484–491.

How do I store them?

Dry legumes will keep indefinitely if they are kept dry, cool, and in a tightly covered container.

Always refrigerate leftover cooked beans immediately, as they will spoil if left at room temperature. You can also freeze cooked beans.

BLACK BEANS

What are they?

If you've ever been to Mexico, you have undoubtedly seen or eaten black beans, or *frijoles negros.*

Also called *turtle beans,* the black bean is a member of the kidney bean family. As a plant it is characterized by the formation of three-leaflet patterns on the plant stalks and white, pealike flowers that form tough pods.

Black beans are medium-sized and very hard when dry. The seed coating is black to purplish in color, but the inside of the bean is creamy white. The beans are slightly square shaped rather than round or oval like most beans, and their flavor is hearty and robust.

Between one and four million pounds of black beans are grown in the United States every year.

How do I use them?

A popular use for black beans is in turtle (bean) soup. They are also great as refried beans to use in tortillas

COOKING CHART

1 cup, **soaked**	Regular		Pressure*	
	Water (cups)	Time (hours)	Water (cups)	Time (minutes)
Black	4	1½	to cover	20
Blackeyed peas	3	¾	to cover	20
Chickpeas	4	3	to cover	25
Fava	3	1½	to cover	20
Lentils	3	¾	to cover	15
Limas, large	2	1½	to cover	15
Limas, baby	2	1½	to cover	10
Mung	3–4	3	to cover	20
Peas, whole	2–3	1½	to cover	20
Pinto	3	2	to cover	10
Red beans:				
Aduki	3	3	to cover	20
Kidney	3	1½	to cover	20
Small	3	3	to cover	20
Soybeans	3	3	to cover	30
White beans:				
Great Northern	3½	1½	to cover	20
Navy	2	1½–2	to cover	20
1 cup, unsoaked				
Black			3	35
Blackeyed peas	3	1	to cover	35
Chickpeas			3	40
Fava			—	—
Lentils	2½–3	¾	to cover	24
Limas, large			to cover	25
Limas, baby			to cover	20
Mung			to cover	35
Peas, split	2–3	¾	1–1½	10
Peas, whole			3	35
Pinto			3	25
Red beans:				
Aduki			3	35
Kidney			3	35
Small			3	35
Soybeans			—	—
Soy grits	4	¼	—	—
White beans:				
Great Northern			3½	35
Navy			2	30

*Time listed refers to after full pressure is reached. **Note:** Cooking times are approximate.

or taco shells. Try black beans in a bean salad for a colorful change from red kidney beans.

Black beans should be cooked (after soaking overnight) in four times their volume of water for $1^1/_2$ hours. With a pressure cooker, add water to cover the soaked beans and cook for about 20 minutes after full pressure is reached.

How nutritious are they?

Black beans contain high amounts of potassium and phosphorus. They are a good source of calcium and contain iron. Also present are vitamins A, B-complex, and protein. This bean is deficient in certain amino acids, so eat it in combination with a grain product such as rice or corn tortillas for more complete utilization of the protein. (See Protein Complementarity, pages 71, 112.)

✦ Nutritive Value: Appendix, 279.

BLACKEYED PEAS

What are they?

What southern cook hasn't prepared blackeyed peas? Also called *cowpeas, blackeyed beans,* and *china beans,* this legume is popular not only in the southern United States but also in Latin American countries, where it is eaten as both a fresh and dried bean. It is white, of medium size, and has a black "eye." The flowers of the plant are yellow or purple and pealike. The pods grow to a length of six to twelve inches, and each pod contains about ten peas.

How do I use them?

Try blackeyed peas with greens for traditional Southern dishes. These beans are an attractive addition to casseroles and salads.

Blackeyed peas are considered to be a soft bean and therefore do not have to be soaked before cooking. They cook faster than most beans, taking only about 1 hour in an open kettle, using 3 parts water to 1 part beans, and 10 to 20 minutes in a pressure cooker, once full pressure has been reached.

How nutritious are they?

Blackeyed peas are a good source of vitamin A. They also contain B-complex vitamins and vitamin C, calcium, magnesium, phosphorus, potassium, and a small amount of iron. They are low in fat.

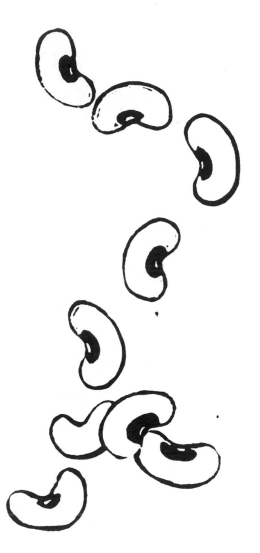

The protein in blackeyed peas is about average for a legume. For more complete utilization of the protein, eat the beans with grains, dairy products, fish, fowl, or dark leafy green vegetables. (See Protein Complementarity, page 71.)

✦ Nutritive Value: Appendix, 288, 357, 358.

Where do they come from?

Blackeyed peas are believed to have originated in Asia, and they are an important food in China, India, and Africa. The plant was brought over by slaves to the West Indies in the seventeenth century, then brought to North America about one hundred years later.

Blackeyed peas are now grown in the southern United States, with much of the crop being produced in California. About one billion pounds of blackeyed peas are grown every year in the United States.

CHICKPEAS (GARBANZOS)

What are they?

One of the more interesting looking beans, chickpeas have been used for centuries in the Middle East as a staple food. They are also known by their Spanish name, *garbanzo beans,* and in India as *grams.*

Chickpeas are large—about three-eighths inch in diameter—and are said to resemble a ram's head. The bean's Latin name, *arietinum,* means "like a ram." They can be red, black, or tan in color, although tan chickpeas are by far the most commonly grown.

The plant is a hairy, bushy annual that is related to the garden pea. It grows to a height of about two feet. The leaves are compound, with nine to fifteen pairs of small, round leaflets. The flowers are white to pink, and pods form from these flowers. The rectangular pods grow to one-inch long and each contain one or two seeds.

How do I use them?

Cooked chickpeas can be eaten whole, mashed, or shaped into balls. Because they are quite hard, they need to be soaked for at least 8 hours before cooking. Cook the beans for 3 hours in a regular pot, using 4 times as much water as you have beans. With a pressure cooker, add water to cover and cook for 25 minutes after full pressure is reached. If you prefer, you can pressure cook chickpeas without soaking, using 3 to 4 parts water to 1 part beans. Cook for 40 to 45 minutes at full pressure.

Whole, cooked chickpeas are nearly a meal in themselves with the addition of tamari or cheese sauce. They are delicious in bean salads and can be added to soups and casseroles. Try roasting them to make a crunchy, nutlike snack.

Raw, whole chickpeas can also be sprouted like other seeds. Soak them overnight, drain and rinse, cover the jar with a screen, and then rinse 3 or 4 times a day for 3 days until sprouts form.

Mashed, cooked chickpeas make a wonderful base for dips, spreads, and bean burgers. Mix them with sesame oil or olive oil, lemon juice, and seasonings to make hummus, a staple food of Lebanon. Another Lebanese dish, falafel, is made by mixing the mashed beans with spices, rolling or shaping the mixture into balls, and deep-fat frying them until golden brown. The falafel balls are typically stuffed into pita (pocket) bread and have a sauce made from sesame butter or tahini poured over them. Topped with sprouts or lettuce, falafels and pita bread make a tasty sandwich.

How nutritious are they?

According to Collier's Encyclopedia, chickpeas are "one of the most nutritious of leguminous seeds." They are high in calcium, phosphorus, and potassium. Also present are iron, vitamin A, and some of the B-complex vitamins. They are high in fat for a bean, but most of the fat is unsaturated.

The protein content of chickpeas is high—about 20 percent—but like most legumes it is incomplete and should be complemented by nuts and seeds or grain products. A good example of a complete-protein dish is chickpeas with sesame seeds or tahini. (See Protein Complementarity, pages 71, 112.)

✦ Nutritive Value: Appendix, 296.

Where do they come from?

Chickpeas are thought to be native to southwest Asia. They are commonly grown and used in southern European and Mediterranean countries, as well as in India, Africa, Central America, Mexico, and the southwestern United States. They grow best in dry soils.

In the United States, annual production of chickpeas is usually less than one hundred million pounds. Much of the crop is from California.

CRANBERRY BEANS

Cranberry beans, also called *October beans* and *Tennessee beans,* are rounded, grayish, maroon-striped legumes similar to pinto beans. When cooked, their texture is mealier than pintos, however.

Many of the cranberry beans that are grown in the United States come from Michigan. Most of these are exported to Italy, although some are sent to South Africa and some are used in the southern United States.

Use cranberry beans as you would kidney beans or pintos. Cook and mash them for bean patties or serve them with cooked pasta.

FAVA BEANS

What are they?

Fava, faba, broad, horse, Windsor, Scotch, English—these are all names for a bean that has been eaten since the earliest days in Europe.

Fava beans resemble lima beans in flavor and size, but they are of a different species of legume—they are in the vetch family. The plants have big,

---

BROWN BEANS

A cousin of black beans, called *Swedish brown* or just *brown beans,* is available in some parts of North America. The beans are occasionally imported from Sweden, where they are popular.

Brown beans are similar in size and taste to Great Northern beans, but they are tannish or rusty brown with a small white "eye." The beans are easy to grow in northern climates. If you plant them early, you may be able to get a picking of snap beans in early summer and another crop for dry beans later in the season.

Brown beans should be soaked before cooking, just as you would black beans or Great Northerns. Use them in casseroles and soups, and for baked beans.

rounded leaves and pretty pink or white flowers with purplish blue or black markings in the center. The broad pods form from the flowers and grow to a length of six to ten inches. Each pod contains several tannish brown beans.

In the United States, fava beans are relatively unknown. In Canada, however, they are grown as a forage or green manure crop. The plants prefer cooler climates.

How do I use them?

Fava beans can be cooked and served as other beans—add them to soups, casseroles, or stews. Before cooking, soak them overnight in about 3 times as much water. Drain off this water and add fresh water. Cook for about 1½ hours or until tender. With a pressure cooker they take only 20 minutes at full pressure. Add fresh water just to cover the beans in the pot.

The taste of fava beans is hearty and "beany." The skins are quite thick, so you might want to remove them before eating to make them more appealing. Try pureeing cooked fava beans and adding seasonings to make a sandwich spread. In Japan, dry fava beans are reportedly popped like popcorn and eaten as a snack or appetizer. The beans can also be eaten green (not dried), but they should be cooked first to destroy a toxin that could cause an allergic reaction if they were consumed raw.

How nutritious are they?

Fava beans are a good source of calcium, iron, and phosphorus. They also contain vitamin A and B-complex vitamins. Their fat content is low.

Fava beans are fairly high in protein. To better utilize this protein, however, you should eat them with bread or other grain products. (See Protein Complementarity, pages 71, 112.)

✦ Nutritive Value: Appendix, 484.

LENTILS

What are they?

The lens-shaped seeds known as lentils are also members of the vetch family. They are rather flat and can be green, yellow, brown, or red in color.

The lentil plant grows to a height of twelve to eighteen inches. Six pairs of oblong lanceolate leaflets grow on each plant. The lavender or white pea-like flowers become short, flat pods that contain two or three lentils each.

Lentils are popular in India, where they are called *dal*. Some cultures refer to them as *pulses*.

How do I use them?

Use lentils for soups, stews, or gravies. They go well with most vegetables and can be a pleasant variation in bean salads. Lentils are easy to sprout—see page 145 for directions.

Because they are quick and easy to prepare, lentils may have been the first convenience food. Presoaking is not necessary. Just add 2½ to 3 parts water per 1 part dry lentils and cook for 30 to 60 minutes, until tender. They take only 15 minutes to cook in a pressure cooker at full pressure.

Cooked lentils are an important part of most East Indian meals. They are usually spiced (curried) and served as a side dish.

Parched lentils are sold as a snack in some areas of the Mediterranean. They are an ideal food for long trips. To make them, briefly cook the lentils, drain off excess water, then toast them in your oven until they are brown and crunchy.

How nutritious are they?

Cooked lentils are high in calcium, phosphorus, potassium, zinc, and iron. They contain vitamin A and B-complex vitamins. Only a trace of fat is present.

Sprouted lentils contain calcium, iron, B-complex vitamins, and vitamin C. They are 90 percent water.

Both cooked and sprouted lentils contain protein. For more complete utilization, eat them with grains, nuts and seeds, or dairy products. (See Protein Complementarity, pages 71, 112.)

✦ Nutritive Value: Appendix, 302, 485.

How do I store them?

Lentils were found in pottery jars in ancient Troy, a city in Greece, where they had been buried for thirty-four centuries. So if you keep them in an airtight container in a cool, dry place, your lentils may last just as long!

Where do they come from?

Lentils are the main commercial crop of Egypt. They are found in other countries of the Middle East, where they are believed to have originated. Lentils are grown in northern Africa, southern Asia, and Europe.

Although lentils used to be imported to North America, production in the United States has increased to the point where it is now the world's largest exporter of this bean. Much of the crop is from the Palouse Hills in northern Idaho and eastern Washington, an area that is ideal for growing lentils.

LIMA BEANS

What are they?

Known as the "aristocrat of the bean family," lima beans are cream colored and mellow tasting. They are sometimes called *butter beans.*

Lima beans are in the kidney bean *(Phaseolus)* family. Two main types are available: the large, thick-seeded *potato limas,* and the small-seeded *baby lima beans.* The seeds have fine ridges, which come out from the "eyes," and they are rather flat.

Another type, called *Christmas limas,* are large, reddish brown speckled beans that are mild and creamy tasting when cooked.

The plants of lima beans grow best in warm, long-season climates and take about four months to mature. Although they are naturally a perennial, lima beans are grown as an annual.

How do I use them?

Cooked lima beans are good in soups, salads, and casseroles. Mash and eat them like mashed potatoes.

To cook, soak dry beans overnight in 4 times as much water as you have beans. Replace the water with fresh water or stock (2 parts water to 1 part soaked beans), then cook for 1½ hours. With a pressure cooker, use less water and cook for 10 minutes after full pressure is reached.

How nutritious are they?

Like most beans, limas are high in iron, potassium, and phosphorus. They contain B-complex vitamins. Commercially canned lima beans are usually somewhat lower in these same nutrients and also have salt added.

Lima beans have a good amount of protein, which is best utilized by eating the beans with rice, corn, or other grains.

◆ Nutritive Value: Appendix, 281, 346, 347.

Where do they come from?

Lima beans are thought to be native to South America and may have originated in what is now Peru. (The capital of Peru is Lima.) They are grown and eaten in Central and South American Countries.

In the United States, lima beans are grown in states along the Gulf of Mexico, the Eastern Seaboard, and in California. From five hundred million pounds to one billion pounds of baby limas and four hundred to seven hundred million pounds of large limas are produced in the United States every year. Most lima beans for domestic consumption are from California.

MUNG BEANS

What are they?

These small green beans are rather unfamiliar to many people in North America. Mung beans are used extensively in East Asian countries, where they are eaten as a fresh vegetable in the form of sprouts. Greeks call mung beans *kalamata beans.*

Mung beans are in the kidney bean family, but they grow in a unique way. Although the plants look similar to the other beans in this clan, the pods grow in clusters that resemble chicken feet. Each of the long, slender pods turns from green to dark purple and contains ten to fourteen little green seeds.

How do I use them?

Mung beans are great for sprouting—see page 145 for directions. Mung bean sprouts are excellent in Chinese entrees and other Oriental dishes. Add them to salads and sandwiches, or saute them with other vegetables. Put mung sprouts in egg rolls.

Dry mung beans can also be cooked as you would other beans, although their taste is less delectable. Use them in soups or casseroles. To cook, use 3 to 4 times as much water as you have beans, and cook for 3 hours (30 to 35 minutes in a pressure cooker once full pressure is reached). For quick meals and to complement the protein, cook mung beans with millet or rice.

How nutritious are they?

Raw mung bean sprouts are a good source of vitamins A, C, and B-complex. They also contain phosphorus, potassium, calcium, and iron. Cooked mung beans contain the same nutrients as sprouts with the exception of vitamin C. Both cooked and sprouted mung beans contain protein and are low in fat and calories.

✦ Nutritive Value: Appendix, 351, 352.

How do I store them?

Dry mung beans will keep indefinitely if they are stored in an airtight container in a cool, dry place. Mung bean sprouts should be refrigerated and used within a week to ten days.

Where do they come from?

Although mung beans are native to India, they are produced mainly in the Far East. In the United States, they are grown in Oklahoma and other south-central states. They can be grown successfully in northern gardens.

PEAS

What are they?

Peas, both dried and fresh, are among the most popular edible legumes. They have been a staple food for centuries; the Greeks and Romans learned about dried peas from the Aryans. During the same period, the Chinese were eating green peas as a fresh vegetable. If you have ever planted peas in your garden, you know how the pea plant twines and climbs. Once the whitish purple flowers blossom, the pods start to grow and mature, reaching two to four inches in length. Although garden peas are usually eaten when the pods are still tender, peas may be kept on the vine until the pods become gray-green or brown and the peas become wrinkled and hard.

Dried peas are sold in various forms. Whole green peas are those that have been shelled from the pod and dried. Green split peas have the outer seed coat removed and are then divided in half. Also available are whole yellow and yellow split peas, which are milder in flavor than green peas.

How do I use them?

Dried peas are good in soups, casseroles, and salads. Some people cook whole green dry peas and eat them as they would fresh peas. They taste starchy compared to fresh or frozen peas.

Before cooking whole peas, soak them in 3 to 4 times as much water as you have peas until they swell—for several hours or overnight. Drain this soaking water, add 2 to 3 parts fresh water or soup stock to 1 part peas, and cook for 1 to 1^{1}/$_{2}$ hours.

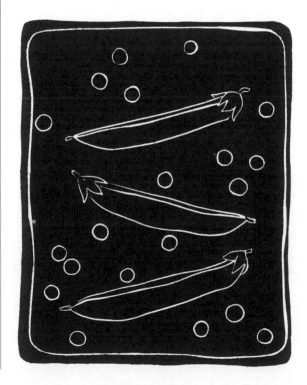

With a pressure cooker, use 1 to 1$^1/_2$ parts water or stock to 1 part peas and cook them 10 to 20 minutes after full pressure is reached.

Split peas take less time to cook and need no presoaking. Use approximately the same amount of water as for whole peas and cook for 30 to 60 minutes with the regular method, or 10 minutes in a pressure cooker at full pressure. For both time savings and protein complementarity, cook split peas with millet or rice.

Cooked peas may be pureed and used in dips or soufflés. You can also grind dry uncooked peas into a flour to be used as a nutritious supplement to breads or other baked goods.

How nutritious are they?

Peas are a good source of vitamin A and have a fair amount of B complex vitamins. They are high in iron, phosphorus, potassium, and calcium.

The protein in peas is lower than other dry edible legumes, but if you eat them with grains, you can get a more complete protein.

✦ Nutritive Value: Appendix, 310, 417, 418.

Where do they come from?

Peas are believed to have originated in the Mediterranean Sea region. Garden peas were brought into North America in the 1800s. The United States now grows over five hundred thousand tons a year on a commercial basis—95 percent is canned or frozen. Wisconsin, Washington, and Minnesota are the main pea-producing states.

PINTO BEANS

What are they?

A beige-colored seed with brown speckles, the pinto bean is related to other beans in the genus *Phaseolus*. It is popular in Mexico and the southwestern United States, and has been used for a long time in Latin America.

Pinto beans are fairly large—about the size of red kidney beans. The plant also looks similar to the kidney bean plant. Pinto bean pods, however, are speckled and grow to a length of four to ten inches. Each pod contains five to ten seeds.

How do I use them?

Pinto beans make delicious *frijoles refritos*—refried beans—a traditional Mexican dish. They are good in chili and salads, and they can be combined with other beans or grains for casseroles and soups.

To cook pinto beans, first soak them for about 8 hours or overnight in 3 to 4 times as much water as you have beans. Or, if you prefer, bring the beans and water to a boil for about 5 minutes, then allow them to soak. This method reduces cooking time. Cook for 2 to 2$^1/_2$ hours or until tender, using 3 parts fresh water or soup stock to 1 part beans. If you have a pressure cooker, cover the beans with water and cook for 10 minutes after full pressure is reached. You can cook them without presoaking: use the same proportion of water to beans and cook for 20 to 25 minutes in a pressure cooker at full pressure.

For refried beans, simply mash the cooked beans and reheat or fry them in a skillet with onions, garlic, seasonings, tomato sauce, and other vegetables. Add them to tortillas to make burritos or enchiladas.

How nutritious are they?

Pinto beans are quite high in calcium, iron, phosphorus, and potassium. They also contain a fair amount of B-complex vitamins.

The protein content of pinto beans is high, but like most legumes it needs to be complemented with grains, dairy products, or nuts and seeds. Combining refried pinto beans and corn or wheat tortillas is a simple way to get complete protein. (See Protein Complementarity, pages 71, 112.)

✦ Nutritive Value: Appendix, 283.

Where do they come from?

Pinto beans probably originated in Mexico, but they are now grown commercially in Idaho and Colorado. Total United States production of pinto beans varies between seven and fourteen billion pounds—more than any other dry, edible bean.

Red Beans: Aduki, Kidney, Small

What are they?

Anyone for chili? Well, you'll need some red beans.

The large red kidney bean is one of the more popular dry edible beans in North America. Its cousin, the small red bean, is less common but not much different in nutritive value or in its appearance as a plant. Another cousin, the aduki bean (also spelled adzuki, adsuke, and azuki), is one of the lesser known dry beans in North America but is second in popularity only to soybeans in Japan. Aduki beans taste less "beany" than other legumes but have a distinct flavor.

Kidney beans, small red beans, and aduki beans are bush-type beans with smooth-bordered, heart-shaped leaves and white, yellow, or purple flowers. They are in the *Phaseolus* family and are called *haricots* in France. In England, kidney beans are called French beans.

How do I use them?

Red beans are a colorful addition to three-bean salad and of course are perfect for making chili and other soups. Kidney beans are used as baked beans in New England. Small red beans and rice are combined for traditional Southern dishes in the United States, as are aduki beans and rice in the Far East.

Red beans are hard and are best soaked for 8 hours or overnight before cooking. Cook them with 3 parts water to 1 part beans for 1 to 1½ hours for kidney beans, and about 3 hours for small red and aduki beans. With a pressure cooker, cook the soaked beans for about 20 minutes at full pressure. You can cook them without presoaking in a pressure cooker: Use the same proportions of water and cook about 30 minutes at full pressure.

A paste can be made by mashing cooked aduki beans and adding flavorings. This paste may be used as a substitute for tomato paste on pizzas. Dry, uncooked aduki beans can also be ground into a meal and added to baked goods such as breads or pancakes.

How nutritious are they?

Red beans are good sources of carbohydrates, phosphorus, potassium, iron, and calcium. They also contain some vitamin A and B-complex vitamins.

Red beans are high in protein, but for more complete utilization they should be eaten with grains, dairy products, or nuts and seeds. Bean soup and crackers, or beans and rice, are examples of complementary protein foods.

Canned kidney beans are almost nutritionally equal to home-cooked kidney beans, but the liquid in the can should be utilized so the water-soluble vitamins are not wasted. Canned kidney beans are usually more expensive and often contain more sodium than home-cooked beans.

♦ Nutritive Value: Appendix, 287.

Where do they come from?

Most of the red kidney beans grown in the United States—especially those that are canned—are from New York. Lighter colored (pink) varieties are grown in California. Total United States production is over two billion pounds a year.

Small red beans are grown to a lesser extent in the United States, with four hundred to six hundred million pounds being produced annually.

Many aduki beans are imported to North America from China or Japan, although some are grown in Texas and other southern states.

Soybeans

What are they?

Soybeans are creamy yellow-colored beans of medium size that grow on hip-high plants inside fuzzy green pods. For centuries, they have been the primary source of protein in the Far East and are increasingly being used in North America for both human and animal consumption.

Also available are black soybeans, which are the same as cream-colored beans except for the outside skin. They are often imported from China.

How do I use them?

Soybeans are a very versatile food. They can be eaten as a cooked bean, sprouted and steamed for salads and Asian dishes, ground into flour for baking purposes, and cracked into grits for a cereal.

Whole Soybeans

To cook whole soybeans, soak them for several hours or overnight in 4 times as much water as you have dry beans. Replace the water with fresh water or soup stock, then cook the beans for at least 3 hours. Cook them very thoroughly to improve their digestibility.

Pressure cooking soybeans saves time and generally cooks them more completely. After soaking and draining the water, add just enough fresh liquid to cover the swelled beans and cook for 30 minutes at full pressure. They have a tendency to foam, so add a tablespoon of cooking oil to the water to prevent a clogged vent.

The test for doneness with soybeans is to put one in your mouth and press it against the roof to mash it with your tongue. If the bean is still hard, continue cooking until tender.

Sprouted Soybeans

Soybean sprouts can be grown in the same way as other sprouts. They can become moldy quite easily, however, so pay close attention to them. (See sprouting directions, page 145.) Soybean sprouts are ready in 3 to 4 days, or when the sprout is the same length as the bean. Never eat raw soybeans—steam or saute them for at least 5 minutes before serving.

Soybean Flour

Soy flour is available in three forms:

Full-fat soy flour is made from whole soybeans that have been hulled, cracked, and heat-treated to remove the beany flavor, as well as to increase the value of the protein and deactivate certain enzymes that cause deterioration in storage. The beans are then cooled and ground into a flour that contains about 20 percent fat and over 35 percent protein.

Low-fat and *defatted soy flours* are made from the meal that remains after soybean oil is extracted from whole soybeans. Low-fat soy flour is from soy meal left by the expeller method of extraction. It has 6 percent fat and 45 percent protein. Defatted soy flour is from soy meal left by the chemical solvent method of extraction and contains less than 1 percent fat and 50 percent protein.

Soybean flour can be used as an addition to or substitute for some of the flour in baked goods and pancakes. It contains no gluten so it must be used with wheat flour in breads that require rising. Soy flour can also be added to soups, cereals, and casseroles. It has a fairly strong soybeany flavor, so use it sparingly until you get used to it. For a change in taste, try toasting the flour in a dry skillet before adding it to your recipe.

Soy Grits

Soy grits, also called *soy granules,* are made from either whole soybeans or soybean meal. Whole-bean soy grits are made from raw or partially cooked soybeans that have been cracked into eight or ten pieces. Defatted soy grits are similar to defatted flour, but they are more coarsely ground.

Soy grits can be added to almost any dish. They cook quickly: use 4 parts water to 1 part grits and heat for 15 minutes. For better texture and digestibility, allow them to soak for a few minutes in boiling water before adding to other food.

For soups and stews, just sprinkle soy grits into the broth as you would vegetables. Try adding soy grits to spaghetti sauce—they will add a hamburgerlike texture and will complement the protein in the noodles. In hot cereals, substitute 2 tablespoons soy grits for 2 tablespoons of uncooked grain. For a delicate crunch and nutlike flavor, add soy grits to breads, muffins, and cookies.

Texturized Vegetable Protein (TVP)

TVP is made from either defatted or full-fat soy flour that is compressed until the protein fibers change in structure. This results in a fibrous-textured product that resembles meat. TVP can be used on its own or can be flavored and colored to simulate ham, beef, bacon, or any other meat product. The "bacon bits" in restaurant-made salads and om-elettes are often made from TVP. Processed products may list TVP as "hydrolyzed" or "isolated" protein, or simply as "soy protein."

Chunk-style TVP must be cooked with liquid before eating. Add it to stew, vegetable pies, or soup stock as it boils. Granulated TVP may be used dry: mix it with hamburger or other raw meat to extend the protein value while decreasing the cost per serving. To hydrate the granules, add 7/8 cup boiling water to 1 cup TVP. This will yield about 2 cups hydrated TVP. Stir until all the water is absorbed and let it soak for 10 minutes.

When browning TVP, stir it often to prevent it from sticking or burning. If you shape the mixture by hand, keep your hands wet so it doesn't stick to you.

Soy Nuts

Soy nuts are whole soybeans that have been soaked, then roasted in a pan or oven until crunchy. They are a nutritious snack and can be made at home.

Start with well-soaked or partially cooked soybeans that have been drained well. Spread the beans onto an oiled baking sheet, one layer deep, and bake at 350°F for about 30 minutes or until brown and crunchy. Add salt to taste, if desired, and store in an airtight container.

If you prefer, deep-fat fry the soaked beans by heating oil to 350°F in a fryer or heavy saucepan, then adding beans in a fryer basket and frying 6 to 8 minutes, until the beans are light brown and crispy. Drain them on absorbent paper and add salt or seasonings to taste, if desired.

How nutritious are they?

Soybeans are high in B-complex vitamins, calcium, phosphorus, and potassium. Also present are vitamin A and iron. Soybeans are 20 percent fat, most of which is polyunsaturated.

Soybean sprouts provide vitamins A, B-complex, and C.

The nutritional value of full-fat soy flour and soy grits is very similar to that of whole soybeans. They are high in protein, B-complex vitamins, vitamin A,

calcium, iron, and phosphorus. Defatted soy products (low-fat or defatted soy flour, defatted soy grits, and TVP) have a similar protein and mineral content as whole soybeans, but much less fat. Some TVP, especially the bacon- and ham-flavored kinds, have extremely high salt contents.

Soybeans contain all eight essential amino acids, the substances of which protein is comprised. This protein is not quite as high in quality as that of animal products, although it is very close. When combined with grains or dairy products, however, soybeans are a very high quality protein source.

Raw soybeans contain trypsin inhibitors (TI), substances that interfere with the action of trypsin. Trypsin is an enzyme in the intestine that digests protein. Laboratory tests have shown that 70 to 80 percent of all TI present in soybeans must be destroyed before the body can make use of all the bean's protein. TI is deactivated only by heat, and this is why it is important to cook soybeans thoroughly. Soaking and grinding whole soybeans greatly reduces the cooking time needed to destroy TI. Thus, soy flour, soy grits, and soybean sprouts need less cooking time than do whole soybeans.

✦ Nutritive Value: Appendix, 318, 486–490.

How do I store them?

Store whole soybeans and soy grits in airtight containers in a cool, dry, place. They will keep for up to one year. Older beans usually take longer to cook than young ones.

Soybean sprouts should be refrigerated and will keep for about a week.

Soy flour must be refrigerated to prevent rancidity and should be used within a few months.

Dehydrated TVP has a long shelf life and needs no special storage.

Where do they come from?

Soybeans were popularized by a Chinese emperor in 2800 B.C. and thereafter became a principal food in China. They were introduced to Japan about one thousand years later and became equally popular in that country.

Soybeans were brought to North America in the 1800s but were not widely grown until after 1920. Today, the United States is the world's largest producer of soybeans, growing about two-thirds of the total crop. Brazil is the second largest soybean-producing country, followed by China.

Soy Milk

What is it?

Soy milk is a beverage derived from soybeans. It can be obtained by finely grinding soaked soybeans, mixing them with water, straining off the "milk" and then heating it, or by blending soy flour with water and heating it.

Soy milk has been popular in Japan for many years, while in North America it has traditionally been consumed by vegetarians who choose to avoid dairy products. Since the mid-1980s, however, soy milk has become a popular beverage in natural food stores throughout North America.

Many brands of soy milk are made from United States-grown soybeans that are shipped to and processed in Japan. The soybeans are dehulled, quartered, steam heated, ground with water, homogenized, pasteurized, flavored, packed in aluminum foil, and shipped back to the United States. Some soy milk brands are processed domestically and are usually less expensive than the Japanese imports.

Soy milk is available either plain (unflavored) or flavored with malt, carob, vanilla, strawberry, almond, coffee, chocolate, or cocoa-mint. To achieve the consistency of cow's milk, some brands of soy milk contain vegetable oil.

How do I use it?

Soy milk can be used interchangeably with cow's milk in most recipes. It may have a "beany" flavor—especially if it is homemade—although this can be masked with honey, maple syrup, carob, or other flavorings, or deactivated by using hot water when making it. Packaged soy milks are ready to drink; some have malt added and taste like milkshakes.

Make Your Own Soy Milk

To make soy milk at home, use large, vegetable-type soybeans available in many natural food stores. For 2 quarts of soy milk, soak 1 pound (2¹/₂ cups) dry soybeans in four times as much water, either overnight or by the rapid method: Boil beans and water for 2 minutes, remove from heat, and let stand 1 hour. Remove the skins if desired, then grind the soaked beans in a blender with some of the water for 2 minutes, or until very fine. Repeat until all the beans have been ground and 3 quarts of water have been used. Next strain the ground beans through two layers of cheesecloth into a large cooking pot. Wring as much liquid from the beans as possible. Boil the liquid for 30 minutes, stirring occasionally to prevent scorching. If it starts to foam, reduce heat to a simmer. While the milk is warm, add sweetener or flavorings. The mash (called okara) can be used as an extender in meat dishes, added to casseroles or baked goods, or used to make tempeh.

Homemade soy milk may be used to make tofu, soy yogurt, soy ice cream, or soy cheese.

How nutritious is it?

Soy milk is sometimes substituted for cow's milk, although the two vary nutritionally in that cow's milk has more calcium, saturated fat, and sodium than soy milk. Cow's milk also contains cholesterol. Plain soy milk has less fat than cow's milk, although some brands of flavored soy milk have nearly twice as much fat per ounce as cow's milk. The protein content of cow's milk and soy milk is about the same: approximately 1 gram per ounce. Soy milk may be fortified with vitamins and minerals to more closely resemble the composition of cow's milk.

How do I store it?

Soy milk, unless packaged in aseptic containers, should be refrigerated and used within seven to ten days. Homemade soy milk may develop a surface skin, so strain it before using.

TEMPEH

What is it?

Tempeh (pronounced **tem**-*pay*) is a food made by combining cooked soybeans, grains, seeds, or a mixture of them with *Rhizopus oligosporus* mold culture, packing it in special bags, then incubating the beans on trays at about 90°F for 18 to 24 hours. The result is a white, distinct-smelling, chunky-textured cake about 3/4-inch thick.

Long used in Indonesia as a daily staple, tempeh is gaining popularity in North America as a meat substitute. With certain seasonings and methods of preparation, tempeh can taste similar to fish sticks, veal cutlets, or fried chicken.

How do I use it?

A common way to serve tempeh is to fry and use it like a hamburger patty. You can cube it and add it to sauteed vegetables or mock chicken salad. Crumble it for "tempeh Joes" (like sloppy Joes), on pizza, or in tacos.

Tempeh is also good with tempura—batter-dipped, fried, and served with spicy sauces, mustard, or other condiments. Try it fried in strips as soy spare ribs and serve with barbeque sauce.

How nutritious is it?

Tempeh is high in protein, is a good source of vitamin B12, and contains other B-complex vitamins. The fermentation process helps break down the gas-producing oligosaccharides (complex carbohydrates) that are normally found in whole beans.

How do I store it?

Store tempeh in your freezer or refrigerator until you are ready to use it. Remove it from the freezer about 45 minutes ahead of time to allow it to thaw. Tempeh will keep for about a week in the refrigerator and for several months when frozen.

Where does it come from?

The origin of tempeh is unknown. It is thought that it was used thousands of years ago in Java. The first United States tempeh shop opened in Los Angeles in 1962, but it wasn't until the late 1970s that the food caught on in North America, particularly among vegetarians.

TOFU

What is it?

Tofu, also called *bean curd* or *soy cheese,* is fast becoming a popular food item in supermarkets and continues to be a big seller in natural food stores.

Tofu is made by pureeing soaked soybeans with water, straining them to extract soy milk, cooking the soy milk, and adding a solidifier to produce curds and whey. The solidifier can either be a salt—such as nigari (mineral flakes that remain when sea water is evaporated), calcium sulfate, magnesium chloride—or an acid such as lemon juice or vinegar. The soy curds are then pressed until they become a firm, custardlike, creamy white cheese.

How do I use it?

Like yogurt and dairy cheese, tofu can be eaten uncooked and by itself. Fresh tofu has a delicate sweetness and a marvelously smooth, soft texture.

In Far Eastern countries, tofu is typically bought very fresh from small shops and eaten plain or with various seasonings and sauces, or in miso soup. In the West, tofu is usually served cooked and mixed with other foods.

Tofu soaks up the flavors of any food with which it is cooked. It is very good mixed with seasoned stir-fried vegetables, crumbled into casseroles, or scrambled with eggs.

In order for it to cook well, water-packed tofu should be dried out a bit. Remove it from its storage water, wrap it in a clean towel, and press it with a weighted dinner plate for 15 to 30 minutes. Well-pressed tofu can be sliced and fried in butter or oil, and seasoned with tamari or a spicy sauce such as Worcestershire or ketchup. It also broils well and is delicious with slightly sweetened miso.

Tofu can also be pureed for dressings, spreads, and dips; cubed for salads, soups, and sauces; mixed with egg, vegetable, and grain preparations; or blended to make creamy pies and other desserts.

How nutritious is it?

Tofu is very high in protein—7.8 percent—and it is nearly nutritionally complete. An 8-ounce serving of tofu has all the usable protein of a $5^1/_2$ ounce hamburger, and far less fat. Tofu contains a high amount of lysine, the amino acid in which most grains are deficient, so it is an excellent complementary food with grains.

The fat in tofu (4.2 percent) is mostly unsaturated. Tofu is also low in carbohydrates. It is about 85 percent water.

Tofu is an excellent source of calcium (if it is made with a calcium salt solidifier) and a good source of iron, phosphorus, and B-complex vitamins.

Due to its precooked nature, tofu is exceptionally easy to digest, so it is a first-rate baby food. It is also easily digested by people who are unaccustomed to beans.

♦ Nutritive Value: Appendix, 320.

How do I store it?

Keep tofu refrigerated and submerged in fresh water. If the water is changed daily, tofu can be successfully stored in the refrigerator for a week, although it will lose some flavor and texture.

As it gets older, tofu begins to develop a sour taste and smell, but it can be refreshed by parboiling it for several minutes or by deep-fat frying. When tofu spoils, you will know it by its bad smell and slimy feel.

Fresh or deep-fat fried tofu can be frozen and stored indefinitely.

MISO AND SHOYU

Miso and shoyu are closely related soybean products that have been indispensable parts of the Far Eastern diet and culture for hundreds of years. The traditional production of these foods is comparable to the Western craft of fermenting milk to form cheese and yogurt, or of fermenting grapes to produce wine. Soybeans are fermented to produce miso (soybean paste) and shoyu.

Both miso and shoyu are used to enrich the flavor and aroma of foods. They can replace salt in many recipes. One tablespoon of sweet miso, $1^1/_2$ teaspoons of salty miso, or 1 teaspoon of shoyu equals $^1/_4$ teaspoon of salt.

Miso and shoyu contain a high amount of protein—7 to 18 percent, depending upon the amount of soybeans used in production. They are both very high in sodium; miso contains an average of 12 percent, and shoyu 18 percent.

Miso and shoyu also contain iron, calcium, potassium, and phosphorus. Miso is over 50 percent water, and shoyu is over 60 percent water.

Miso

What is it?

Like fine wines and cheeses, miso is available in a vast array of colors, textures, flavors, and aromas. Its color ranges from warm, earthy tones to light yellow. The texture may resemble chunky or smooth peanut butter, or it can be as firm as cottage cheese. The flavor of miso ranges from salty to sweet, and its aroma can be heavy to light.

TYPES OF MISO

Name	Also Called	
Barley	Mugi miso	
Rice	Light-yellow	
	Mellow or sweet white	
	Red	Aka
	Genmai	Kome
	Shinshu	Shiro
Soybean	Hatcho miso	
Finger Lickin'	Kinzanji	
	Moromi	
	Natto	
Modern	Akadashi	
	Miso shiru	
	Dehydrated miso (for instant soup)	
Sweet simmered	Peanut	
	Tekka	

The characteristics of miso are determined by the duration and temperature of fermentation, the relative proportions of mold and salt, the particular strain of mold, the type of grain used, and the cooking methods employed.

How is it made?

Miso, or fermented soybean paste, has traditionally been made in huge cedar vats in which cooked soybeans, salt, a grain such as rice or barley, and a mold are mixed and fermented.

Miso is available in its traditional, or natural, form as well as in "quick" form. Natural miso has the finest flavor and can usually be identified by its distinctive chunky texture of whole soybeans and mold-covered grain *(koji)*. Quick miso does not have the fullness of flavor, aroma, deep color, or storage qualities of natural miso because it is fermented for only a short time—3 days to 3 weeks—in a temperature-controlled, heated environment. Various chemicals and additives (bleaches, food colors, sweeteners, vitamins, and monosodium glutamate) are occasionally added, along with preservatives (ethyl alcohol or sorbic acid). Quick miso may also be pasteurized. This prevents the microorganisms in miso from producing carbon dioxide, which would swell the plastic bags in which miso is sometimes packaged. Pasteurized miso has even less flavor and aroma, and it is also less nutritious due to the heat-induced killing of the microorganisms.

How do I use it?

Miso has an extensive range of uses, from casseroles to soups to sandwiches to seasoning.

Any soup with a vegetable stock base can become miso soup by adding $1/4$ cup miso to each quart of soup. Dissolve the miso in a small amount of soup stock removed from the pot just before serving. Add this mixture to the soup, but do not allow it to boil, because high temperatures will kill the essential enzymes in miso.

Miso can be added to any grain, vegetable, fish, or tofu dish as a condiment. It is generally best to dilute it or to make a paste by adding a small amount of water and stirring it until the miso is dissolved.

To make a nutritious spread, combine 1 part miso, 1 part water, and 2 parts tahini (sesame seed spread). Use it on crackers, bread, or raw vegetables.

To make a delicious sauce for hot, fried tofu (soybean curd), substitute white wine or sake for the water and add a small amount of honey and minced onion to the miso spread recipe above. A 1-to-2 mixture of miso and butter is excellent on sweet corn.

How do I store it?

Natural misos packaged in plastic bags are usually pasteurized and can be kept at room temperature almost indefinitely. Misos packaged in bulk containers are typically not pasteurized and should be refrigerated, as this prolongs the enzyme activity. Keep nonpasteurized miso cool and in an airtight container to prevent the formation of surface molds. If mold does form, either scrape it off or mix it into the miso, just as you would a cheese mold.

Saltier varieties of miso, such as hatcho miso, are fairly stable, although mold may form on them. The sweet or light-colored miso will change in taste and/or color if the miso is not kept sealed and in a cool place.

♦ Nutritive Value: Appendix, 319.

Shoyu

What is it?

Shoyu, a salty liquid seasoning, is produced by mixing soybeans, salt, wheat, and sometimes mold with water. This mixture is fermented for a specified period of time to achieve a desired flavor.

The types of shoyu most commonly available in North America are:

Natural shoyu—Made from whole soybeans in the traditional Japanese manner and fermented naturally for 12 to 18 months. Natural shoyu is imported to North America from Japan.

Shoyu—Made from defatted soybean meal, which is cheaper than whole soybeans. It is made under conditions where the temperature and humidity are carefully controlled. The manufacturing techniques are based on traditional methods, and the characteristics of this product are similar to natural shoyu. It is allowed to ferment for 4 to 6 months.

Shoyu is manufactured in the United States as well as in Japan.

Synthetic (chemical) soy sauce—This product is made from defatted soybean meal—the solids that remain after soybean oil has been chemically extracted from soybeans—which reacts with hydrochloric acid and becomes hydrolyzed vegetable protein. Caramel coloring and corn syrup are usually added to give it color and flavor. Some brands contain sodium benzoate as a preservative. Synthetic soy sauce is comparatively inexpensive, since it takes only a few days to make. It is generally marketed under Chinese-sounding brand names such as Kikkoman® and LaChoy®.

Tamari A salty liquid that is left over and drained off soybean miso after fermentation. The word *tamari* is sometimes used to describe shoyu or soy sauce.

How do I use it?

Shoyu is typically added to Asian foods; however it is also an excellent condiment that adds a unique flavor to Western-style dishes that use vegetables, grains, beans, or eggs.

In Japan, shoyu is the traditional seasoning used with tofu. It can be served as the only condiment for raw or cooked tofu, or as the base for sauces used for dipping.

To make a basic Japanese dipping sauce, combine 1/4 cup shoyu and 1 cup vegetable stock made from sea or land vegetables. Add grated horseradish and grated ginger (or ginger powder) to taste. This sauce is delicious with fish, tofu, or batter-fried vegetables (tempura). A sharp hot sauce can be made from 3 tablespoons shoyu, 1/2 teaspoon dry mustard, 1/2 teaspoon sesame oil, and 2 teaspoons vinegar.

How do I store it?

Synthetic soy sauce will keep at room temperature almost indefinitely. Shoyu and natural shoyu are usually flash-pasteurized at low temperatures, while synthetic soy sauce generally contains preservatives to keep it from spoiling.

✦ Nutritive Value: Appendix, 491.

WHITE BEANS: NAVY, GREAT NORTHERN

What are they?

Navy beans and Great Northern beans are so similar that you may get them confused. Just remember: navy beans are the little ones.

Navy beans are sometimes referred to as *pea beans* because they are about the same size as peas. Great Northern beans—popular in northern areas—are about the same size as blackeyed peas. Less commonly available are flat white beans.

Navy and Great Northern beans are both in the Phaseolus family, and are related to kidney beans and pinto beans.

How do I use them?

Baked beans and pork 'n beans are generally made from navy or Great Northern beans. These beans are also great in soups.

To cook them, first soak the beans for several hours or overnight in about 3 times as much water as you have beans. If you plan to bake them, add a pinch of baking soda to the soaking water, as this will help keep the skins from breaking. Discard soaking water, add fresh water or soup stock (3 1/2 parts water to 1 part Great Northern beans, or 2 parts water to 1 part navy beans), then cook for 1 1/2 to 2 hours. With a pressure cooker, add water to cover and cook 20 minutes after full pressure is reached. If you plan to bake them, pressure cook them first for 10 minutes. You can also pressure cook unsoaked beans, but increase cooking time by 10 to 15 minutes.

A convenient way to have a meal prepared is to cook soaked beans throughout the day in a slow cooker (crock pot). Add seasonings and vegetables at any time up to 20 minutes before serving.

How nutritious are they?

White beans contain small amounts of B-complex vitamins, calcium, phosphorus, potassium, and iron. They are good sources of carbohydrates and protein.

Because the protein is incomplete, these beans

should be eaten with grains (such as crackers or bread) or nuts and seeds, as these foods contain amino acids which complement those of the beans.

✦ Nutritive Value: Appendix, 280, 282.

How do I store it?

Store navy beans and Great Northern beans in an airtight container in a cool, dry place. They will keep almost indefinitely.

Where do they come from?

The production of navy beans is second only to pinto beans in the United States, with an annual crop of five to seven billion pounds. They are grown mainly in Michigan.

Great Northern beans are the third most commonly produced dry edible bean in the United States, where two to three billion pounds are grown every year. Most Great Northern beans are from western states.

NUTS AND SEEDS

What are they?

While North Americans tend to consider nuts and seeds as snack foods or condiments, they are the primary protein foods for many cultures around the world. Nomadic people of ancient times relied on nuts and seeds as dietary staples.

All *seeds* are embryonic plants that contain the nourishment needed to feed new plants through the first stage of life. The foods we call seeds grow on vegetative plants, such as flowers or legumes. They have softer, sometimes edible hulls. *Nuts* are the seeds of trees and are characterized by a hard, removable outer shell and a softer, edible, inner kernel.

Buying tips

Nuts and seeds are marketed in a variety of forms. They may be shelled or in the shell; raw or roasted; salted, spiced, or unseasoned; prepackaged or in bulk. In general, the more processing and packaging a nut has been subjected to, the higher the price will be.

When shopping for shelled nuts and seeds, avoid those that are limp, dark, shriveled, or rubbery. Packaging is an important consideration: Nuts and seeds in clear containers, such as glass jars and cellophane bags, are subject to degradation by light. Clear containers, however, also allow you to check for quality. The vacuum-packed can is an excellent storage container, but it leaves you blind to the contents.

Nuts and seeds in the shell are oftentimes the best buy. With the exception of peanuts they are generally not roasted, and they usually cost less than shelled nuts and seeds. The shell or hull also protects the kernels from spoilage, preserves the nutri-tional value, and shields the kernels against exposure to chemicals. Some nuts are treated with lye and gas to soften and loosen the shells. The shells may also be bleached with hydrochloric acid (household bleach), colored, or waxed. Yet as long as the shells are not cracked, these treatments will not penetrate to the edible nut inside. An exception to this is pistachios: because pistachio shells open easily, those that are dyed red may be exposed to the chemicals in processing.

When buying nuts and seeds in the shell, look for clean ones with bright, well-shaped shells. They should feel heavy, as this indicates fresher, meatier kernels. Those that are dirty, stained, cracked, broken, or very lightweight (dried up) should be avoided. Never buy or eat moldy nuts and seeds.

One type of mold to especially look out for is aflatoxin. This highly carcinogenic substance may grow on peanuts and other nuts or grains. The United States Food and Drug Administration routinely tests batches of commercial nuts—both domestically produced and imported—to find out if the level of aflatoxins present in the food is below acceptable limits for human consumption. The current acceptable limit is 20 parts per billion. In recent years there have occasionally been recalls of peanut butter or other nuts and grains due to aflatoxin contamination above this level.

Shelled nuts are often roasted or dry roasted. One roasting process called french frying involves frying the nuts in oil that has been continually heated. If the nuts appear or taste oily and are not very crunchy, they are quite likely nuts that have been fried. The nuts sold as cocktail nuts are often heavily salted. Some roasted nuts are called fancy mixed nuts.

Dry-roasted nuts are cooked without additional oil. They are heated in huge, drum-shaped roasters, usually for 20 to 30 minutes at 275°F. Many commercially available dry-roasted nuts also contain sugar, salt, starch, monosodium glutamate, vegetable gums, spices, or preservatives.

How do I use them?

Nuts and seeds are very versatile foods. They can be ground into a meal or paste and added to baked goods, chopped or ground slightly and mixed into casseroles, tossed into salads, or browned and served with cooked or raw vegetables. Seeds can be sprouted and used as a green vegetable. Nuts and seeds with high levels of oil—such as sesame seeds, cashews, and sunflower seeds—can be ground or pureed into smooth butters.

For a refreshingly different but slightly filling beverage, finely grind nuts or seeds in a blender, then add about twice as much water as you have nuts. This nut milk is a good substitute for milk or soft drinks. You can use blanched almonds, cashews, or sunflower seeds. Add sweetener if desired.

Nuts and seeds are, of course, popular as snack foods, but the amount of them that you should eat depends on the rest of your diet. If, for example, you eat mostly whole or unprocessed foods with only a moderate amount of animal fats, you can afford to eat larger quantities of nuts and seeds. If your diet is rich in meats, cheeses, and other foods high in fat, you may wish to cut down on these foods in order to incorporate nuts and seeds into your meals. In general, nuts should be eaten in moderation—not by the handful. It is also better to eat them as part of a meal rather than as a snack between meals.

It's easy to roast nuts and seeds at home: Spread them on a baking sheet one layer deep and bake at 350°F until lightly browned. Bake shelled nuts for 5 to 10 minutes; nuts and seeds in the shell for 15 to 20 minutes. Be sure to not over roast them, as they will continue to bake for a short time after they are removed from the oven. Taste-test them for doneness.

How nutritious are they?

Most nuts and seeds are between 12 and 29 percent protein. Pumpkin seeds and peanuts are the most protein rich of the group. This protein is incomplete, so nuts and seeds should be eaten with grains, dairy products, or legumes for better protein utilization (see Protein Complementarity, pages 71, 112).

Most nuts and seeds are high in fat. They range from 45 to 70 percent oil, and most of this is unsaturated fat. They also provide lots of calories—30 to 60 calories per gram of protein.

Nuts and seeds are good sources of calcium, phosphorus, magnesium, and potassium. Most contain B-complex vitamins, and some raw nuts and seeds supply vitamin E. A few contain vitamins A and D.

In order to utilize the nutrients in nuts and seeds, it is important to chew them well or eat them in the form of nut butter, paste, or nut meal. Nuts that are swallowed whole or in big pieces will not be digested—they will pass through the body unchanged. Nuts and seeds are also more easily digested if they are eaten when the stomach is not full rather than right after a large meal.

✦ Nutritive Value: Appendix, 277, 278, 289, 291–295, 297–301, 303–309, 311–315, 317, 321, 323–326, 493–497.

How do I store them?

Keep nuts and seeds in a tightly covered container in a cool, dark, and dry place. If stored properly, they will keep for several months. Some nuts and seeds may be frozen in airtight containers for longer storage.

Whole nuts and seeds in the shell will remain freshest for the longest period of time. But once they are removed from the shell—especially if they are chopped, ground, or roasted in oil—they will be more prone to spoilage or rancidity and should therefore be refrigerated.

ALMONDS

What are they?

Almonds are the fruits of sweet almond trees. The popular soft-shell almonds are easy to crack, fun to eat, and nutritious.

Almonds are in the rose family and are first cousins to peaches. In fact, the outer fleshy hull of an almond resembles a dry, green peach. And the kernel of a peach pit, as you may know, looks like an almond.

Almond trees are small compared to other nut trees. New trees take four or more years to bear fruit. The blossoms are large white and pink flowers that, if they are not damaged by cold weather, will produce fruits—the almond nuts.

Buying tips

Almonds are marketed in several forms: raw and in the shell, or shelled raw almonds; sliced, slivered, or blanched (brown skins removed); roasted and salted; dry roasted; and smoke flavored.

About half the weight of almonds in the shell is the shell. But you can usually save money and have fresher nuts if you buy them this way and crack them yourself as you need them. One pound of almonds in the shell will yield 1 to 1½ cups of shelled nuts.

Generally, the more that almonds are processed, the more likely they are to contain excess oil, salt, sugar, or preservatives and the more they will cost. Commercially roasted almonds are often fried in oil, whereas dry-roasted nuts are not. Dry-roasted almonds, however, usually contain unnecessary additives. To be sure of what you are eating—and to possibly save money—buy raw almonds and roast them at home. If raw almonds are not available, look for dry-roasted, unsalted nuts without extra additives or preservatives.

How do I use them?

The mild flavor and high nutritional value of almonds make them appropriate for more than just an occasional snack or dessert.

You can chop or slice whole almonds, toast them slightly, and mix with green beans for a special dinner treat. Wild rice casserole with almonds is absolutely divine. Add them to any vegetable loaf or cookie recipe for a pleasant crunch.

Have you ever had almond milk? It is easy to make and quite delicious. Grind 1 cup blanched almonds in a blender. Add 2 cups water and blend until creamy. Add a small amount of sweetener, if desired. Strain the milk to remove the particles of nuts—this nut meal is great for recipes that call for almond paste, or for any baked goods and confections. Almond milk can also be coagulated and made into cheese. Commercial mozzarellalike almond products are available in many natural food stores.

Blanched almonds have had the brown skins removed. You can do this at home by allowing the nuts to simmer in water until the skins wrinkle or puff up. Then, one at a time, pop the nuts out of the skins by pressing your thumb and index finger together with the nut in between. Discard the skins.

To roast almonds at home, simply spread whole raw almonds on a baking sheet and bake them at 350°F for 5 to 10 minutes.

How nutritious are they?

Almonds are about 18 percent protein. This protein is incomplete by itself, but if you eat almonds with beans or cheese, you will get a good supply of high-quality protein (see Protein Complementarity, pages 71, 112).

ALMOND EXTRACT

This liquid flavoring is used in baking and is made from the oil of the bitter almond, a cousin to the sweet almond. The oil, in concentrated form, contains a poisonous substance called prussic acid. To make almond extract, the oil is diluted with water and alcohol.

ALMOND OIL

The oil of sweet almonds is used in cosmetics, some food products, as a nutrition supplement, and occasionally as a cooking oil. It is made by crushing and pressing raw almonds to extract the oil.

Almonds are also high in unsaturated fat. Commercially roasted almonds usually contain even more fat, so almonds should be eaten in moderation, not munched down by the handful.

As a source of minerals, almonds rank high in calcium, iron, magnesium, phosphorus, and potassium. Raw almonds have magnesium, manganese and selenium, as well as vitamins E and B-complex.

✦ Nutritive Value: Appendix, 277, 278, 492.

Where do they come from?
Almonds were first found in parts of Asia and the Mediterranean. They are still grown in Spain, Italy, Iran, and Morocco.

In 1843 almonds were brought to California, and today that state is the world's leading almond producer. From five hundred to six hundred million pounds of almonds in the shell are grown there every year.

BRAZIL NUTS

What are they?
From the wilds of the Amazon River Valley forests come Brazil nuts, fruits of the broad-leaf evergreen trees. They have also been called *cream nuts* and *para nuts*.

The huge Brazil nut trees grow to 150 feet high and produce yellowish white blossoms. They bear two hundred to four hundred large fruits per tree every year. The hard-husked fruits look somewhat like coconuts, and inside the fruits are clusters of seeds—the Brazil nuts—which resemble orange segments within the rind.

Buying tips
The Brazil nuts to buy are ones that feel heavy and solid when shaken and that have no signs of blemish. Avoid those with cracked shells or a dry rattle. Some Brazil nut shells may be dyed reddish brown for cosmetic purposes.

If you are buying shelled Brazil nuts, keep an eye open for signs of staleness or rancidity. Those that are slightly darkened, bruised, moldy, or rubbery are probably rancid and should not be used.

PROTEIN COMPLEMENTARITY

Protein is a nutrient made up of twenty-two amino acids, eight of which our bodies cannot produce. We must get these eight essential amino acids from the foods we eat, and we need to have them all together and in certain proportions. When they are, the food is referred to as a *complete protein*.

Nuts and seeds contain most or all of these essential amino acids, but not in the right proportions. They are called *incomplete protein*.

By eating nuts and seeds with other foods that are high in the amino acids that nuts and seeds lack, you can get a high-quality or complete protein. A peanut butter sandwich on whole wheat bread is an example of complementary protein. Another is the popular Middle Eastern combination of sesame products and chick-peas.

Brazil nuts that are commercially roasted tend to be extremely high in fat and salt, and they are often rancid. Dry-roasted nuts do not contain extra oil, but they may have excessive salt, preservatives, sugar, or starch added. Look for dry-roasted nuts without additives—or better still, buy raw Brazil nuts and roast them at home.

How do I use them?
Like all nuts, Brazil nuts are quite versatile. Chop them, toast them, and add them to casseroles, vegetables, or grain dishes. Try them as filling in baked apples.

If you have a nut butter machine, food grinder, or blender, you can grind Brazil nuts into a creamy, rich-tasting spread. This is good on breads or mixed into sauces or soups as a thickener.

Roast Brazil nuts by spreading them in a pan and

baking them at 350°F for about 10 minutes if shelled, or for 15 to 20 minutes if in the shell.

For easier shelling, steam the nuts in a vegetable steamer for a few minutes, or freeze them and allow them to defrost slightly before cracking. These methods will help in getting the whole nut in one piece.

How nutritious are they?

Brazil nuts are very high in fat—65 percent—and most of that is unsaturated. They provide a high amount of calories.

Brazil nuts are also high in protein, which is incomplete. If you eat them in combination with beans or dairy products, the protein will be more complete (see Protein Complementarity, pages 71, 112).

Brazil nuts contain calcium, iron, magnesium, phosphorus, potassium, and selenium. Raw nuts also contain zinc. Some B-complex vitamins and vitamin C are present.

✦ Nutritive Value: Appendix, 289.

How do I store them?

Because of their high oil content, shelled Brazil nuts can become rancid easily. They should always be refrigerated and eaten within two to three months.

Store Brazil nuts in the shell in a cool, dry place, and use them within six months. It may be wise to refrigerate these also.

Where do they come from?

Native to and still growing in Brazil and Bolivia, Brazil nut trees are reportedly so abundant that only a fraction of the nuts produced are even harvested—almost all of them from wild trees. An estimated fifty thousand metric tons are marketed every year.

Harvesting is done by hand by native South Americans during the month of January. After being dried in the sun, the nuts are placed in baskets and submerged in the Amazon River. Any hollow or light nuts will float away, leaving the marketable nuts in the baskets. The good nuts are sold to traders.

About one-fourth of the commercial Brazil nut crop is shelled in Brazil. The rest are shipped in the shell to the United States, Canada, and Europe.

CASHEWS

What are they?

Curvy, crunchy cashews—the ones you like to pick out of the bowl of mixed nuts because they taste so good—have uses far beyond the nut bowl.

The cashew tree is native to the tropics and grows to a height of forty feet. Red and yellow pear-shaped "apples" form on it, and at the bottom of the fleshy fruits grow the kidney-shaped nuts. These nuts have hard shells with two layers. Between the layers is a black, resinous liquid called cardol, which is caustic and can form blisters on the skin if attempts are made to crack the shells by hand or by biting them.

In commercial processing, the cashew nuts are separated from the apples and dried in the sun. After being moistened and softened, the nuts are roasted at 350 to 400°F to release the cardol. This by-product is used to make paints, varnishes, and insecticides. The nut kernels are extracted from the shells and are again heated to remove a membrane.

The cashews are then graded according to size and packed into tightly sealed tin cans for export. They are considered to be raw at this stage, even though they have been heated during the shelling process.

Buying tips

Cashews are the only nuts that are not commercially available in the shell. They can be obtained in their raw form, however.

Commercially roasted cashews are generally quite oily or salty. Dry-roasted cashews have no extra fat, but they usually contain added salt, sugar, starch, and preservatives. You can, of course, roast them at home to be sure that no unnecessary additives are present.

How do I use them?

Cashews are fun and crunchy additions to salads, casseroles, muffins, and stir-fried vegetables. They add a nutty flavor, subtle richness, and a good supply of nutrients.

For a special main dish, try mushroom and

cashew stroganoff. Use cashews in the stuffing of birds at holiday time, or in stuffed green peppers with rice. They make nut burgers something to talk about.

Cashew butter, made by grinding toasted or raw cashews in a blender or food grinder, can be used as a spread for crackers and bread. This butter is also a delicious thickener for sauces or soups; use it instead of flour. You can also make another type of cashew butter by melting regular butter, adding seasonings, and mixing this with cashew pieces. Use this as a sauce with vegetables.

How nutritious are they?

Cashews contain a healthy amount of protein—about 20 percent. This protein is not as high-quality as that of animal products, but when cashews are eaten with grains, dairy products, or beans, they provide a more complete protein (see Protein Complementarity, pages 71, 112).

About 45 percent of the cashew is oil, or fat, and most of that is unsaturated. This is a lower level of fat than most nuts, but it may be high enough to discourage one from eating large amounts of them as a snack.

Cashews have high levels of calcium, iron, magnesium, phosphorus, potassium, and zinc. Also present are B-complex vitamins.

✦ Nutritive Value: Appendix, 291–294.

How do I store them?

Cashews should be stored in a tightly covered container in a dry, cool place away from heat and light. They will keep in the refrigerator for up to six months. Chopped, ground, or commercially roasted cashews are highly prone to rancidity, so they should be stored carefully and only for short periods of time. Cashew butter should always be refrigerated.

Where do they come from?

Cashews originated in Brazil, but the trees were planted in other countries with tropical climates. Today, about 90 percent of the world's supply of cashews comes from India. The rest is from Brazil and Mozambique.

CHESTNUTS

Known to many as sweet, brown holiday nuts, chestnuts are unique in the nut group because of their high starch content and low percentage of fat.

Chestnuts are in the beech tree family and are related to the small, triangular-shaped and less-available beechnut. Their other cousin, the chinkapin, has been eaten by Native Americans for centuries.

Chestnuts grew abundantly in the United States until about ninety years ago, when some diseased trees imported from Asia spread a fungus that nearly wiped out all of the existing chestnut trees. Some varieties are resistant to this fungus, and new stocks have been planted, but most of the chestnuts sold for eating today are imported from Italy and Japan.

Fresh chestnuts are quite starchy and not very sweet, so they should be allowed to age and dry before eating. As the nuts lose some of their moisture, sugars develop and their flavor improves. The nuts are cured when they feel soft if lightly pinched with your fingers. They will have a crumbly texture and a light, sweet flavor.

Chestnuts are made even more delicious by roasting. Cut deep slashes through the shell of each nut to form a cross. Use a small knife with a sharp point. Then spread the nuts one layer deep in a shallow baking dish. Cover the pan tightly with a lid or foil and place it in a 450°F oven for 30 minutes, occasionally shaking the pan to turn the nuts inside. Reduce the heat so the nuts will stay warm, and remove only as many nuts as you can peel and eat at one time. One pound of chestnuts in the shell will yield about 2 cups of nut meats.

Pre-peeled, canned chestnuts are often available in food stores year-round. Look for them in the Asian foods section.

For use in cooking, fresh chestnuts can be boiled for 10 minutes and then peeled. The cooked nuts can then be pureed or chopped and used in many ways. Europeans incorporate them into soups, vegetable casseroles, and desserts. Because of their high starch content, they are often used as a substitute for potatoes or noodles.

Fresh chestnuts are about 50 percent water and mostly carbohydrates. Once dried, they provide not only carbohydrates but protein, fat, B-complex vitamins, and the minerals calcium, iron, phosphorus, and potassium.

Store chestnuts in a dry, cool place or refrigerate them to prevent rancidity. Canned chestnuts will keep for about a year.

✦ Nutritive Value: Appendix, 295, 494, 495.

Coconut

What is it?

The coconut grows on a palm tree in tropical climates. Each nut is encased in a large, fibrous husk that is removed when the nut is ripe.

The round, hairy nuts are shipped whole or split open to remove the meat—the half-inch wide white band inside each coconut shell. This nut meat is scraped from the shells and dried in the sun to produce copra—flaked or shredded coconut as we know it.

The center of a coconut is filled with a white fluid called *coconut milk,* which is sometimes drunk as a beverage. Another kind of coconut milk is made by mixing freshly grated coconut meat with water, straining it, and adding a vegetable gum or sweetener. The liquid inside a coconut is quite watery in comparison. In some places, coconut is eaten while it is "green"—when all of the inside is a creamy liquid.

Buying tips

If you want really fresh and tasty coconut, buy the whole nuts in season, from October through December. Shake them and listen for lots of liquid, and check to make sure they feel heavy and have no soft or moldy spots.

Commercially shredded or flaked coconut is often stale or flat tasting. Although coconut meat has its own natural sweetness, some commercial shredded coconut makers add extra sugar and propylene glycol to retain moisture. If you cannot get whole fresh coconut, try to find unsweetened shredded or flaked coconut without additives. One pound of shredded coconut equals 6 cups.

How do I use it?

Coconut is an important ingredient in the spicy dishes of South Indian cuisine, such as curries, chutneys, and stews. The nuts are also a basic food in the Polynesian lands where they grow.

Shredded or flaked coconut is a wonderful garnish for cakes and candies, and is the basic flavor ingredient in other baked goods, such as macaroons and coconut cream pie. Mix it with granola, trail mixes, and fruit salads. Sprinkle shredded coconut on vegetable and rice dishes.

To crack a whole coconut, first use a sharp, pointed tool, such as an ice pick, to pierce the "eyes" (the three small circular spots at one end). Drain the milk from one of the holes, then heat the nut in an oven for 20 to 30 minutes at 325°F. Wrap the nut in a towel, then tap all around the outside with a mallet or hammer to loosen the meat from the shell. Pound it hard with the hammer to break it open, and peel off the skin with a vegetable peeler. The skin is actually edible, for those who don't mind the texture. The white meat can then be chopped or grated with a cheese grater.

Another shelling method is to freeze the whole, drained coconut, then allow it to defrost. The nut meat should pop out of the shell when you crack it. Fresh coconut meat usually sticks to the shell when it is broken open at room temperature.

How nutritious is it?

Coconut is very high in fat—up to 60 percent—so it should be eaten in moderation and not as a big part of your diet. It is one of the few plant foods that contains mostly saturated fat rather than unsaturated fat.

Coconut is relatively low in protein compared to other nuts and seeds. It provides calcium, iron, magnesium, phosphorus, and potassium, as well as small amounts of B-complex vitamins.

✦ Nutritive Value: Appendix, 297–299.

How do I store it?

Fresh whole coconut will keep for one to two months at room temperature, but an open or cracked coconut should be refrigerated and used within a week. Shredded or flaked coconut should also be refrigerated or frozen until it is to be used.

Where does it come from?

Coconut is thought to be native to Polynesia and southern Asia. It grows where it is hot, humid, and rainy. Much of the world's production is from wild groves and plantations in the Philippines, Indonesia, and other islands in the South Pacific.

FILBERTS (HAZELNUTS)

The squirrels love them, they grow on small trees or bushes, they have easy-to-crack shells and they are ready to eat in early autumn. What are they?

Hazelnuts! Or filberts, as they are more commonly known. These seeds of a tree in the birch family have been eaten for thousands of years, by squirrels and humans alike.

Although filberts and hazelnuts are virtually identical in taste, they are distinguishable by the size of the plant and by the way they are grown. Hazelnuts are wild shrubs that grow in woods along fence rows. They form hard-shelled seeds within husks that don't quite conceal the nuts. Filberts, on the other hand, are short, domesticated trees that are planted in groves for commercial purposes. Their fringed husks grow around and beyond the nut shells. These shells are usually larger and more oblong than hazelnuts. Both are ready to harvest when the hazel-colored shells fall to the ground.

Buying tips

When shopping for filberts in the shell, look for clean nuts with no cracks or pinholes. They should feel relatively heavy and should not rattle when shaken.

Shelled filberts have a pleasantly sweet smell when they are fresh. Those that have a peculiar, unpleasant odor may be rancid or moldy and should be avoided. Also pass by nuts that are limp, rubbery, shriveled, or visibly moldy.

Commercially roasted filberts usually contain high amounts of fat and salt. Dry-roasted nuts are also usually high in salt and may have sugar, starch, and preservatives added.

Whenever possible, buy fresh, raw filberts in the shell. Approximately $1\frac{1}{2}$ pounds will yield 1 pound (about $3\frac{1}{2}$ cups) shelled filberts. If you prefer roasted filberts, buy them raw—in the shell or shelled—and roast them at home. Or look for dry roasted filberts with no salt or other additives.

How do I use them?

Filberts and hazelnuts are, of course, fun to crack and eat as a snack. You may have also seen or eaten them as garnishes in drinks such as martinis and grasshoppers.

Chopped filberts add a delicious and unusual flavor to casseroles, grain dishes, and cookies. Have you ever tried hazelnuts in the stuffing of wild birds? How about using filbert halves as big eyes of gingerbread people?

Roasting filberts or hazelnuts at home is simple. Just spread the raw nuts one layer deep in a pan and bake at 350°F for 5 to 10 minutes if they are shelled, or 20 to 25 minutes in the shell. Add salt to taste, if desired.

You can also make filbert butter by grinding the nuts in a grinder or blender. This creamy, rich-tasting butter is good with bread or crackers, or it can be mixed into the batter of baked goods.

How nutritious are they?

Filberts and hazelnuts are about 12 percent protein—not exceptionally high, but good for complementing with beans or dairy products. They are high in fat (over 60 percent), and most of the fat is unsaturated.

Other nutrients found in filberts include calcium, iron, phosphorus, potassium, zinc, magnesium, and the vitamins A, B-complex, and E.

✦ Nutritive Value: Appendix, 300, 301.

Where do they come from?

Hazelnuts and filberts were found growing in eastern Europe about three thousand years ago. They prefer northern temperate climates and grow well in many different areas of North America.

Large-scale commercial production of filberts in North America is limited to Oregon and Washington, where about 25,000 tons are grown annually. Some filberts are imported from Turkey, Italy, and Spain.

FLAX SEEDS

Flax seeds are shiny, oval shaped, and golden brown in color. The small seeds are edible and are an important element in the diets of people in eastern Europe.

Flax seeds are rich in oil, which is used as a cooking oil; as a nutritional supplement; in making paints, lacquers, and varnishes; and for linseed oil, the type used on woodwork.

The flax plant grows from one to four feet high. Its tall stems contain fibers that can be cleaned and woven to produce linen as well as fine, high-grade paper and cigarette papers.

Flax seeds can be eaten in a number of ways. Add them to granola or hot cereal (1 to 2 teaspoons per serving) during or after cooking. Try flax seeds in casseroles, sauces, and salads. They can be used like cornstarch as a thickening agent in gravies and dressings. For proper digestion, it is best to grind the seeds into a paste or meal before mixing with other ingredients.

In Germany, a delicious bread called *Leinenbrot* (linen bread) is made with flax seeds. To make it, knead approximately 1/4 cup flax seeds into whole wheat bread dough prior to forming it into a loaf.

A tea made from flax seeds is reputedly soothing to the intestines because of its mucilaginous qualities; that is, it becomes jellylike and sticky.

Flax seeds are best kept in a cool area away from excessive light and moisture. It is good to refrigerate or freeze them for long-term storage.

Although Russia, Belgium, and France all cultivate flax for linen, the flax grown in the United States is almost exclusively for linseed oil. Most of the domestic flax seed is from North and South Dakota, Minnesota, Montana, and Texas.

MACADAMIAS

Also called *Queensland nut,* this rich and tasty seed originated in Australia and grows in other areas of the South Pacific, especially the Hawaiian Islands.

The nuts form on macadamia trees in clusters of about twenty seeds. They have leathery husks that split when they are ripe, which causes the nuts to fall. A hard shell protects the round white kernels.

Macadamias have a mild, sweet flavor. Add them, chopped, to baked goods and casseroles, or use them to garnish fruit salads.

These nuts are extremely high in fat—over 70 percent, most of which is saturated. They should not be eaten in large quantities as a snack food. They also contain protein, some B-complex vitamins, and the minerals calcium, phosphorus, and iron.

Keep macadamia nuts refrigerated to prevent rancidity. Store them in an airtight container and use them within a month.

✦ Nutritive Value: Appendix, 303, 304.

PEANUTS

What are they?

Peanuts, ground nuts, goobers—they are all names for one of the most popular nuts in North America. Funny thing is, the "all-American nut" didn't originate in this country, and it's not really even a nut!

Peanuts are believed to have originated in South America. They migrated to Africa with Spanish and Portuguese explorers and were then brought to North America by slaves in the eighteenth century.

Peanuts are legumes, like beans and peas. But the pods grow underground, much like potatoes. The plants resemble clover and grow to a leafy one and one-half feet high. After their pretty yellow blossoms appear, ovary pegs form and grow from the principal plant stem into the soil. These pegs form peanuts—as many as thirty to forty pods per plant. In the fall, or after the plant withers, the peanuts are dug and hung to dry. After they are cured, they are ready to eat.

Three varieties of peanuts are grown:

- Spanish—Small, roundish nuts
- Valencia—Medium-size, oval-shaped nuts often used for salted-in-the-shell peanuts
- Virginia (or Jumbo)—Large nuts typically added to mixed (cocktail) nuts

All three can be used for peanut butter, candies, and snacks or home use.

How do I use them?

Peanuts go well with just about everything. Eat them roasted or raw; whole, chopped, or ground; cooked or baked. Add them to soups, cookies, casseroles, or stir-fried vegetables. Poke them into bananas to make a funny-faced food for kids.

You can cook and use raw peanuts as you would other beans—Spanish and Valencia peanuts are the best for this. Soak the nuts overnight, then drain off water. Cover with fresh water, bring the nuts to a boil, then simmer for 2 hours or until tender. With a pressure cooker, cook unsoaked peanuts for 20 to 25 minutes after full pressure is reached.

Peanuts can be eaten raw, but they are somewhat softer and taste less nutty than roasted peanuts. To roast them at home, spread the nuts—shelled or unshelled—on a baking sheet one layer deep. Bake at 350°F for 10 minutes if shelled, or 20 minutes if in the shell.

Have you tried making your own peanut butter? It's easy—just put peanuts in a blender, food grinder, or special peanut butter machine. Grind them, then add salt, honey, extra oil to improve the spreadability, or nothing at all—and eat!

How nutritious are they?

Peanuts are more than 26 percent protein, but it is incomplete. You can complement the protein by eating peanuts with bread or crackers, sunflower seeds, or milk products (see Protein Complementarity, pages 71, 112).

Peanuts are also high in fat—nearly 50 percent. This fat is mostly unsaturated. Commercially roasted peanuts may contain even higher levels of fat unless they are dry roasted.

Niacin, a B-complex vitamin, is abundant in peanuts. Also present are thiamine and riboflavin (B_1 and B_2), calcium, iron, phosphorus, and potassium. Many commercial peanuts and peanut butters have salt and sugar added.

✦ Nutritive Value: Appendix, 307–309, 497.

Aflatoxin

One potential problem with peanuts is their susceptibility to a cancer-causing substance called aflatoxin. Aflatoxin comes from the mold *Aspergillus flavus,* which can appear on just about all vegetables, fruits, and grains. Peanuts are prime targets because of the way they are grown, harvested, and stored.

Mold grows best in warm, damp places, so if the peanuts aren't properly dried after being dug from the ground, aflatoxin can form.

To minimize the risk of consuming aflatoxin, never eat peanuts (or other foods) with traces of mold on them. Contact the peanut packer or peanut butter manufacturer to be sure they test their products for aflatoxin contamination, and that they don't sell any that contain aflatoxin at levels above twenty parts per billion.

How do I store them?

Keep natural peanut butter refrigerated to prevent rancidity and oil separation. Cooked peanuts can be frozen.

Where do they come from?

Peanuts are ranked as one of the six basic farm crops by the United States Department of Agriculture. Peanut farmers in the United States produce three to four billion pounds of peanuts every year. Most peanuts are grown in Georgia, Alabama, New Mexico, Texas, and other southern states.

PECANS

What are they?

Mmm . . . pecan pie, the pride of Southern bakers. What would it be without the nuts?

But pecans are good for more than just rich desserts. American Indians used pecans and their cousins, hickory nuts, to make a milky beverage by pulverizing the nuts and mixing them with water.

Pecans grow on huge trees that can grow as tall as 150 feet, with trunks reaching seven feet in diameter. Mature trees will produce as much as two hundred pounds of nuts every year. Pecans are the most popular nut produced in the United States.

Buying tips

When shopping for pecans, check the color of the shells. Their natural color is a spotty, dull brown. Shiny, reddish brown shells have been bleached and dyed. Those processes do not affect the nut meats inside, as long as the shells are not cracked, but they are unnecessary. The shells should be free of holes and cracks, feel heavy, and sound solid when shaken. Stale pecans will feel light and have a dry rattle. Two to three pounds of pecans in the shell will yield 1 pound (4 cups) of nut meats.

Shelled pecans should be hard, not rubbery or shriveled. Never buy or eat nuts with mold on them, as they may contain aflatoxin or other dangerous molds. The best time to buy fresh pecans is in the fall.

Commercially roasted pecans often contain high amounts of fat and salt. Dry-roasted nuts do not contain extra fat but usually have salt, sugar, starch, and preservatives added.

How do I use them?

Pecans are good with almost any food, especially casseroles, stuffings, baked goods, and confections. You can substitute them for walnuts in most recipes.

Try mixing chopped pecans into your favorite nut loaf or bean burgers, or hide a few in sandwiches at lunchtime for a crunchy surprise. They are great in fruit salads and, if toasted slightly, are a delicious topping for cooked grains or steamed green vegetables.

If you want roasted pecans, simply spread the raw nuts on a cookie sheet and bake in a 350°F oven. Shelled pecans take 5 to 10 minutes to roast, while pecans in the shell require 20 to 25 minutes.

How nutritious are they?

Pecans are more than 70 percent fat, and most of this is unsaturated. Because of this high fat content, pecans should not be eaten in large quantities as a snack. A few nuts will curb your appetite or desire to chew something crunchy.

Pecans are comparatively low in protein for a nut—about 10 percent. They also contain calcium, iron, magnesium, phosphorus, potassium, and se-lenium. Vitamins A, B-complex, C, and E are present in small amounts.

♦ Nutritive Value: Appendix, 311, 312.

How do I store them?

Pecans in the shell will keep for up to three years if stored at 30°F. Shelled pecans, however, will become rancid within four months at room temperature. Keep them refrigerated or frozen until ready to use.

Where do they come from?

Pecans are native to the Mississippi River Valley and grow from Iowa to Texas. Georgia, however, is the state that leads in production, followed by Texas and New Mexico. From two hundred to three hundred million pounds of pecans are produced annually in the United States.

HICKORY & HICAN

Smaller but more flavorful cousins of pecans are hickory nuts, the seeds of shagbark or shellbark hickory trees. Hickories grow in the same areas as pecans, although they can withstand slightly colder climates.

The availability of these tasty nuggets is limited, as they are too hard to grow on a commercial basis because of the long time between planting and bearing a sizable crop. It is also hard to crack and remove the nut meats.

A natural hybrid nut, called hican, is produced by crossing an edible hickory variety with a pecan tree. The result is a nut larger than the pecan but still as tasty as a hickory. These special trees are not abundant, although tests have been conducted to assess commercial viability.

Use hickory nuts or hicans as you would pecans in cooking, snacks, and baked goods.

Hickory nuts are high in fat—over 68 percent. They also contain 13 percent protein, which is incomplete and should be combined with beans, grains, or dairy products. Also present are iron and phosphorus. No nutritional data was available for hicans.

Like all nuts, keep hickory nuts and hicans in

their shells for maximum freshness. Refrigerate cracked nuts or freeze them for long-term storage.

✦ Nutritive Value: Appendix, 496.

PINE NUTS

Pignolias, piñons, pinyon nuts—whatever you call them, these nuts are actually seeds inside the pine cones of certain pine trees. About one hundred nuts, each ³/₄ inch long, can be found in large, four- to six-inch cones. The cones are dried in the sun to separate their scales, then the nuts are removed by hand. The hard nut shells are usually cracked mechanically.

Pine nuts are extremely versatile. Their small size and mild flavor make them suitable for almost any recipe. Mix some toasted pine nuts with steamed fresh vegetables just before serving. Add them to casseroles or thick stews and soups. Pine nuts are often used in spicy East Indian curries. The native Pueblo Indians of the southwest United States have been eating them for centuries in stews, cakes, and cookies.

Raw pine nuts may have a "piney" or turpentine taste, but this will dissipate if you roast the nuts. Just bake them in the oven at 350°F for about 10 minutes.

The nutritional value of pine nuts varies considerably with the species of tree from which they come. Pignolias imported from Spain are lower in vitamins and fat but contain over twice the protein of piñons from the southwest United States. Piñons, on the other hand, are richer in vitamin A, B-complex vitamins, and the minerals calcium, iron, and phosphorus.

Store pine nuts, like all seeds, in a tightly closed container in the refrigerator to maintain freshness.

✦ Nutritive Value: Appendix, 313.

PISTACHIOS

What are they?

Pistachios, or *green almonds* as they are sometimes called, are popular because of their small size, green color, and easy-to-open shells.

Pistachios have been eaten for over four thousand years and are an important food crop in Middle Eastern countries. The nuts grow on trees that are related to both the common sumac and the tropical cashew. They prefer a dry, hot climate and do well in rugged soil.

Pistachios grow in clusters and are beaten off the trees when ripe. Then they are hand husked and sun dried. The shells of these nuts will change from a natural light brown to a pinkish color. Some are stored and later are soaked in water to remove the husks; these nuts are mechanically dried instead of sun dried, so the shells are artificially dyed red.

Buying tips

If possible, buy raw pistachios and roast them yourself. Avoid those with dyed shells, as the dye may be harmful, especially if the shells are partially open or cracked. Also avoid those that are heavily salted.

Two pounds of pistachios in the shell will yield about 1 pound (3 cups) of nut meats.

How do I use them?

Pistachios, like other nuts, have a variety of uses besides as a snack. The unsalted nuts can be added to any kind of grain dish, casserole, or loaf. Their distinctive green color will blend well with many other foods.

A delicious nut and cheese ball can be made with pistachios and Camembert cheese. Serve the mixture with crackers or French bread and steamed broccoli for an elegant and nutritious light supper.

Have you ever tried pistachio pudding or pistachio bread? Experiment with these nuts, or use them in place of other nuts in your favorite recipes. Early Persians used to grind pistachios and other nuts and use the paste as a thickener.

To roast your own pistachios, spread the raw nuts one layer deep on a baking sheet and bake at 350°F for 5 to 10 minutes.

How nutritious are they?

Pistachios are fairly high in protein—about 19 percent. This protein is incomplete, but if the nuts are eaten with beans or dairy foods, they will provide complete protein (see Protein Complementarity, pages 71, 112).

Pistachios are over 50 percent fat, and most of that is unsaturated. Because of this high fat level, they provide energy and are high in calories, so be careful that you don't overeat them when snacking.

The nuts also provide calcium, iron, magnesium, phosphorus, and potassium, as well as vitamin A, thiamine, and niacin.

✦ Nutritive Value: Appendix, 314.

How do I store them?

Like other nuts, pistachios are best left in the shell and used as needed. Those that have been shelled or that have open shells should be kept cool or refrigerated. They will stay fresh for about three months. Freeze them for longer storage (up to one year).

Where do they come from?

Pistachios originated in the area called Asia Minor. They now grow there and in countries along the Mediterranean Sea, including Syria, Italy, and Turkey. Iran has historically had a near monopoly on the pistachio export market, but commercial production in California has increased in recent years.

PUMPKIN SEEDS

What are they?

Pumpkins aren't just for jack-o'-lanterns and creamy pies. Hidden within the orange flesh of these vegetables is a treasure trove of crunchy, nutritious gems—pumpkin seeds!

The best way to get pumpkin seeds is fresh from the pumpkin. You can grow your own pumpkins—they're an easy garden crop—or buy them in the fall when they abound at roadside stands and food stores.

All pumpkin and squash seeds are edible. Some pumpkin varieties have hull-less seeds and are grown specifically for the seeds, but the pumpkin flesh reportedly tastes inferior to other pumpkins.

In Mexico, *pepitas* have been eaten for centuries as a nutritious snack, and they can still be purchased there in outdoor markets. Many pumpkin seeds sold in the United States come from Mexico, although some are produced domestically.

How do I use them?

To harvest your own pumpkin seeds, just cut open a pumpkin and scoop out the seeds and stringy pulp. Separate the seeds from the pulp, rinse well, and spread them on a pan to dry. Stir them occasionally so they don't stick together. In a few days they will be dry.

Unhulled pumpkin seeds are a great snack food. Crack them open with your teeth as you would sunflower seeds and eat the kernel.

Hulled or hull-less pumpkin seeds can be used just like any other nuts and seeds. Mix them into casseroles or stews, toss them into a green vegetable salad or fruit salad, or sprinkle them on top of cottage cheese. Make a hearty trail mix by combining pumpkin seeds with dried fruits and other seeds.

Both unhulled and hulled pumpkin seeds can be ground into a meal and added to pancakes, muffins, or other breads. Try mixing pumpkin seed meal with peanut butter to make a protein-rich spread.

If you like them roasted, spread the pumpkin seeds on a baking sheet one layer deep and bake at 350°F for 10 to 15 minutes, stirring occasionally. If you prefer salted seeds, soak them in a mixture of tamari and water for about 20 minutes before roasting.

How nutritious are they?

Pumpkin seeds are higher in protein than almost any other nut or seed—a whopping 29 percent—but the protein is incomplete. If you eat them in combination with beans, peanuts, or dairy products, however, the protein will be complemented and of high quality (see Protein Complementarity, pages 71, 112).

Pumpkin seeds are about 46 percent fat, and most of that is unsaturated. Commercially roasted pumpkin seeds may contain additional fat.

Besides being an excellent source of iron and phosphorus, pumpkin seeds contain calcium, vitamin A, and several B-complex vitamins.

✦ Nutritive Value: Appendix, 315.

How do I store them?

Pumpkin seeds should be stored in a tightly covered container in a dark, cool place. Make sure they are dry, as mold grows easily on these seeds.

SESAME SEEDS

What are they?

Sesame seeds have been known since ancient times as a staple food, a delicious flavoring, and a prolific source of cooking oil. They are still a major protein source in many cultures, especially in Africa and the Middle East.

The sesame plant is a rough, hairy, and gummy annual. Its rose-colored flowers become four-celled capsules that contain many tiny black and white seeds. Because the capsules of sesame seeds do not ripen at the same time, most of the sesame seed crop is harvested by hand rather than mechanically.

In North America, sesame seeds are primarily used for cooking oil and animal feed. Only about 10 percent of the two hundred million pounds produced annually is for human consumption as seeds, mainly as a condiment or seasoning.

Buying tips

Sesame seeds packaged in small jars or cans sold in supermarkets are extremely high-priced and are usually hulled. For the best economical and nutritional buy, look for whole (unhulled) sesame seeds at your food co-op or natural foods market.

How do I use them?

Don't let you imagination be stifled by the typically limited use of sesame seeds as a coating on hamburger buns. Sesame seeds can be added to cereals, spreads, drinks, casseroles, granola, and desserts.

For a delicious nutty flavor, toast sesame seeds in a dry skillet over medium heat for 2 to 5 minutes. Sprinkle the toasted seeds on yogurt or cottage cheese and on steamed vegetables. Toasted or untoasted, sesame seeds are excellent additions to soups, salads, fish, and baked goods.

Make a flavorful and refreshing drink by mixing bananas, sesame meal (ground sesame seeds), and ice-cold water in a blender. To make halvah, a traditional Middle Eastern candy, grind a cup of sesame seeds and add a tablespoon of honey. Mix well and roll into small pieces or press into a pan and cut into bars.

Another common way to use sesame seeds is as tahini or sesame butter. Tahini is made by finely grinding hulled sesame seeds and adding oil and water until the desired consistency is reached. Sesame butter is made in the same way, but with unhulled sesame seeds instead. The seeds may be roasted or raw in either product.

Both tahini and sesame butter are good as a spread on crackers or bread, used in salad dressings or sauces, or added to casseroles and baked goods. Since tahini and sesame butter are about half oil, use twice as much as you would other fats if you are using them as a substitute for fats in baked goods.

How nutritious are they?

Whole sesame seeds are 18 percent protein. This protein is not complete, but if the seeds are eaten with whole grains, dairy foods, or beans, a high-quality protein can be obtained (see Protein Complementarity, pages 71, 112).

Sesame seeds are about 50 percent fat, which is mostly unsaturated.

Unhulled sesame seeds contain a high amount of calcium. Because it is in the form of calcium oxalate, however, this calcium cannot be utilized by the human body and may even be toxic. Hulled sesame seeds, however, have only one-tenth the amount of calcium and therefore have a lower amount of the toxic substance.

The nutrients present in sesame seeds are iron, phosphorus, and B-complex vitamins. Unhulled sesame seeds also contain potassium, sodium, and vitamin A.

It is important to chew sesame seeds well or eat them as sesame meal, tahini, or sesame butter. Whole seeds cannot be digested.

✦ Nutritive Value: Appendix, 317, 322.

How do I store them?

Store sesame seeds in an airtight container in a cool, dark place. Once the seeds are ground or are in the form of tahini or sesame butter, they should be kept under refrigeration.

Where do they come from?

About half the world's production of sesame seeds comes from India, where they are a main crop. Most sesame seeds consumed in the United States, however, are grown in Latin American countries. Some are also grown in Texas and Arizona, where they were first planted commercially in 1953. The United States imports between thirty-five and forty thousand metric tons of sesame seeds every year.

SUNFLOWER SEEDS

What are they?

Often thought of as simply a bird food, sunflower seeds are great eating for humans, too. Some people have maintained that this useful, attractive plant should be declared the United States national flower!

The sunflower plant is a member of the daisy family and grows to heights of up to seventeen feet. Its tall stalk is topped by a head that can reach thirty-three inches in diameter—a ring of bright yellow petals surrounding a central spiral of black seeds. Within the shells of these teardrop-shaped seeds are edible kernels.

Until the mid-1960s, about 65 percent of domestically grown sunflower seeds was sold as birdseed, and the remainder was used in the confectionary trade. Since then, sunflower seeds have gained popularity both as a snack food and as an important element in meals.

Other varieties are grown specifically as oil seeds, yielding edible oil and oils for varnishes and soaps. See page 34 for more information on sunflower oil.

How do I use them?

Sunflower seeds are perhaps the most versatile of all the nuts and seeds. Their mild flavor and pleasant crunch are great in many recipes. They are good

raw or roasted, whole, or ground into a meal or butter, or sprouted like other seeds.

You can substitute whole or chopped sunflower seed kernels for other nuts in any recipe. Sprinkle a few on top of a casserole before baking, or mix them into vegetable or fruit salads. Saute sunflower seeds with chopped onion until the onion is tender and the seeds are brown, then toss with a cooked vegetable just before serving—a great way to serve green beans! Or throw some seeds into your stuffing mixture, whether you're stuffing turkey or tomatoes.

Grind sunflower seed kernels to a fine meal and use it as a substitute for some of the flour in bread, pancakes, or other baked goods. It is best to use a grain grinder to make sunflower meal, but you can also try a meat grinder on its finest setting or a blender at high speed. If you prefer, toast the seeds before grinding them and sprinkle the toasted meal on hot cereal or yogurt, in casseroles or in vegetable burgers.

Hulling Sunflower Seeds

There are several ways to remove the shells from whole, unhulled sunflower seeds.

Use a grain mill with its settings as far open as possible. Put the unhulled seeds through the mill—they should all break open and most kernels should remain intact. Now stir the mixed kernels and hulls around in a pan of water, so the hulls will float to the top and can be skimmed off. Drain the water and dry the seeds.

If you don't have a grain mill, try putting the unhulled seeds, $1/4$ to $1/2$ cup at a time, in an electric blender. This method, however, will break more kernels than the grain mill. Buzz them at the lowest speed for about 10 seconds—experiment for best results. Separate the hulls from the kernels as described above.

How nutritious are they?

Sunflower seeds are said to be a good survival food because they contain so many important nutrients. They contain an average of 27 percent protein and 50 percent fat, most of which is polyunsaturated. The protein in sunflower seeds is incomplete, but if the seeds are eaten with grains, legumes, or dairy products, they provide complete and high-quality protein (see Protein Complementarity, pages 71, 112).

Sunflower seeds provide the minerals calcium, iron, magnesium, phosphorus, and potassium. They are also good sources of several B-complex vitamins and vitamins A and D. Sprouted sunflower seeds have all the nutrients of raw seeds and also contain vitamin C.

✦ Nutritive Value: Appendix, 321.

How do I store them?

Whole, hulled sunflower seeds should be stored in tightly sealed containers in a cool, dry place, where they will keep for several months. Sunflower seeds that have been chopped or ground into meal or butter should be refrigerated and used within a few weeks.

Whole, unhulled seeds will keep for a year or longer if packed in airtight containers, and they may be frozen for long-term storage.

Where do they come from?

The sunflower plant is native to North America and was first cultivated by the American Indians. It was introduced to Europe in the 1500s and soon spread to Asia, where the seeds became very popular.

Most of the sunflowers grown in the United States are from the Red River Valley in Minnesota and North Dakota. Some are produced in California.

WALNUTS

What are they?

English, Persian, Carpathian . . . by whatever name you preface them, walnuts are probably the most popular nuts throughout the world.

The *wal* of walnut is thought to be a derivation of *wealh,* an Old English word meaning "strange." Their shape may be odd, but their flavor and versatility have been prized for centuries.

Walnut trees are grown in groves. They will bear fruit in three to five years after planting and will continue to produce for another ten to twenty years or more. The nuts are hand picked or shaken off and gathered by special machines.

Each walnut is surrounded by an outer hull or shell that can be easily crushed and discarded. Commercial shelling machines can crack fifteen hundred pounds of nuts in an hour. Walnuts in the shell are sometimes bleached during processing, then stamped with a brand mark. The bleach will not penetrate the shell unless it is cracked.

Buying tips

Walnuts in the shell are generally fresher and less expensive than shelled nut meats. Check for cracks or other defects, and be sure the nuts feel relatively heavy and don't rattle when shaken. Pinholes, cracks, and rattles are all indicators of stale or damaged nuts. Two pounds of walnuts in the shell will yield 1 pound, or 4 cups, of nut meats. And cracking them is good exercise for your hands!

Look for fresh shelled walnuts—they are brittle and will snap if broken. Shriveled or rubbery nuts are stale or rancid and should be avoided. Never buy or eat moldy nuts.

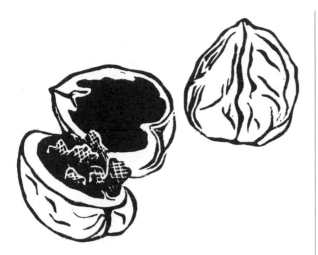

How do I use them?

The only limit to uses for walnuts is your imagination. They can be incorporated into salads, casseroles, spreads, grain and vegetable dishes, and baked goods.

Walnut milk—made from pulverized walnuts soaked in water—was drunk in many European households that had no cow. Early Greeks used to extract the oil from walnuts and use it in cooking.

Walnuts, rice, and cheese make a wonderful dinner loaf. Lentils, walnuts, and vegetables mixed together make a tasty veggie burger. These nuts add special crunch to holiday stuffings and cookies.

How nutritious are they?

Walnuts have a fairly high protein content—about 15 percent. This protein is best complemented by eating walnuts with beans, cheese, or grain products.

About 60 percent of the walnut is fat, mostly unsaturated. Because of this high fat level, they should not be eaten in large quantities as a snack. A few nuts will curb your appetite between meals.

Walnuts contain notable levels or iron, magnesium, phosphorus, potassium, and zinc. Vitamins A, B-complex, and E are also present.

✦ Nutritive Value: Appendix, 325, 326.

How do I store them?

A cool, dry cupboard is the best place to keep walnuts in the shell. Shelled, chopped, or ground nuts, however, are susceptible to rancidity and should always be refrigerated. They may be frozen for long-term storage, but they should be used within a year to assure good quality.

Where do they come from?

Walnuts are probably native to the area called Persia (now Iran), but they grow in many parts of the world, including China and the Carpathian mountains of eastern Europe.

The name "English" walnut was given to these nuts because English merchants in past centuries shipped the nuts to all of the colonies. Few walnuts even grow in England, however, and none are produced there on a commercial basis.

Walnuts were introduced to California in the 1700s. And today, of the two hundred thousand tons of walnuts grown commercially in the United States every year, 95 percent are from California, while most of the other 5 percent are from Oregon.

Black Walnuts and Butternuts

Two distinctive-tasting relatives of the English walnut are the *black* (or *American*) *walnut* and the hardy *butternut* (also called *white walnut*).

The nuts are encased in hard, protective, and sticky hulls that are difficult to remove. Mechanical walnut hullers are sometimes available at hardware stores.

Once the hulls are removed, there are still the nut shells to tackle. A hammer and a hard surface, or a vice grip, usually does the trick. Hitting the pointed end works the best. Butternuts are easier to crack if they are first soaked in hot water for about 20 minutes.

After the hard work of cracking is done, you can settle back to enjoy these unusual nuts. Black walnuts add a unique flavor to casseroles, stuffings, and baked goods. You can acquire a taste for them as a snack. Butternuts can also be used like any other nut. Their high oil content makes them easy to grind into a nut butter to spread on bread or blend into soups or sauces.

Both of these nuts contain a fair amount of protein,

Oil Separation and Hydrogenation

The oil in nut butters tends to separate and float to the top. This is caused by gravity: oil is lighter than the solids, which sink to the bottom.

There are two easy ways to deal with oil separation. One is to simply stir the oil back into the butter. The other method is to keep the stirred or freshly made nut butter in the refrigerator or a cool place (50°F or cooler). You can also pour off the oil and save it for cooking, although the nut butter will be made drier or thicker by doing so.

Many manufacturers add hydrogenated (hardened) vegetable oil to nut butters.

Hydrogenation is a process whereby hydrogen gas is added to a liquid vegetable oil, which causes a change in its chemical structure. That is, it causes the unsaturated oil to harden and become a saturated fat. Saturated fats are thought to contribute to the buildup of deposits in the bloodstream, which could lead to circulatory difficulties.

When a small amount of hydrogenated oil, often called "partially hardened oil" on package labels, is added to peanut butter, the spread keeps its creamy, uniform appearance no matter how long it sits on the shelf. The addition of hydrogenated oil does *not* affect the freshness of peanut butter, just the consistency.

as well as a large proportion of fat—about 60 percent.

Black walnuts have only a trace of calcium but are high in vitamin A, while butternuts are high in iron.

Store these nuts as you would other nuts: in a tightly sealed container in a cool, dry place. Be sure to remove the hulls before storage, and keep the nuts away from squirrels.

Black walnuts and butternuts grow well in northerly climates, from eastern and central Canada down to Arkansas and Georgia. Many black walnuts grow in the central Mississippi River Valley and the Appalachian Mountains region.

✦ Nutritive Value: Appendix, 323, 324, 493.

Nut Butters

What are they?

Nut butters are nuts that have been ground into a thick paste. The most familiar and popular nut butter in North America is, of course, peanut butter. But cashews, hazelnuts, walnuts, almonds, pecans, and sunflower seeds—almost any nut or seed—make delicious and unusual butters.

Raw sesame seeds, for example, can be ground to make tahini. Toasted and ground sesame seeds produce sesame butter. These sesame products are commonly used in Middle Eastern and Indian cooking.

Buying tips

Nut butters are freshest and often taste best when you make them at home. All you need are fresh nuts and a grinding machine, and possibly some extra oil to improve the texture.

When you buy ready-made nut butters, however, it is important to read the labels. Many commercial nut butters—notably peanut butter—contain sugar and salt. Stabilizers, such as mono- and diglycerides and hardened vegetable oil, are added to prevent the natural oil from separating and to maintain uniform spreadability. Nut butters that are sold in tubs or buckets should smell nutty and not have large amounts of oil floating on the top. This excess oil separation results from prolonged storage.

How do I use them?

Nut butters can be used in a variety of ways besides the traditional use as a sandwich spread. Mix them with dried fruit and nuts for delectable confections. Add them to cookies, pancakes, or muffins. Try nut butters in frostings and sauces.

Most nut butters, especially tahini, can be used

as a partial or full substitute for milk in sauce and pudding recipes. For a unique salad dressing, blend lemon juice, yogurt, herbs, and nut butter. Toss with vegetable or fruit salads.

When you substitute nut butter for shortening, butter, or margarine in recipes for baked goods, keep in mind that nut butters are about one-half oil. You may need to use twice as much or may want to alter your recipe.

Homemade Nut Butter

To make nut butter, use a grain grinder, blender, nut butter machine, or a meat grinder with its finest attachment. Never use a stone-wheel grain grinder, as the oil from the nuts would coat the stone, making it smooth and useless.

Grind the seeds or nuts until they form a paste. If the paste seems too dry, add a small amount of oil. If you use a blender, grind them at high speed, about 1 cup at a time. Mix in a small amount of salt, if you desire. A little goes a long way, so taste the nut butter as you sprinkle in the salt.

How nutritious are they?

Nut butters made with nuts only are as nutritious as the nuts or seeds from which they are made. Most nut butters are good sources of protein, but they should be eaten with grains, legumes, or dairy products to maximize their protein value. A combination of peanut butter and sesame tahini will make a complementary protein, as peanuts are technically legumes, not nuts (see Protein Complementarity, pages 71, 112).

Because of their high oil content, nut butters are very concentrated forms of food energy. An ounce of peanut butter, for example, has more than three times the calories of an ounce of bread.

Nut butters also contain important minerals, such as calcium, phosphorus, potassium, and magnesium, as well as B-complex vitamins. They are more digestible than whole nuts and seeds because it is harder for your body to break down larger, hard pieces.

✦ Nutritive Value: Appendix, 309, 322.

How do I store them?

Store nut butters in tightly covered jars in a cool, dark place. They will usually keep for about a month without becoming rancid. For maximum freshness, however, you should refrigerate or freeze them. Cool temperatures will cause nut butters to become stiff, so to improve spreadability, let them stand at room temperature (70°F) for about 5 minutes before using.

SWEETENERS

The words *sweeteners* and *sweets* bring to mind sugar, honey, candy bars, ice cream, soft drinks, and pastries. But did you know that sweeteners are added to such foods as salad dressings, canned soups, canned meat, frozen dinners, fruit drinks, crackers, and nondairy creamers?

Although it is hard to imagine a diet without sweeteners, they are a relatively recent addition to the human diet. Essentially all of the sugar consumed by our early ancestors came from fruits and vegetables. Refined sugar was virtually unknown to the populace until the fifteenth century.

Today, the annual consumption of sweeteners in the United States is 145 pounds per person—up dramatically from the 15 pounds per person in 1815, and even up from the 125 pounds per person during the mid-1970s. With all the media attention and warnings by health professionals advising people to cut down on sweeteners, and with the upsurge in the natural foods business, one may wonder *who* is eating all that sugar!

What are they?

All sweeteners are forms of sugar. Sugar is manufactured by green plants during their conversion of sunlight into food, a process called photosynthesis. Except for their mineral content, all components of plants are derived from this sugar.

A *refined sugar* is one that is separated from the rest of the food substances in a plant—sucrose from sugarcane, for example. Sweetener is a descriptive term that refers to refined sugars used as additives in the processing or preparation of foods for human consumption.

The most common sweetener is sucrose, or white sugar. Other popular sweeteners include molasses, brown sugar, honey, corn syrup, malt syrup, sorghum, date sugar, and turbinado, or "raw" sugar. Highly refined sweeteners are often added to processed foods; these include fructose, maltose, dextrose (or glucose), and lactose. Synthetic sweeteners derived from coal tar and other sources are also available; these include saccharin, aspartame, mannitol, sorbitol, and xylitol.

How nutritious are they?

Chemically speaking, sugars are carbohydrates (an exception to this is aspartame; see page 130). Carbohydrates are foods that are composed of glucose molecules, the substances that produce energy in the body. Carbohydrates are present in large quantities in fruits, grains, and vegetables.

There are three main types of digestible carbohydrates, all of which occur in plant foods. A simple carbohydrate is called a *monosaccharide,* or single sugar, because it is composed of one glucose molecule. A *disaccharide,* or double sugar, is composed of two glucose molecules. Starches or *polysaccharides* are referred to as "complex carbohydrates." They are composed of many glucose molecules arranged in a chainlike manner. The specific carbohydrates and the foods in which they commonly occur are:

- Monosaccharides:
  Glucose (also called dextrose)—corn syrup, grape sugar, vegetables, honey
  Fructose (also called levulose)—honey, fruits, corn syrup, vegetables
  Galactose— product of lactose after digestion

- Disaccharides:

  Sucrose (glucose + fructose)—cane sugar, beet sugar, maple sugar, sorghum syrup, fruits and vegetables

  Lactose—milk and milk products

  Maltose (glucose + glucose) sprouted grains, beer

- Polysaccharides:

  Starch—grains, legumes, vegetables

✦ Nutritive Value: Appendix, 329–337.

What do carbohydrates do in the body?

Single or double sugars break down quickly into glucose molecules, which are simultaneously and rapidly absorbed into the bloodstream to supply energy to the body. This speedy burst of energy may, however, be followed by a drop in energy and a craving for more sugar, especially if the food contains only or mostly carbohydrates. Such foods include candy bars, soda pop, and cookies.

Complex carbohydrates, such as potatoes and oatmeal, are composed of chains of glucose molecules that steadily release glucose to the body over a longer period of time and thus provide sustained energy.

Too many sweets?

There is much controversy over the harmful effects of too much sugar in the diet. The opinions range from sugar having no unique harmful effects to it directly causing a multitude of diseases, including obesity, hypoglycemia, diabetes, and arteriosclerosis. The documentation of these effects has been disputed in the health fields for quite some time, and very few claims have been conclusively proven. Substantial scientific evidence, however, supports the following statements:

1. *Refined sugars are "empty calories."* They supply very little or no nutrients. Even the so-called health-food sweeteners—honey and maple syrup—have levels of nutrients so negligible as to be insignificant. Because refined sugars supply no nutrients other than calories, their consumption may lead to two health problems:

- Nutrient deficiency—The calories from refined sugars can displace those from more nutritious foods. That is, if you attempt to maintain a fixed intake of calories while eating sweets, you may be cutting out foods that could supply the nutrients you need.

- Obesity—If you attempt to maintain a nutritionally balanced diet while consuming sweets, you may be taking in too many calories, which contributes to obesity. The amount of sweeteners that a person can consume without gaining weight or cutting out nutrients depends on many factors, including individually varying metabolic rates, level of physical exercise, and composition of the entire diet.

2. *Consuming too much refined sugar may lead to tooth decay and possibly hypoglycemia and diabetes in genetically predisposed persons.*

- Tooth decay—This is the only effect of sugar that everyone agrees on, even those in the sugar industry. The mouth normally contains bacteria that feed on sugar and as a side product the bacteria produce a thick substance that sticks to the teeth and encourages the buildup of plaque. This process also forms acids that collect under the plaque and attack the teeth, causing dental caries or cavities. The rate of decay is greatly influenced by how much sugar gets stuck to the teeth, for how long, and how frequently. For example, sticky candies that adhere to the teeth and that are eaten between meals cause more trouble than sugary foods eaten as part of a meal when other foods and liquids help dislodge the sweet particles from the teeth. Other factors that affect tooth decay are hereditary resistance and the frequency of brushing and flossing the teeth.

- Hypoglycemia and diabetes—There has been a lot of speculation but little conclusive evidence about the relationship of sugar consumption to hypoglycemia and diabetes. Most arguments center around the idea that excessive sugar consumption strains the ability of the pancreas to accurately regulate the amount of glucose in the bloodstream. Ultimately, then, the regulating mechanism breaks down completely, causing either hypoglycemia (low blood sugar) or diabetes (high blood sugar). Research results suggest connections between obesity and diabetes, and since excessive sugar consumption can contribute to obesity, it can be claimed to indirectly lead to diabetes.

How do I use them?

Even though refined sugars are nutritionally unnecessary and more stressful to the body than complex carbohydrates, the fact is that sweets and sugared foods are widely available and enormously appealing. Practically speaking, the critical questions become: Even if we don't need refined sugar, can we eat it without harmful effects? How much can we eat?

Probably the best answer to this second question is: Eat it in moderation. The dietary guidelines suggested by the United States Department of Agriculture recommend decreasing the level of sugar in the diet. The goals also suggest eating less of all types of sugar and foods containing sugar. This means not only cutting down on the sticky, gooey sweets, but also on foods with added sugar, such as presweetened cereals, sweetened canned fruits, imitation fruit drinks, frozen desserts, and ketchup.

A safe rule of thumb is to plan your meals to get the needed nutrients from whole foods or highly nutritious sources, then add sweets. The question of how much should be answered by each person paying attention to how he or she feels physically and by watching his or her own weight variances. If you notice, for example, that you experience an energy drop at midday, one of the factors to look at is your intake of refined sugar. Did you eat a sweet roll and coffee with sugar for breakfast, or did you eat a "real" breakfast? Remember, grains are composed of complex carbohydrates, so a whole-grain cereal for breakfast will provide a gradual release of sugar into the bloodstream for longer lasting energy. Also, pay attention to whether you really are hungry before you eat. Sweets sometimes serve emotional and social needs, so try to eat only to satisfy your hunger.

ASPARTAME (NUTRASWEET®)

Aspartame is a combination of aspartic acid and phenylalanine, two amino acids (the substances that make up protein) that occur naturally in some foods. Aspartame is not derived from these sources, however. The amino acids are synthesized from hydrocarbons or by fermentation.

The sweetener was, like saccharin, an accidental discovery. In 1966 James Schlatter, a chemist employed by G. D. Searle Company, was testing aspartame as a possible treatment for ulcers and for some reason licked his fingers and found the taste sweet.

Aspartame has the same number of calories per gram as white sugar, but it is nearly two hundred times as sweet. One packet has about 4 calories, compared to 32 calories in the equivalent 2 teaspoons of white sugar. Because of its composition, the body metabolizes aspartame as a protein rather than as a carbohydrate.

Aspartame breaks down and loses its sweetness when subjected to heat, so it is useful only in cold and uncooked foods. It is added to chewing gums, preserves, dry cereals, dry beverage mixes, and dry table sweeteners (Equal®). Its shelf life is about one year, after which time it decomposes into methanol, a potentially toxic alcohol.

The safety of this product has been under investigation by the Food and Drug Administration (FDA) since 1974. It is suspected of having the potential to alter brain chemistry and thus affect mood and behavior, particularly when it is combined with carbohydrates. The decomposition of aspartame may also result in products that can cause cancer, mental retardation, and brain lesions when consumed in large quantities. The FDA approved the use of aspartame in dry foods in July 1981, and further approved of it as a sweetener in soft drinks in July 1983. It has also been "legal" in Canada and other countries for several years.

CORN SYRUP

You may be a big user of corn syrup and not even know it. This sweetener has replaced maple syrup as the main ingredient in most commercial pancake and waffle syrups. It is also used as a filler in processed foods, from bouillon to ketchup to peanut butter. The consumption of corn syrup in the United States has risen dramatically in the last thirty years, from about ten pounds per person in 1960 to more than seventy pounds per person in 1990.

What is it?

Corn syrup is a highly refined sweetener made from the endosperm (the starchy middle part) of the corn kernel. The starch is mixed with water and hydrochloric acid or sulfuric acid, then steamed to convert it to commercial glucose. This dark and odd-smelling substance is deodorized and filtered to produce the odorless, clear, and virtually tasteless liquid called corn syrup. So-called dark corn syrup is often artificially caramel colored.

Corn sugar—also called solid glucose, dextrose, or starch sugar—is made in the same manner as corn syrup, although more acid is used and the product is steamed for a longer period of time.

Another sweetener derived from corn is high fructose corn syrup. For more information on this product, see page 132.

How is it used?

Corn syrup and corn sugar are mostly sold as ingredients in commercially processed foods. They are used as sweeteners, but are also used to thicken foods (such as ketchup), to add body, to prevent crystallization in frozen foods and ice cream, and to retain moisture.

When corn syrup is made into pancake or waffle syrup, small amounts of other sweeteners, artificial colors and flavors, and preservatives are added.

Corn syrup solids that are dried into a powder are found in nondairy creamers, imitation fruit drinks, and pudding mixes.

WAYS TO REDUCE YOUR SUGAR INTAKE

1. *Read the ingredient lists on product labels.* Look first for ingredients labeled "sugar," "sucrose," "dextrose," "fructose," "corn syrup," "honey," "maltose," "sweeteners," and "natural sweeteners." A general guideline is that anything ending in *-ose* is a sugar. Also look for the number of times different sugars appear in the ingredients list. Often a product will contain three or four different forms of sugar. Ingredients are listed in order of proportion by weight of the product; be aware of the high sugar content of any product that lists a sweetener as one of the primary ingredients.

2. *Eliminate or severely reduce your consumption of soft drinks.* When you are thirsty, drink water. For a refreshing and flavorful beverage, try herbal tea, unsweetened fruit juice (in moderation), or mineral water.

3. *Reduce your intake of highly sweetened snacks.* Instead, eat snacks that are high in protein and starch, such as cheese and whole grain crackers, toasted seeds and nuts, hard-boiled eggs, fruits, vegetables, and unsweetened yogurt. Eat dried fruits in moderation, as they have high concentrations of fructose.

4. *Cut the quantity of sweeteners in homemade desserts and baked goods by one-third to one-half the amount called for in a recipe.*

5. *Eat sweets with other foods.* This will slow down the digestion of the sugar, insure intake of needed nutrients, and decrease your craving for sweets. If you make sweet treats at home, use nutritious foods such as nuts, seeds, peanut butter, wheat germ, or milk powder with the sweeteners.

6. *Try eating sweets only after a meal, but wait fifteen minutes.* You may decide that you are full enough and really don't want that dessert anyway!

Corn syrup that is produced and sold as a separate product often contains added sucrose. By itself, corn syrup is about half as sweet as sucrose. If you use it in baking and cooking as a substitute for white sugar, reduce other liquids in the recipe by ¼ cup for every cup of syrup used. Before pouring corn syrup, rub oil in the measuring utensils to prevent the syrup from sticking to them.

How nutritious is it?

Corn syrup and corn sugar are high in carbohydrates and calories. They contain very small amounts of calcium, iron, phosphorus, vitamin C, riboflavin, and niacin.

Like other refined sugars, corn syrup and corn sugar may have a harmful effect on your health. Be sure to read labels of processed foods to see how much of the product is made of corn syrup. If corn syrup is one of the first ingredients listed on the label, it is one of the main ingredients, and so you can bet that the product may contribute carbohydrates to your diet, but little else.

✦ Nutritive Value: Appendix, 337.

How do I store it?

Corn syrup has a long shelf life and will keep well in a dry area. It can become moldy, however—sometimes even if preservatives are added—so store it in a tightly capped jar in a cool place.

Where does it come from?

The original corn syrup made by Peruvians and Mexicans was made from the stalks of the corn plant rather than the kernels. The juice from the stalks was pressed out and then boiled down to a sweet syrup, similar to the process used for sorghum.

Commercial corn syrup made from the kernels was first marketed in the early 1900s under the name *glucose.* (Corn syrup is almost pure glucose.) The name didn't catch on, though. Apparently, consumers thought the syrup was made from glue.

Today, much of the corn syrup produced in the United States is from Iowa and other midwestern Corn Belt states.

FRUCTOSE

Fructose has been touted as a simple, natural, and miracle sweetener; that is, more healthful than white sugar. It is also promoted as an aid to weight loss because it is sweeter than white sugar, enabling one to get the same sweetness with less sweetener.

Although fructose is a naturally occurring simple sugar found in fruits and honey, that which is sold commercially is highly refined and is no more natural than white sugar.

Two types of fructose are available: liquid and crystalline. *Liquid fructose* is made by adding enzymes to corn syrup and heating it to convert some of the glucose to fructose. The resulting sweetener is sometimes called *high fructose corn syrup.* The final product still contains 10 to 50 percent glucose.

Crystalline fructose is made by chemically splitting sucrose into its two components, glucose and fructose, and then separating out the fructose. This powder, sometimes called *levulose,* is presently manufactured in Finland and imported to the United States. It is more expensive than liquid fructose.

Fructose has the same number of calories per gram as sugar, but it is up to one and one-half times as sweet. The sweet taste, though, depends on temperature and acidity. It tastes sweeter than white sugar in cold, slightly acidic foods such as lemonade, but when it is heated it has about the same sweetness as white sugar.

Fructose is metabolized somewhat differently than sucrose. It is absorbed more slowly, stimulates fewer insulin secretions, and is processed by the liver before reaching other organs. Because of these differences, fructose has less impact on blood sugar levels than does sucrose. Thus, it is used as a sugar substitute by people with diabetes.

GRAIN SYRUP

A sweet liquid can be made from sprouted barley or other sprouted grains and cooked rice. The mixtures of these will convert the starch in the grains to sugar, or *maltose.*

Use grain syrup as you would maple syrup, molasses, or sorghum—on pancakes or in baking. If you want to use it as a substitute for granulated white sugar, use half as much grain syrup as sugar and decrease other liquids in the recipe by ¼ cup per cup of grain syrup.

This is how you make it: Soak 3 tablespoons barley, wheat, oats, or rice in warm water in a quart jar overnight. Cover the mouth of the jar with cheesecloth or screen and attach a rubber band or metal canning jar ring.

After 12 hours of soaking, drain off the soaking water, rinse the seeds with clear water, and drain off the water again. Rinse the grain twice a day to keep it moist and prevent mold. After 3 to 5 days there will be sprouts that are about the same length as the seeds.

When the sprouts are ready, boil 2 cups of rice in 6 cups water for 45 minutes, or pressure cook the mixture for 15 to 20 minutes. Do not drain off excess water. Allow the rice to cool to 140°F—test it with a candy thermometer to be sure—then add the sprouted and crushed grain. Mix well, cover the pot, and put it in a pan of hot water or on a stove at low heat, so a temperature of 130 to 140°F is consistently maintained.

After about 5 hours, taste the mixture to see if it is sweet. If it is not, let it sit a few more hours, and taste it occasionally to see if it is as sweet as you want it to be.

Place cheesecloth in a colander and pour the mixture into it. Squeeze out the liquid, saving the grain residues for other foods such as bread or pudding. Now pour the liquid back into the cooking pot and boil it until it becomes a syrup.

HONEY

What is it?

Honey is one of the oldest sweeteners known to humans. People collected and ate this sweet, golden substance before they knew how to raise cereal grains or keep dairy animals.

Honey is composed mostly of the sugars glucose and fructose. It is manufactured by honeybees who

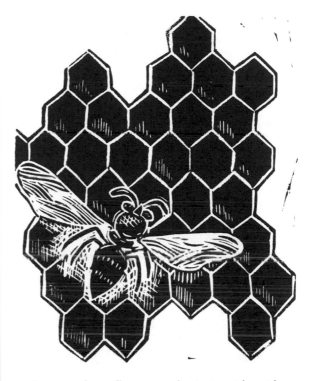

suck nectar from flowers and mix it with acid secretions from the glands at the base of their tongues. The mixture is then temporarily stored in the bees' stomachs, where the sucrose is broken down into glucose and fructose. After they return to the hive, the bees transfer the honey to wax cells, or honeycomb, where the temperature is a constant 93 to 97°F. Here the water evaporates and the honey thickens until it reaches the consistency with which we are familiar.

Bees produce honey in a wide variety of flavors and colors, depending on the geographic location and the type of plant on which the bees have fed. Honeybees tend to stick with one type of flower in their nectar gathering. This not only produces distinctive flavors of honey but also makes the bees excellent pollinators, as they fly from one plant to another, inadvertently picking up pollen on their legs and depositing it onto the next plant.

The three most commercially prevalent types of honey are alfalfa, clover, and buckwheat. Alfalfa honey and clover honey are usually light-colored and mild-flavored. Pure buckwheat honey is dark brown and strong-flavored, similar to sorghum. It is less popular now than it was a few decades ago. Also available in certain parts of the United States are orange blossom honey and tupelo honey.

How do I use it?

A teaspoon of honey tastes sweeter and has more calories than a teaspoon of white sugar because the liquid honey is more dense than dry sugar crystals. So if you substitute honey for sugar in a recipe, replace 1 cup of sugar with ³/₄ cup or less of honey, and reduce the amount of liquids in the recipe by ¹/₄ cup or more (proportional to the amount of honey used).

When using honey in baked goods, reduce the oven temperature by 25°F to prevent over browning. It is sometimes suggested that ¹/₂ teaspoon of baking soda should be added to baked goods for every cup of honey used, in order to neutralize the acid, but this is not absolutely necessary.

For better measuring and to prevent sticking, rub a small amount of oil on the insides of measuring cups and spoons before pouring in honey.

How nutritious is it?

Honey has been promoted by some people as a healthy alternative to white sugar because it is natural. This claim leads people to believe that they can merely substitute honey for white sugar to avoid the potentially harmful effects of sugar. However, honey can be abused in the same way as sugar, and may have similar effects on the body. Like other sweeteners, honey is an empty-calorie food, and if it is eaten in excess, it may lead to obesity and contribute to tooth decay.

Honey is a concentrated and refined sugar—refined by bees and further clarified by the beekeepers who extract it. It is 77 percent sugar—a combination of sucrose, fructose, and glucose—and 17 percent water.

In comparison to sugar, which is 99.9 percent sucrose, honey has some minerals and B-complex vitamins. But these nutrients are in rather insignificant amounts, and you should not rely on honey as a source for them.

✦ Nutritive Value: Appendix, 329, 330.

How do I store it?

Store honey in a tightly sealed jar in a warm, dry, dark cupboard. It will stay fresh indefinitely. Be sure to keep the honey jar clean of sticky drippings so ants or other insects are not attracted to it.

Honey may crystallize after a long or cold (less than 60°F) storage. To reliquefy it, place the honey jar in a pot of hot water and heat the pot slowly until all the crystals are completely dissolved.

Surprisingly, honey will quickly crystallize if it is refrigerated, but it will stay liquid if it is frozen at 0°F or below.

Where does it come from?

Centuries-old tombs in Egypt bear wall paintings of beekeepers and contain sealed jars of honey. The ancient Mayans of southern Mexico and Guatemala kept large numbers of bee colonies, as do their modern descendants.

In the United States today, the main areas of honey production are in California, Florida, and the Midwest. From thirteen to eighteen million gallons—one hundred fifty to two hundred million pounds—of honey are produced every year by more than eight hundred thousand beekeepers. Some is imported from Canada and Australia.

MALT SYRUP

What is it?

Malt syrup is a sweet liquid made from malted barley. Raw, unhulled barley is soaked in drums of cold water for two or three days and allowed to sprout in temperature- and humidity-controlled chambers. The sprouted grain is then kiln dried at 120 to 180°F, and the rootlets are removed; this is malted barley. Finally, the malted barley is ground and is briefly dipped in an acid solution, then it is heated with water to form the mildly sweet, concentrated liquid we know as malt syrup.

If this liquid is subjected to further heating and evaporating, it will become malt extract and maltose (malt sugar), a crystalline, colorless powder.

Malt syrup is about 65 percent maltose. Maltose

tastes about 30 percent as sweet as sucrose (white sugar). Some malt syrups are made from a combination of barley and corn grits—usually one part barley to four parts corn. These syrups are sweeter than pure barley malt syrup because they contain glucose as well as maltose.

How do I use it?

Malt syrup is often used for making homemade beer. It can also replace other sweeteners in cooking and baking. Malt syrup adds subtle sweetness and color to breads and is a flavorful substitute for brown sugar in cookies or cakes.

Try experimenting with malt syrup when making baked goods and confections. Mix it with honey and use it on pancakes or French toast. Make barley pudding (like rice pudding), using malt syrup for extra flavor.

Do you like malted milk? Malted milk powder is made by mixing milk with malt syrup and heating the mixture to evaporate the moisture. You can concoct your own malted milk by adding malt syrup to instant nonfat dry milk powder.

How nutritious is it?

Malt syrup is mostly carbohydrates and contains small quantities of calcium, iron, phosphorus, potassium, B-complex vitamins, and vitamin C. Like other sweeteners, however, a normal serving of malt syrup contains only scant amounts of these nutrients.

How do I store it?

Keep malt syrup in a tightly capped jar away from ants. Canned and unopened malt syrup will keep indefinitely.

MAPLE SYRUP

What is it?

Maple syrup—the rich-tasting sweetener made from the sap of sugar maple trees—was used by native North Americans, from whom the early white colonists learned the techniques of tapping maple trees. It is still popular today, although it is one of the most expensive sweeteners available.

In the early spring, sap starts flowing from the trees' roots to the branches, bringing nourishment for budding leaves. To gather the sap, collectors drill holes into the tree trunks and insert a spout into each hole, which diverts the sap from the trees into buckets. One maple tree can supply 10 to 25 gallons of sap—a clear, tasteless, and watery liquid.

The maple sap is then collected and boiled in a large vat to evaporate the water. It takes 35 to 50 gallons of sap (about three trees' worth) to produce 1 gallon of maple syrup. It is this energy-intensive aspect of maple syrup production that makes the sweetener so costly in comparison with other sweeteners.

The unique flavor of maple syrup comes from trace amounts of minerals, sugars, and other substances in the syrup. It is very difficult to synthesize this flavor artificially.

To make maple sugar, a crystalline sweetener, maple sap, is boiled until virtually all the water is evaporated. One gallon of syrup yields about 8 pounds of maple sugar. What remains is nearly all sucrose—essentially the same as cane sugar or beet sugar, except for a subtle maple taste.

How do I use it?

Maple syrup is, of course, favored as a syrup for pancakes, waffles, and French toast. When it is used in baked goods and confections, maple syrup adds a pleasant flavor to the foods.

To make a delicious upside-down cake, pour a small amount of maple syrup over chopped nuts and pineapple rings that have been put in muffin tins or a cake pan. Spread your favorite cake batter on the top, and bake it.

If you substitute maple syrup for sugar, use $3/4$ cup syrup to 1 cup sugar, and reduce the liquids in the recipe by 3 tablespoons for every cup of syrup used.

How nutritious is it?

Maple syrup is about 60 percent sucrose, so it is high in carbohydrates. It supplies 50 calories per tablespoon of syrup. The remaining portion is mostly water, with small amounts of calcium, potassium, phosphorus, iron, and sodium.

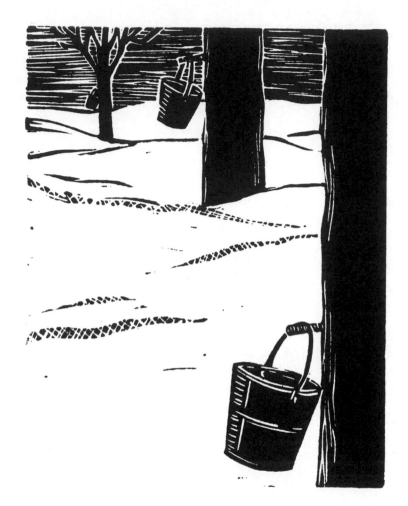

Various techniques are employed to speed up or increase the collection of maple syrup. Pellets made of paraformaldehyde are frequently inserted into the tap holes, which act as a germicide and prevent sap from clotting and clogging the holes. Some residues of this poison may be present in the maple syrup, and the treatment may also shorten the lifespan of the maple trees.

Another potential hazard in maple syrup is excess lead concentration. Maple sap collectors often use metal pans and buckets whose seams and patches are soldered with lead. The syrup can also pick up lead from the seams of metal containers used for storage and packaging.

To avoid possible lead contamination, ask your co-op or grocery store to contact the suppliers to see what types of equipment are used for collecting and storing their maple sap. Are they metal or stainless steel? The latter is safe but also more expensive, so some maple syrup producers do not use it. If the syrup is sold in glass or plastic bottles, the risk will be minimized.

✦ Nutritive Value: Appendix, 337.

How do I store it?

To prevent crystallization, mold, and fermentation, store maple syrup in a place that is cool and dry and that has an even temperature. Do not freeze it.

If maple syrup does crystallize, place the jar in a pan of warm water and heat it gently until the crystals dissolve.

Where does it come from?

Most of the maple syrup produced in North America is from Quebec. In the United States, Vermont leads production, followed by New York. About three billion gallons of maple syrup are consumed annually in the United States.

POLYALCOHOLS

Mannitol

Mannitol is a centuries-old sweetener that is either derived from plants such as seaweed or synthesized from sugar. It has about half the calories of sugar, but it is only two-thirds as sweet. Besides its main use as chewing gum dust or sweetener, and its addition to some foods as an antisticking agent, mannitol is popular for cutting heroin. Much of the heroin sold on the streets contains eight times as much mannitol as the drug itself.

Mannitol is metabolized by the body like other sugars and is generally considered safe, but kidney diseases and gastrointestinal disturbances may be aggravated or caused by an excess of mannitol.

Sorbitol

Sorbitol is a relative of mannitol and is present in many fruits, algae, and seaweed. It is quite costly to isolate this sugar from natural sources, however, so commercial quantities are obtained by processing glucose, the sugar in corn syrup.

Sorbitol is sometimes used in soft drinks, in candy to thicken it, in frozen desserts to stabilize and sweeten them, in shredded coconut to add texture and control moisture, and in printing inks and resins.

This sweetener is about 40 percent as sweet as sugar but contains virtually the same amount of calories per gram. It is absorbed slowly by the body and therefore is used as a sugar substitute by people with diabetes or those on a low-carbohydrate diet. Some vitamin and mineral supplements and pharmaceutical preparations contain sorbitol, as it helps increase the absorption of nutrients. It may also alter the absorption of medications or drugs if it is obtained from a source other than the prescription.

Too much sorbitol—one ounce or more—can cause diarrhea or digestive problems. Sorbitol sometimes produces these effects even in smaller quantities.

Xylitol

Xylitol is made from wood or other plant by-products. It has about one-fourth the calories of sugar, but at the present time costs about ten times more to process. Tests in Finland, where xylitol is manufactured, have shown that it may prevent or even reverse tooth decay if it is eaten in high concentrations (that is, if it makes up about 60 percent of the product). Xylitol is used in chewing gum and jams.

SACCHARIN

Saccharin is a coal-tar derivative that was accidentally discovered by a chemist at Johns Hopkins University in 1879. About twenty years later it became a commercial sweetener and was used extensively by diabetics.

Saccharin has no nutrients and little or no calories, and for the most part it passes through the body unchanged. It is three hundred to four hundred times as sweet as white sugar, although it has a bitter aftertaste which is often masked by another sweetener such as aspartame. Saccharin costs twenty times less than white sugar to produce.

Saccharin is used mostly in diet soft drinks or other low-calorie foods. About five million pounds of saccharin are made every year in the United States. The Food and Drug Administration requires that products containing saccharin have a warning label advising consumers to restrict their usage of this sweetener. Tests have found saccharin to cause cancer, birth defects, and kidney damage in test animals.

SORGHUM

What is it?

Sorghum syrup is made from sweet sorghum, a grain related to millet and similar in appearance to corn. Sorghum has long been used for adding flavor to foods and still has devoted consumers in areas where it is made.

There are actually four types of sorghum: *sweet,* used for sorghum syrup; *grain,* grown for the seed heads and fed to livestock; *grassy,* also called Sudan grass; and *broomcorn,* the source of fiber for brooms.

The sweet sorghum plant grows to a height of fifteen feet and forms a juicy stalk (cane) that is topped by clusters of seeds. In the fall, ripe canes are cut and pressed through rollers to extract the juice, which is then boiled down to a thick, mildly sweet syrup. It takes 8 to 12 gallons of sorghum sap to make 1 gallon of finished syrup.

Good quality sorghum is a clear amber color with little sediment and no gritty or grainy feel in the mouth. Darker or thicker syrup may have more trace nutrients.

How do I use it?

Traditionally, sorghum syrup is used on pancakes, corn muffins, and other breads. But sorghum is also a suitable substitute for other sweeteners in most recipes.

Sorghum can be used to make popcorn balls. It adds a unique taste to granola and is good in puddings, toppings, and frostings. It can also replace molasses in sauces and baked beans.

Try sorghum instead of sugar in baking or cooking. You can substitute it for other sweeteners as follows:

- For honey—Substitute one for one, unless the recipe is for a baked good calling for baking powder. In that case, don't substitute.
- For sugar—Use one-half to three-quarters the amount called for in baked goods, depending on the recipe. For uses other than baking, increase sorghum by one-third of that listed for sugar, and reduce liquids by one-third.
- For molasses—Substitute one for one. For baked goods, also reduce the amount of any other sweeteners in the recipe by one-third.

How nutritious is it?

Like all sweeteners, sorghum is high in carbohydrates and calories. It also contains iron, calcium, and phosphorus, and it has small levels of the B-complex vitamins riboflavin and niacin. Don't rely on sorghum syrup as a source for these minerals and vitamins, however, as you would have to consume an excessive amount of the sweetener in order to get any appreciable amount of these nutrients.

How do I store it?

Keep sorghum syrup in a cool, dry place, preferably in a glass container. The syrup may, after several months, crystallize or become jellylike. These changes aren't harmful, just slightly inconvenient. Heat the syrup by placing the jar in a pan of water over low heat to rid it of crystallization. (Some commercial sorghum is processed with enzymes called carbohydrases, invertase, or diastase to prevent crystallization.)

Sorghum can ferment, so refrigerate it if you do not use it often.

Where does it come from?

Sorghum is thought to be native to Egypt, where it has been grown for thousands of years.

The grain was probably introduced to North America in the 1700s. It is now grown mainly in the southeastern United States, although it is also found in parts of the Midwest.

SUGAR PRODUCTS

What are they?

You've probably heard sugar tagged with all sorts of names, from "nature's quickest energy food" to "killer white." Besides the sweet white crystals that bear these names, there are also brown sugar, molasses, and raw or turbinado sugar. All these sweeteners come from the same plants: sugarcane or sugar beets. Sugarcane is a tall, tropical stalk, whereas sugar beets are eaten as vegetables. Both sugarcane and sugar beets are grown specifically for sugar.

How do I use them?

Sugar is used in many foods and beverages. One scoop of ice cream has four teaspoons of sugar in it. A twelve-ounce glass of cola contains about

SUGAR REFINING

Sugar cane and sugar beets are subjected to the same refining processes and produce identical products.

First, canes or beets are crushed and flushed with water to extract a syrup, which is 13 to 15 percent sucrose. The syrup is heated until some of the water evaporates and the sugar begins to crystallize, then it is spun in a centrifuge to separate the crystals from the liquid (molasses). This process of heating, crystallizing, and centrifuging is repeated two more times to get as much sugar as possible from the syrup. The sugar crystals are then cleaned, clarified, filtered, and dried.

eight teaspoons of sugar, as does a four-ounce piece of chocolate candy. Many breakfast cereals are presweetened and contain 20 to 60 percent sugar.

Besides adding sweetness, sugar helps foods such as pudding and jelly to thicken or become firm. It provides the nourishment for yeast to grow in breads, and it makes the crust brown and crumbs tender.

Granulated white sugar was (and still is) a staple item on pantry shelves. It is used for nearly all foods that require sweetening.

Brown sugar is popular for cookies and candies, as it makes them chewy.

Confectioner's sugar (powdered sugar) is used mainly for frostings and glazes or as a dust on cookies, cakes, and doughnuts.

Molasses has a robust aroma and adds a distinctive flavor to baked beans, gingersnap cookies, and anadama bread. Historically, molasses was called *treacle*. As described in Lewis Carroll's *Alice in Wonderland,* treacle wells were left on dining tables to pour or spoon molasses onto breads, porridges, and puddings. It is not as sweet as dry sugar, so it is typically added to a recipe with some other sweetener. You can substitute molasses for brown sugar in many recipes. Be sure to reduce

MOLASSES

Most molasses is a by-product of the sugar-refining process. It varies in color and sweetness.

Light molasses is what remains after the first extraction of sugar crystals, and it is quite sweet.

Medium or dark molasses is obtained from the second extraction and is moderately sweet.

Blackstrap molasses is the liquid left after the third extraction. It is slightly sweet and very aromatic.

Some manufacturers produce a light or medium molasses that is extracted from cane for the molasses only, in a process similar to that of sweet sorghum. This molasses is referred to as *unsulfured;* it contains sucrose, glucose, and fructose.

Molasses contains minerals and trace elements such as iron, calcium, zinc, copper, and chromium. Since sugarcane and sugar beets leach minerals from the soil, the mineral content of molasses will depend on whether the soil was adequately fertilized. Cane and beet sugar plants may also absorb other elements, such as lead and pesticides. These, too, can concentrate in the molasses. In addition, molasses may contain by-products of the sugar-refining process, such as sulfur.

TURBINADO (RAW) SUGAR

Technically, raw sugar is the light brown crystalline substance that is separated from molasses in the first extraction. This sugar is banned from sale in the United States because it often contains insect parts, molds, bacteria, soil, or waxes. If it is sanitized by steaming, it can be sold as turbinado sugar.

Turbinado is marketed as a minimally processed, natural, and nutritious sweetener. Actually, this sweetener, like its white cousin, is a highly processed product, having gone through all but the final filtration of sugar refining. It contains 95 percent sucrose. Traces of a few minerals may be present but in such small quantities as to be nutritionally insignificant.

WHITE (GRANULATED) SUGAR

This sweetener is produced by further refining turbinado sugar. After being washed and centrifuged, then clarified with lime or phosphoric acid, the sugar is filtered through charcoal to whiten it and to remove any calcium or magnesium salts. Finally, it is crystallized and dried into granules that are pure (99.9 percent) sucrose. *Everything* in the original sugarcane or beet has been removed, except the sucrose.

CONFECTIONER'S (POWDERED) SUGAR

This product is made by pulverizing white sugar until it becomes a powder. Antica-king agents may be added to the product to prevent it from forming lumps. It is nutritionally the same as granulated white sugar.

BROWN SUGAR

Where does brown sugar fit in the processing, then? It's the last step: Brown sugar is made by adding a small amount of molasses to refined white sugar. Sometimes caramel coloring—burnt white sugar—is added instead. Brown sugar is about 96 percent sucrose.

---

the liquids called for in the recipe by about ¼ cup per cup of molasses when you do substitute.

How nutritious are they?

Sugar supplies carbohydrates, but it contributes little or no other necessary nutrients. Blackstrap molasses has notable levels of iron, calcium, magnesium, and potassium.

There is a great deal of controversy about the extent of harmful effects caused by the consumption of too much sugar. There is conclusive evidence relating sugar to tooth decay, and substantial support for its relation to obesity and to short-term peaks and drops in an individual's energy level. The links between sugar and diabetes, hypoglycemia, heart disease, and other disorders are less documented. See page 129 for more information on the health effects of eating sugar.

✦ Nutritive Value: Appendix, 331–336.

How do I store them?

Store white, brown, turbinado, and powdered sugars in tightly sealed containers. They will keep indefinitely, although they may become lumpy.

Molasses may become moldy if it is stored in a warm, damp place, so keep it in a sealed jar in the refrigerator. This will thicken it, however, so remove it and keep it at room temperature before using it. Wipe up any spills or drops on the molasses jar, especially around the cover, for easier handling.

Where do they come from?

Nearly 2,500 years ago, residents of India obtained a crude sugar from the evaporated juice of sugarcane. Cultivation of the plant slowly spread to the Mediterranean, China, and other areas, but sugar remained a scarce luxury until the fifteenth century.

When Christopher Columbus and his crew

landed in the West Indies, they found a perfect environment for cultivating sugarcane. Huge sugar plantations were soon built, and slave labor kept them going, just as low-paid indigenous workers provide the labor for sugarcane production today.

Much of the sugar consumed in the United States comes from the Philippines and Latin America. The farmland in these countries was once used to grow a variety of crops. Now much of it is devoted to cultivating sugarcane. Staple foods must then be imported, often at prices beyond the means of the workers in the sugarcane fields. The plantations are owned by foreign (largely United States) interests, so the industry returns very little to the local economy.

Besides the sugar that is imported, there is a good share of domestic sugar produced by sugar beet farmers in the Red River Valley area of Minnesota and North Dakota, as well as sugarcane farmers in the Gulf states.

VEGETABLES

What are they?

Vegetables are the edible portions of plants—namely, the leaves, stems, tubers, roots, bulbs, berries, and seeds.

There are hundreds of types of vegetables and thousands of varieties from which to choose. They are available fresh, frozen, canned, dehydrated, powdered, and juiced. This chapter deals primarily with fresh vegetables, but it also provides information on some processed items.

Buying tips

Generally, the freshest, tastiest, most nutritious vegetables are those that are consumed raw immediately after picking or harvesting. Locally grown produce from a farmers' market or roadside stand is often superior to vegetables that are shipped from long distances.

Look for crisp, healthy-colored vegetables with no signs of decay, wilt, major insect damage, bruises, or odd shapes. Bulk displays allow you to examine and pick out the vegetables you want. Plastic wrapping and wax prolong the shelf life of vegetables by preventing dehydration, but both result in waste.

The chart on the following page lists the most common vegetables, their availability and months of peak supply, and from which country they are imported to the United States.

How do I use them?

First and foremost, all vegetables should be washed in water or wiped clean. Leafy greens are usually quite dirty and may require several thorough rinsings. Tubers and root vegetables should be scrubbed with a vegetable brush, but do not peel them (unless they are waxed) because many nutrients are found in the peels.

Preparing vegetables can be a very creative process. You can juice them; pickle them; combine them for soups, salads, and casseroles; add them to breads, muffins, and cakes; bake them in pies; or eat them raw as snacks or dipped into fondue and creamy dips.

Chop, slice, grate, or tear vegetables right before you serve or cook them to preserve nutrients. Use a sharp knife for trimming and chopping. A dull knife can actually reduce the amount of vitamins A and C in the vegetables you cut by bruising the vegetable tissues.

Vegetables cook best when the pieces are of similar size; however, nutrients and flavor are depleted relative to the amount of surface area exposed to air and water. So it is best to cook vegetables whole or in large pieces—and in only as much water as you need to prevent scorching—or steam them in a rack. Do not add salt to the cooking or water, as it will draw out even more of the nutrients and may make the vegetables tough. Save any remaining cooking water for soup stock, gravy, or omelettes. Always use kettles with tight-fitting lids, and cook only as many vegetables as you expect will be eaten at that meal. Leftover, refrigerated vegetables are less nutritious than freshly cooked ones.

Oil used to saute or stir-fry vegetables will coat the pieces and thus conserve some of the nutrients, flavor, and color.

Pressure cooking vegetables reduces the time and energy expended by about half; microwave cooking even more. Consult your appliance instruction manual for proper procedures. Vegetables cooked in a pressure cooker can easily be overcooked if cooking time is not monitored. An energy-saving method of pressure cooking vegetables is to turn off the heat and remove the pressure cooker from the burner as soon as full pressure is reached. Then allow the kettle to cool down on its own rather than cooling it under tap water.

When baking vegetables, rub the skins with oil to keep them moist and prevent dehydration, then pierce them with a fork to allow steam to escape and prevent explosions. Although it is common practice to wrap vegetables in foil for baking, this results in a steamed product, and steaming could be done more quickly in a pan on the stove than in the oven. For home canning, freezing, and pickling vegetables, consult a food preservation manual or your county or provincial home economist.

Some raw vegetables, while providing nourishment, are also excellent cleansers of the teeth. These vegetables include cauliflower, carrots, and celery.

How nutritious are they?

Most vegetables are good sources of vitamins A and C, potassium, and fiber. Some vegetables provide notable amounts of B-complex vitamins, calcium, iron, magnesium, protein, and carbohydrates. Most are low in calories and fat. They have a high percentage of water.

Generally speaking, the longer time vegetables are exposed to air, heat, and water, the less nutritious they will be. "Fresh" vegetables shipped from long distances and displayed for several days in a store may actually be less nutritious than frozen vegetables that were quickly cooked and frozen shortly after harvesting.

Canned vegetables (both home canned and commercial) are usually packed in water—which many people pour off—and are heated to high temperatures. They are consequently lower in nutrients than fresh or frozen vegetables. Approximately 50 percent of the vitamin C in vegetables is destroyed by canning.

Dehydrated and powdered vegetables are even lower in nutrients than canned ones, because of the lengthy exposure to air or heat.

Freshly made vegetable juices provide essentially all of the nutrients found in whole raw vegetables, except for fiber.

Pickled, french-fried, and many commercially canned vegetables are usually very high in sodium.

✦ Nutritive Value: Appendix, 338–459, 498–507.

How do I store them?

Each vegetable has an optimal temperature and relative humidity for maximum storage time. In general, however, keep fresh vegetables refrigerated in a tightly sealed plastic bag or crisper to prevent moisture loss. Use them within a week. Consult the chart on page 144 for specific storage requirements.

Canned vegetables should be stored in a dark, cool (65°F) place. If they are stored for a year at warm temperatures (80°F or higher), the vegetables may lose up to 25 percent of the vitamin C and thiamine.

Where do they come from?

The various vegetables we eat originated in countries all over the globe.

Most of the *Brassica* vegetables (cabbage, broccoli, et al.) originated in the Mediterranean region of Europe. Squash, corn, potatoes, tomatoes, and peppers are native to North, South, and Central America. Radishes, onions, garlic, and cucumbers originated in China and India.

Vegetables sold in North America come from nearly every state and province. However, many of the large commercial vegetable farms are in California, Texas, Florida, and Mexico. People in the United States eat, on average, about 260 pounds of fresh and processed vegetables every year.

ALFALFA SPROUTS

What are they?

One of the newest vegetables on the market, alfalfa sprouts have quickly gained popularity because of their delicate taste and attractiveness.

Alfalfa is a legume that is typically grown as a forage crop. Human beings cannot digest fully grown alfalfa leaves and stems, although a tea made from them is pleasant. But the sprouted seeds of alfalfa are not only digestible; they are also delicious and nutritious.

GUIDE TO VEGETABLES

Name	Availability	Peak	Imported from	Storage Temp °F	Special Conditions
Alfalfa sprouts	all year	—		35	keep sealed
Artichokes, globe	all year	Mar.–May		32–35	
Artichokes, Jerusalem	Oct.–Mar.	—		32–35	
Asparagus	Feb.–July	Apr.–June	Mexico	32–35	
Beans	all year	May–Aug.		45–50	
Beets	all year	June–Oct.		32–35	cut off tops
Broccoli	all year	Oct.–May		32–35	
Brussels sprouts	all year	Oct.–Mar.		32–35	
Cabbage	all year	—		32–35	
Cardoon	all year	—	Europe	32–35	
Carrots	all year	—	Canada	32–35	cut off tops
Cauliflower	all year	Sept.–Jan.		32–35	stem side up
Celery	all year	—		32–35	
Corn, sweet	all year	May–Aug.		32	
Cucumbers	all year	May–July	Mexico	45–50	
Eggplant	all year	Aug.–Sept.	Mexico	45–50	
Garlic	all year	—	Italy, Spain	32	in a dry area
Greens					
Arugula	May–Oct.	Aug.–Sept.		32–35	
Chard	all year	July–Dec.		32–35	
Collards	all year	—		32–35	
Kale	all year	Dec.–Feb.		32–35	
Mustard	all year	Dec.–Apr.		32–35	
Dandelion	all year	May–Sept.		32–35	
Endive, escarole	all year	—			
Belgian endive	seasonal	—	Belgium	32–35	
Watercress	all year	May–Oct.		32–35	
Jicama	all year	—		45–50	
Kohlrabi	July–Nov.	Aug.–Sept.		32–35	
Leeks	all year	Oct.–June		32–35	
Lettuce	all year	—		32–35	
Mushrooms	all year	—		33–40	
Okra	June–Nov.	July		40–50	
Onions, dry	all year	—		65–70	in a dry area
Onions, green	all year	—		32–35	
Parsley	all year	—		32–35	
Parsnips	all year	Jan.–Apr.		32–35	
Plantain	all year	—		60–70	
Peas	Mar.–Sept.	Mar.–June		32–35	
Peppers	all year	June–July	Mexico	45–50	
Potatoes	all year	—	Canada	45–55	dark, dry area
Potatoes, sweet (yams)	all year	Sept.–Jan.		55–60	
Radishes	all year	Mar.–May		32–35	
Rutabagas	all year	Oct.–Feb.		60	
Spinach	all year	Dec.–May		32–35	
Squash, summer	all year	May–July		45–50	
Squash, winter	Aug.–Mar.	Oct.–Dec.		50–55	
Tomatoes	all year	May–July	Mexico	50–70	
Turnips	all year	Oct.–Mar.		32–35	

Buying tips

You can find alfalfa sprouts in the produce section of most grocery stores. Look for fresh, green sprouts that appear vibrant and full of life. Those that are brown or wilted have spoiled and may have a strange odor.

Alfalfa sprouts are one of the easiest foods to grow at home. Buy alfalfa seeds that are not treated with chemicals. Treated seeds are for planting, not eating, so read the label or ask the supplier to be sure. Do not buy large quantities of alfalfa seeds, as you need only a small amount for sprouting. The seeds are generally quite inexpensive, another big plus for growing your own alfalfa sprouts. See below for directions on sprouting.

How do I use them?

Alfalfa sprouts add a fresh crunch to salads, sandwiches, and tacos. Toss them on soups, casseroles, omelettes, and stir-fried dishes right before serving. They are pretty as decorations on hors d'oeuvre trays.

How nutritious are they?

Alfalfa sprouts contain calcium, iron, zinc, B-complex vitamins, and vitamin C. A small amount of protein is present. They are 90 percent water, have very little fat, and are low in calories. Alfalfa (and clover) sprouts contain a substance called canavanine, which may affect digestion.

✦ Nutritive Value: Appendix, 338.

How do I store them?

Alfalfa sprouts should be refrigerated; they will last for about a week. They stay fresh longer in glass jars than plastic containers.

Alfalfa seeds are best kept in a tightly covered container in a dry, cool place. They will last for up to a year.

Where do they come from?

Alfalfa is also called *lucerne* and has been cultivated for centuries throughout Asia, the Middle East, Europe, and Africa. Although Spaniards brought alfalfa

---

SPROUTS

You can have fresh, homegrown produce 365 days a year—and all you need are seeds, water, a jar, and a screen. Voilà . . . sprouts!

Sprouts are very easy to grow in your own kitchen, requiring little labor and few materials. Here's what you need:

- 1 wide-mouth glass jar (quart, half-gallon, or gallon size)
- 1 small piece of cheesecloth, old nylon stocking, or fine-mesh screen
- 1 rubber band or screw-on ring
- 2 tablespoons of seeds per quart

1. Soak seeds in the jar with a cup or so of warm water for 8 to 12 hours or overnight. Cover the jar or opening with the screening material, and hold it in place with a rubber band or ring.

2. Drain off soaking water, rinse the seeds with lukewarm water, and drain again. Repeat this until the water runs clear. (The water from the first rinse is good for your houseplants.) Drain thoroughly, then place the jar, mouth down, on a dish-draining rack or in a bowl. Now put the jar in a warm (70°F) shelf or cupboard away from direct sunlight.

3. Rinse and drain the seeds 2 or 3 times a day—more often in hot, humid weather. When the sprouts are as long as you want them to be, place the jar on or near a sunny window sill. The light will increase the vitamin C in the sprouts.

Sprouts should be refrigerated and used within a week. They will stay fresher a day or two longer if kept in a glass jar rather than a plastic bag or carton.

CLOVER

In some stores you may find clover sprouts, which look and taste similar to alfalfa sprouts.

Although there are some three thousand species of clover throughout the world, the seeds that are used for sprouting are red clover. These tiny, maroon-colored balls look very much like poppy seeds.

You can buy red clover seeds in some natural foods stores or seed and garden outlets. Be sure to obtain untreated seeds, and buy only as many as you plan to sprout within a short period of time—you only need 2 tablespoons of seeds per quart!

to Peru and Mexico during their conquests, the strain grown in most of North America came from German immigrants in the 1800s. Today in the United States, most of the alfalfa produced is grown in the dairy states—Wisconsin, Minnesota, and California—to feed dairy cattle. It is an important forage crop because of its high nutritive value.

Alfalfa sprouts are quite often locally grown and therefore fresh. Some may be shipped in from California or elsewhere.

ARTICHOKES

What are they?

Two vegetables of entirely separate species are named artichoke: globe artichoke, the flower head of a type of thistle; and Jerusalem artichoke, the tubers of a plant in the sunflower family.

Globe Artichoke

Globe artichoke, or simply artichoke, is one of the funniest looking vegetables in the produce coolers. The grayish green scales of what looks to be a reptilian Christmas tree ornament entice you to peel

them to find out what's in the center.

Globe artichokes are sold throughout the year and are in peak supply from March through May. Look for heavy, compact scales and a healthy green color. Fresh globe artichokes will squeak if they are rubbed against each other. Old ones have gray or tannish scales that are separated or opened, and they are often woody and lighter in weight. Check the stem ends for possible worm damage. Those with bronze-tipped scales have been exposed to cold weather ("winter kissed"), but this does not affect their quality.

To cook globe artichokes, first wash them well by spreading the scales under water. Cut off the stem without severing the bottom scales. Trim about 1/2-inch off the scale tips if they are hard. To prevent the flesh from turning brown, dip the scales in a mixture of 2 cups water and 1 1/2 tablespoons lemon juice. Now boil the globe artichokes, completely covering them with water, for 20 to 40 minutes. (Small ones cook more rapidly than large ones.) Insert a sharp knife to test for doneness—it should penetrate easily. Aluminum and iron pans will cause artichokes to turn gray, so use stainless steel, enamel, tinned copper, or earthenware pans to cook them.

Eat globe artichokes by peeling off the scales one by one and dipping them into melted butter, hollandaise sauce, yogurt, or other dips. Scrape off the flesh by pulling the scale through your teeth.

Inside the globe artichoke is the choke, a round, fuzzy center that should be removed either before or after cooking by cutting or pulling it out. Under the choke is the artichoke bottom, sometimes called the artichoke heart, although the latter more correctly refers to younger globes with small or insignificant chokes. To cook artichoke bottoms or hearts, simmer them in water for 10 to 30 minutes or until tender, then serve with butter.

Raw globe artichokes will keep for four to five days under refrigeration. Since they can be eaten cold, cook several at a time and store the extras in your refrigerator for a few days.

Globe artichokes originated in the Mediterranean. The name is derived from the Arabic *al-khurshuf.* Nearly all of the globe artichokes grown in the United States are from Castroville, California, a town south of San Francisco known as the "artichoke capital of the world."

Jerusalem Artichokes

Jerusalem artichokes, or *sunchokes,* are not from Jerusalem. The name is a corruption of the Italian word *girasole,* which means to gyrate or turn to the sun. Jerusalem artichokes are a type of sunflower, and the flower head does indeed turn toward the sun. Sunchokes are native to North America.

The part of the Jerusalem artichoke plant that is eaten is the tuber, which grows underground. These tubers, it was thought, tasted similar to globe artichoke—hence the other part of its name.

Jerusalem artichokes look like ginger root or misshapen potatoes. Their texture and flavor have been compared to water chestnuts. Fresh, firm ones are best. Avoid wilted or limp tubers. One pound of Jerusalem artichokes will serve four people. They are available from October to March.

To prepare Jerusalem artichokes, scrub them thoroughly, then dip them in acidulated water (water with lemon juice or vinegar added) to prevent the flesh from darkening. Do not use aluminum pans for cooking sunchokes, as they will cause the tubers to become black.

You can eat Jerusalem artichokes raw. Slice them into salads or add them to vegetable trays. Try sauteing, broiling, baking, or pickling them as you would other vegetables. Boil them in water for about 15 minutes or until just tender. Overcooking will cause them to become mushy and fall apart.

A nutritious flour is made by grinding dried Jerusalem artichokes. This flour is sometimes added to pasta.

Unless you are accustomed to eating Jerusalem artichokes, you should probably eat only a small portion. Many people, when first introduced to this vegetable, suffer stomach cramps and flatulence after eating a number of them.

The carbohydrate of fresh Jerusalem artichokes is in the form of inulin rather than sugar. They have a caloric value of only 7 calories per 100 grams. If they are stored for a long period of time, however, the inulin converts to sugar and thus increases the calories to 75 per 100 grams. This vegetable also contains vitamins A and B-complex, potassium, iron, calcium, and magnesium.

Store fresh Jerusalem artichokes in a plastic bag in your refrigerator. If you grow or harvest them, keep them in the ground throughout the fall and winter, as they improve in taste when they are frozen. Then dig up the tubers when you want to eat them in the spring.

✦ Nutritive Value: Appendix, 393.

ASPARAGUS

What is it?

Asparagus is one of spring's first vegetables. It is related—believe it or not—to onions, garlic, and other plants in the lily family. It is quite likely

---

BLANCHING

Blanching is a technique employed in the growing of stalk vegetables to cause them to become white or colorless.

To achieve this, sunlight is blocked from the plant, and that prevents photosynthesis (the natural greening process) from occurring. Several methods are used: boards or boxes are placed around the plants; they are wrapped in newspapers; or earth is mounded up around the young stalks for several days or weeks before harvesting, depending on the vegetable.

White (blanched) asparagus is reportedly quite common in Europe, and it tastes rather bland. Blanched or golden celery—not as popular as it once was—is reputed to have a milder flavor than green celery. Blanched asparagus and golden celery have lower amounts of nutrients than the fully green vegetables.

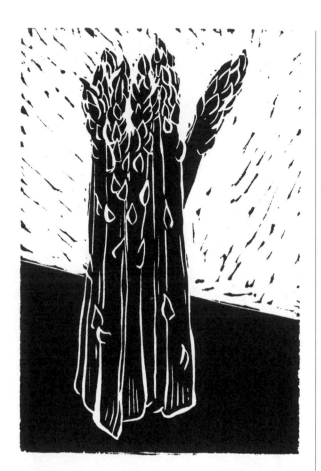

derived from wild asparagus, a plant that foragers of wild foods like to hunt.

The name of this vegetable is from *asparag,* the Persian word for sprout. Asparagus has been used since ancient times by Romans and Egyptians and has remained popular in Arabian countries. Today, nearly two hundred million pounds of asparagus are marketed in the United States every year, mainly from March through July. It is grown commercially in California and Michigan, and some is imported from Mexico.

Buying tips

The selection of asparagus is a matter of personal preference. Some like thin spears; other find the thick ones more tender. In either case, look for bright green, straight, fresh-looking spears with compact tips. Avoid wilted, stringy, woody, or streaked spears, or those with spreading tips. For uniform cooking, select those of similar thickness.

How do I use it?

Prepare asparagus by first rinsing it in cold water, then trimming off the bottoms or woody portions. Peel large asparagus spears if they are tough.

Raw asparagus is fine for salads (cut into $1/2$-inch pieces), for vegetable trays to be eaten with dips, or to eat as is.

To cook asparagus, steam whole spears until just tender. They take only 5 minutes in a vegetable steamer or layered in a large, flat pan with an inch of water.

How nutritious is it?

Raw asparagus contains good amounts of vitamins A, B-complex, and C, as well as potassium and zinc. Cooked asparagus also contains these nutrients, but it has lower levels of vitamins B-complex and C. This vegetable is low in sodium and fat, unless salt, butter, or similar substances are added.

✦ Nutritive Value: Appendix, 340–344.

How do I store it?

Keep asparagus refrigerated in a plastic bag and use it within two or three days. Leftover cooked asparagus should be cooled and placed in a covered container. Refrigerate it for up to two days, or freeze it for future use.

BEANS

Beans are among the most common vegetables grown and eaten in North America. While most vegetables are consumed only when they are at a certain stage of growth, beans are edible when they are fresh or immature as well as when they are allowed to dry or become mature. (See "Legumes" chapter for information on mature beans.)

Green, snap, string, yellow, wax . . . these words refer to beans that are picked while the pods are soft or fleshy and while the seeds are tender. They are—or should be—crisp, firm, long, and slender when they are ready to pick. Beans should also feel velvety and look fresh and bright colored. Very young beans are small and flabby, while old beans are bulging, leathery, and sometimes ridged. Avoid beans with rust spots or broken stem ends, as rotting can result from these defects.

Beans cook in 10 to 15 minutes when they are boiled in water, and 15 to 20 minutes when steamed over water. The beans will retain more nutrients if they are cooked whole rather than cut into strips or pieces. The cooking time is longer for whole beans, however. Cook beans only until tender.

Fresh green or yellow wax beans are excellent as snacks and in salads. You can also pickle them in vinegar with spices.

Unless they are a "rustless" variety of beans, store them unwashed in a plastic bag in your refrigerator. Leftover cooked beans will keep for up to three days if they are covered and refrigerated.

Another popular type of fresh bean is the *lima bean,* which is eaten for its seeds only. The pods are unpalatable.

Fresh lima beans are pale green and rather starchy but are still appetizing when they are properly prepared. Cook and mash lima beans like potatoes, or try them in a baked casserole.

Fresh lima beans are sold in the pods, so you must shell them as you would fresh peas. Store them, unshelled, in your refrigerator.

Fresh beans provide good quantities of vitamin A, calcium, potassium, and B-complex vitamins. Green beans have a higher level of vitamin A than yellow wax beans, but there is no significant difference in the other nutrients. Lima beans contain more protein, carbohydrates, and calories by weight, although their water content is about 67 percent. Green and yellow beans are more than 90 percent water.

✦ Nutritive Value: Appendix, 346–352.

BEETS

What are they?

"Eat your beets," your mom or dad probably used to say. "They're good for you." Beets *are* good, because both the roots and the leafy tops are edible and highly nutritious.

There are actually four types of beets: the *gar-* *den beet;* the *"leaf" beet* (also called *chard,* see page 158); the *sugar beet,* which is processed into refined sugar; and the *mangold beet,* grown mostly in Europe for cattle feed.

Garden beets are red or yellow. There are several shapes of roots: round, flattish-round, and long—up to a foot long. In North America we are accustomed to red, round, or flattish round beet roots. We are also, unfortunately, accustomed to discarding the tops, which are highly nutritious and taste like zesty spinach.

Buying tips

Look for firm, smooth roots with no signs of worm damage. Old beets are wrinkled and flabby. Large beets are sometimes woody or have thick skins; they are usually less tender than small ones *(baby beets).* Beets with round bottoms are reportedly sweeter than flattish round ones. Beet roots are usually okay even if the tops are wilted.

Fresh, vibrant, and crispy beet greens are best. Avoid tough, wilted, slimy, or yellow leaves.

How do I use them?

Beet roots must be cooked or baked to become palatable. For the best flavor, appearance, and nutritive value, cook them whole. Cutting them will cause color and nutrients to leach out into the cooking water. Color leaching can be minimized by adding a small amount of lemon juice or vinegar to the water.

Small beet roots cook in 30 to 45 minutes. Pressure cooking them reduces the cooking time by half. When baking beets, brush the skins with oil to keep them tender. Bake them as you would potatoes— on the oven racks or placed in a casserole dish. Beet roots can also be pickled. They are a colorful addition to relish trays.

Use raw beet tops in salads. Cook or steam them and use as you would spinach.

How nutritious are they?

Beet roots provide notable amounts of calcium, iron, magnesium, phosphorus, and potassium. They also contain vitamins A, B-complex, and C.

Beet tops are an excellent source of vitamin A, and they offer the same nutrients as beet roots in slightly higher amounts. Both beet roots and tops contain fiber. The protein, fat, and carbohydrate levels are low.

✦ Nutritive Value: Appendix, 353–356.

How do I store them?

To maintain the firmness of beet roots, cut off the tops, leaving one to two inches of stalk on the root crown, and refrigerate them in a plastic bag. They will keep for about three weeks. You can also keep them for up to five months in a root cellar or with controlled humidity (90 to 95 percent) and constant temperature (32 to 40°F).

Beet tops will stay fresh for only about a week. They should be stored unwashed and refrigerated in a plastic bag. Blanch and freeze them for long-term storage.

Where do they come from?

Beets were found growing wild in western Europe and North Africa; these had only small roots. Through cultivation, the larger-size root was developed.

Most of the beets grown in the United States are canned or bottled rather than sold fresh.

BROCCOLI

The word broccoli is derived from the Latin term *brachium,* which means "branch" or "arm." Two types of broccoli are commonly available: *sprouting broccoli,* the kind with which most people are familiar; and *heading broccoli,* a type that forms a compact head like cauliflower. A lesser known type is *Gai lon* or *Chinese broccoli,* which is pale green and has large leaves but small flower buds.

Select broccoli that has a fresh smell, bright and compact green florets, and firm, tender stalks. Avoid broccoli that has a pungent odor, yellow florets, and woody or limp stalks; these are overmature. A medium-size branch (about two pounds) will serve three or four people. Broccoli is available all year, and supplies are best from January to March.

Raw broccoli adds variety to salads, and it is good with dips. To cook it, cut off the tough stem ends, then rinse well but do not soak it. Peel the thick stalks and cut several slashes through them so the whole branch cooks evenly. Cut large florets apart, if desired. Boil it in a small amount of water until al dente—tender but fairly firm, not wilted—for 7 to 10 minutes. If you prefer, steam broccoli to preserve nutrients and the bright green color; it will be tender in about 5 minutes. A delicious way to serve broccoli is to squeeze lemon juice over it and top it with grated cheese.

Broccoli stalks can be peeled and eaten as a raw vegetable like carrot sticks, or cut or shredded for sauteed vegetable dishes, soups, and casseroles.

Broccoli has substantial amounts of vitamins A and C, and it provides B-complex vitamins, calcium, phosphorus, and potassium. It also contains protein and fiber. It is low in fat and calories.

Raw broccoli will stay fresh for only a few days. Store it with crushed ice or tightly wrapped in a plastic bag in your refrigerator to extend the storage time to one week. Cooked broccoli will keep for about three days if it is covered and refrigerated.

✦ Nutritive Value: Appendix, 359–363.

BRUSSELS SPROUTS

Brussels sprouts were reportedly first cultivated in Brussels, Belgium, in the thirteenth century. This vegetable is one of the strangest looking plants in a garden: Twenty to forty "baby cabbages" grow on a stalk, with large leaves hanging over them from the top.

Firm, green, compact brussels sprouts are best. Yellow and puffy sprouts, or those with spreading leaves, should be avoided. Brussels sprouts are in good supply during fall and winter. One pound serves four people.

To cook brussels sprouts, wash them right before cooking, and cut off the stems close to, but not flush with, the bottom. Boil or steam them until tender, approximately 5 to 10 minutes. Cutting an X on the top of large sprouts will hasten their cooking time. Add them whole to soups or casseroles.

The nutrients in brussels sprouts are similar to

those in broccoli, except vitamin A and calcium are lower and the protein content is a bit higher.

Refrigerate fresh, unwashed brussels sprouts in a plastic bag, and use them within a few days. Old ones develop a strong odor and lose their color.

✦ Nutritive Value: Appendix, 364, 365.

CABBAGE

What is it?

Cabbage is truly a food for the masses. It is eaten in almost every country in the world. It is the "cole" of coleslaw. (*Cole* is an archaic English term for plants in the genus *Brassica*, which also includes broccoli, brussels sprouts, cauliflower, kale, and kohlrabi.)

Several types of cabbage are available:

- Domestic—The most popular type; has flat or rounded heads with crinkled, fairly compact leaves. It is often used to make sauerkraut. It is pale green in color and is considered an early season cabbage. It does not store well.

- Red or Purple—Similar to domestic cabbage, although it has reddish purple and white streaked leaves. It is frequently used for pickling.

- Savoy—Yellowish green, loose and crinkly leaves form its head. The taste is milder than domestic.

- Danish—Also called Hollander, it is a late-season type with round, oval, or flat heads and smooth, tightly compacted leaves. It will keep longer than other types.

- Chinese cabbages—One type is *bok choy* (or *pak-choi*). It is sometimes called spoon cabbage and resembles chard with its wide, bushy green leaves and thick white stems. Another type, called *celery cabbage* or *pe-tsai,* forms a conical or nearly rect-angular-shaped, fairly compact head and looks similar to romaine lettuce. It has a mild flavor and is favored for stir-fried vegetable dishes.

Buying tips

Cabbage should look fresh and have crisp leaves, heavy and well-shaped heads, and good color. Avoid cabbage with wilted or thinned leaves, puffy or cracked heads, pale color, or signs of severe insect damage. Most types are available all year. One pound serves three or four people or yields $2^1/_2$ cups cooked or shredded cabbage.

How do I use it?

You can cut raw cabbage into wedges for an appetizer, or shred it for salads. Leafy types should be torn like lettuce rather than shredded.

Shredded cabbage will cook in 3 to 8 minutes. Cabbage cut in wedges cooks in about 15 minutes. Boil it in a small amount of water, or steam it to retain nutrients. When cooking red cabbage, add lemon juice or vinegar to the water to retain the color. Chopped cabbage can be sauteed or stir-fried with other vegetables.

Sauerkraut, a popular German dish, is shredded cabbage to which salt has been added. It is allowed to ferment in a large crock. The salt and cabbage juice form a brine, and this causes the distinct smell and taste of sauerkraut.

An old "cure" for hangovers was raw cabbage and vinegar, eaten before and after indulgence.

How nutritious is it?

Cabbage is a good source of fiber. It is over 90 percent water and has negligible amounts of protein, carbohydrates, and fat.

Cabbage also contains moderate amounts of vitamins A, B-complex, and C, potassium, magnesium, and calcium. Raw red cabbage has slightly

---

INSECTS AND VEGETABLES

To remove insects, eggs, worms, or other infestation, soak brussels sprouts and cauliflower in a half-gallon of water, to which 2 tablespoons each salt and vinegar have been added, for 30 minutes. Dip broccoli in the same solution, or rinse it well under hot tap water and swish the stalks around until no insects remain.

more vitamin C than other types, although this nutrient will decrease if cabbage is shredded and stored prior to serving.

✦ Nutritive Value: Appendix, 366–371.

How do I store it?

Keep raw cabbage tightly wrapped in a plastic bag or in a closed container to prevent its odor from permeating other foods in your refrigerator. It will keep for at least two weeks. Do not remove the outer leaves until you are ready to use the cabbage, as they help retain moisture. If you are storing partially used or cut cabbage, rub lemon juice or vinegar on the cut edges to minimize discoloration.

Cooked cabbage should be refrigerated in a covered container and used within four days.

Where does it come from?

Most types of cabbage originated in the Mediterranean region. The Chinese types are, apparently, from Asia.

Cabbage is grown commercially in about twenty-five states, particularly Florida, Texas, California, New York, and North Carolina.

CARDOON

This vegetable is relatively unknown in North America but is quite common in Italian and French cuisine. Cardoon is in the thistle family and is a close relative of globe artichoke.

Cardoon stalks form a bunch similar to celery, and they can be used like celery in casseroles and vegetables dishes. Peel the stalks, slice them, then dip the pieces in lemon juice or vinegar prior to cooking so they do not turn brown.

Cardoon cooks in 10 minutes. You can bread it, fry it, or serve it with cheese sauce to enhance its taste. The roots and leaves of cardoon are also edible. Use them in soups, salads, and casseroles.

Nutritionally, cardoon offers vitamins B-complex and C, some protein, and small amounts of carbohydrates and fat. It is 90 percent water.

Store cardoon in a plastic bag in your refrigerator. It will keep for about a week.

CAPERS

Do you want to make your salads and pasta dishes dance? If you do, then add some capers.

These round, pungent, flavorful little buds of shrubs in the caper family are a mainstay in gourmet kitchens. The dark olive-green capers are usually pickled with tarragon-flavored vinegar and salt brines. Also called *mountain pepper,* the light-sensitive caper buds blossom into a tuliplike flower. The trick in harvesting is to pick them at dawn before they reopen. The smaller the bud, the better the flavor or marketability. Midget capers are called *nonpareils*; the larger buds are referred to as *capotes* and *capuchins.* Reputedly, the best capers are firm and have a piece of stalk attached to the blossom.

The caper plant grows wild in the Mediterranean region, from North Africa to the Sahara Desert, and on archaeological sites in what is now Iran (though capers are not typically used in Middle Eastern cookery). The straggly, prickly bush can reach a height of about three feet, and the white blossoms have been compared to that of passion flowers. To protect themselves from excessive heat, the leaves of the caper plant turn edgeways toward the sun. Capers with thornless bushes are also cultivated commercially in southern Europe, and the pickled buds are sold locally or exported from Sicily, Italy, and France (particularly Toulon) to North America or other countries.

Capers are frequently added to sauces, salad dressings, and appetizers. They are sometimes found in Liptauer, a Hungarian goat cheese seasoned with caraway seeds, chives, capers, and/or peppers. A popular French Provençal dish called tapenade blends capers, anchovies, and ground black olives.

You may find caper substitutes in some markets. False capers or English capers are actually pickled nasturtium buds. Sometimes the buds of buttercup, broom, or marigold are used like capers. Although some gourmands may consider them inferior, these flower buds have their own unique flavors that can be just as appropriate as capers for certain dishes, particularly salads.

Unopened bottles of capers can be kept at room

temperature on a shelf for many months. Refrigerate after opening, or keep them tightly capped or corked in a dry, cool place.

CARROTS

What are they?

Carrots belong to a plant family that has about 2,500 members, including parsley, parsnips, caraway, and celery, to name a few. There are also several hundred varieties of carrots.

Carrots grow in a variety of shapes. They can be short (two inches) to long (twelve inches); cylindrical or tapered; and have squared, rounded, or conical bases. They are often sold with their tops removed because leaves extract moisture from the roots. Carrot tops, when available, can be cooked as greens or dried and used as you would parsley flakes.

Buying tips

Look for smooth, firm carrots that have no cracks, bruises, soft spots, or knobs. Avoid flabby ones or those with deteriorating stem ends. Carrots that have an excessive amount of new sprouts or leaves may have large or hard, woody cores. A deep orange color usually indicates sweetness. Those with green areas on the crown are sunburned, but this does not affect the quality of the rest of the carrots. Carrots are available year-round. One pound serves 3 or 4 people and will yield 3 cups of grated carrots.

How do I use them?

Raw carrots—either cut into sticks or shredded—are excellent for snacks, salads, and appetizers. Shredded carrots will cook in about 5 minutes, sliced carrots take 10 minutes, and whole carrots are done in 15 to 20 minutes.

Carrots will add sweetness and flavor to soups, stews, and casseroles. Try steaming rather than boiling carrots to retain nutrients. Do not peel them, as many of the nutrients are in the peels. Simply scrub off any dirt with a vegetable brush and remove stem ends and rootlets.

A delicious beverage is made by juicing carrots.

Don't drink too much carrot juice, though, or your skin may turn orange!

How nutritious are they?

Carrots contain carotene, a substance that is converted by the body to vitamin A. Carrots are one of the best sources for this vitamin. They also provide fiber, calcium, potassium, and other trace minerals.

✦ Nutritive Value: Appendix, 372–376.

How do I store them?

Keep raw carrots refrigerated in a tightly closed plastic bag or airtight container, where they will keep for up to two weeks. For long-term storage, remove the tops and place them in a root cellar, packed in a bag or tub of moist sand or sphagnum moss.

If you grow carrots, you can keep them in the ground throughout fall and winter. Cover them with a few feet of leaves, a wide layer of plastic, and another pile of leaves. Then dig up the carrots when you need them.

Where do they come from?

Carrots are thought to have originated in Afghanistan and are derived from the wild carrot, Queen Anne's lace. These plants may crossbreed if they are growing near each other, resulting in a whitish-colored root. About three billion pounds of carrots are produced every year in the United States, predominantly in California, Washington, Michigan, Texas, Wisconsin, and Florida. Some are imported to the U.S. from Canada in the fall.

CAULIFLOWER

Mark Twain once referred to cauliflower as "cabbage with a college education." Also called *cabbage flower,* this vegetable is available with white heads (especially in North America) and purple and green heads (in Europe).

Fresh cauliflower has a firm, compact head that is either conical or slightly rounded. It should be creamy white with no major brown spots. Unless the spots are widespread or penetrating, they can be cut out before eating. Avoid old cauliflower—that which has spreading florets or is limp. Cauliflower is on the market all year and in peak supply during the fall. One medium-size head will serve four people.

When cooking cauliflower, allow 15 to 25 minutes for whole heads and 10 minutes for florets. Cook until tender, not mushy. Raw florets are excellent for dips, and they add color and variety to salads.

Raw cauliflower offers vitamins A, B-complex, C, and E, as well as phosphorus, potassium, calcium, and magnesium. Cooking reduces vitamin C and eliminates vitamin E.

Store cauliflower in a plastic bag and keep it refrigerated, stem side up, to prevent moisture from collecting on top, which would speed up deterioration. Leftover cooked cauliflower should be refrigerated and used within two days.

✦ Nutritive Value: Appendix, 377–379.

CELERY

Once upon a time—namely, in sixteenth-century Europe—celery was grown for use as a medicine. It eventually became a foodstuff, and approximately 1.8 billion pounds of it are now sold in the United States every year. That's a lot of celery sticks!

Celery is typically harvested after its first year of growth, when the stalks are thick and leafy. Some plants, however, are allowed to grow a second year, which results in the formation of seeds. Celery seeds, and the dried leaves or celery flakes, are popular as seasonings.

Celery stalks should be firm, stiff, or brittle, with no signs of rotting or damage. Yellow-leaved, woody, spongy, or wilted stalks are old and should be avoided.

Use celery in salads, casseroles, soups, and stews. One stalk of celery will yield about ¹/₂ cup of diced celery.

Raw celery contains vitamins A, C, B-complex, and E, calcium, magnesium, phosphorus, potassium, and sodium. Cooked celery contains these same nutrients, except no vitamin E and lower amounts of B-complex vitamins. Celery is 94 percent water and is low in fat. Raw celery sticks are good for cleansing the teeth and exercising the gums. More calories are expended chewing celery than what one obtains from the celery itself.

Store raw celery in a tightly closed plastic bag in your refrigerator, where it can stay fresh for up to two weeks. Don't break apart the stalks until you are ready to use them, otherwise the bunch will wilt more rapidly. Store cooked, leftover celery in a covered container for no more than four days.

Celery is produced year-round in California and Florida. Together these states account for 80 percent of the United States' celery crop.

✦ Nutritive Value: appendix A, 380, 381.

SWEET CORN

The vegetable that most often typifies summer harvests, roadside stands, and "can't wait for supper" suppers is, or course, sweet corn. It is considered to be the most popular vegetable in the United States, and it is now available year-round, with peak supplies from May to September.

Florida provides about one-third of the annual 1.7 billion-pound U.S. fresh sweet corn crop, mostly in the off months and throughout winter. California, New York, and Pennsylvania also produce large quantities of sweet corn.

For maximum flavor and nutrition, use sweet corn that is freshly picked—the same day, if possible. Look for bright green, compact husks and dark brown corn silk. The ears should feel firm and full. Corn that has been stripped of its husks and has exposed kernels will quite likely be dehydrated. Dried, wilted, or yellow husks indicate prolonged storage and aged corn. Ripe kernels, when they are poked with a fingernail, will be milky, whereas dark yellow or hard kernels are doughy and will taste starchy. Tiny kernels are immature and will usually have no taste. Avoid sweet corn that has excessive insect or worm damage, or mold.

When buying or picking sweet corn, keep in mind that a typical serving is two ears per person.

Have you ever eaten sweet corn raw? It's quite good! Eat it plain or cut the kernels into a garden salad.

When boiling sweet corn, do not add salt to the

water, as it will cause the corn to become tough. Save energy by bringing the water to a boil, adding the corn, and covering the kettle. When the water returns to a boil, remove the kettle from the burner and allow the corn to remain in the water for 5 to 10 minutes. (It can stay in the water for up to 20 minutes, if you have to wait.) Remove corn from the water, and serve it piping hot.

You can roast corn by placing unhusked ears in the oven, on an outdoor broiler, or over a campfire. Roast the corn for 20 to 30 minutes.

If you have leftover ears or corn, cut off the kernels and use them for another meal or add them to cornmeal muffins, fritters, or pancakes. One ear of corn will yield about 1/3 cup of kernels.

Corn provides vitamins A and B-complex, phosphorus, potassium, protein, and carbohydrates. It has more fat than most vegetables but is still low in this nutrient. Be sure to chew corn well—otherwise it will pass through the body undigested.

Use fresh corn as soon as possible. If you must store it, keep the unhusked ears in a tightly closed container, or wrap them in damp paper towels or newspapers to minimize moisture loss. Keep corn in a cold part of your refrigerator.

♦ Nutritive Value: Appendix, 384–388.

CUCUMBERS

What are they?

There are white and yellow-skinned varieties of cucumbers, but green cucumbers are the most popular. Cucumbers are classified as *pickling types*—usually small, prickly, or bumpy; *field grown*—actually the same varieties as pickling types, but they are larger and usually have smoother skins; and *greenhouse grown*—relatively new, long, thin, "burpless" and seedless, sometimes called English or European cucumbers.

"Cool as a cucumber" is not just an expression. The inside of a cucumber can be up to 20 degrees cooler than its outside temperature.

Buying tips

Look for firm cucumbers with bright-colored skins and no wrinkled or sunken spots. Avoid yellowed, puffy, and dull-colored ones, as they will probably be overmature, tough, bitter, watery, or have hard seeds. Some producers add wax to cucumbers to prolong the shelf life; this wax must be peeled off before eating. Cucumbers are available all year.

How do I use them?

Cucumbers are favored for salads, relishes, and pickling. Try cold cucumber and yogurt soup for a refreshing summer lunch, or slice cucumbers for sandwiches. Cut them lengthwise to make "icicles," and eat them as a snack with or without dips.

Most cucumbers—except the long English type—have bitter skins. This bitterness can be eliminated by cutting the cucumber in half and twisting the ends together, each hand turning in opposite directions, until foam appears around the cut edges. Then rinse off the foam and slice the cucumber without peeling it.

How nutritious are they?

Cucumbers are mostly water (95 percent), but they do provide some potassium and vitamin A. They are amazingly high in vitamin E, which may be why cucumber slices are effective as a skin treatment for cosmetic purposes.

Cucumbers have a considerable amount of fiber if they are eaten with the skins and seeds.

♦ Nutritive Value: Appendix, 389.

How do I store them?

Store raw cucumbers in your refrigerator, preferably wrapped in plastic or kept in a covered, airtight container to minimize moisture loss. However, if they are refrigerated at a cold temperature for too long (after a week or so), the insides may become mushy or watery.

Sliced cucumbers may cause a strong odor that can affect other foods, so be sure to keep them tightly sealed.

Where do they come from?

India is credited as the country where cucumbers originated. Today, the United States produces nearly six hundred thousand tons of cukes every year; most are from Michigan, North Carolina, and Wisconsin. Some are imported from Mexico.

Eggplant

What is it?

Eggplant is a cousin of tomatoes and peppers. It is called *aubergine* in Europe, where both purple-black and white-skinned varieties are available.

Nearly all of the eggplant grown and sold in North America is purple in color but comes in a number of shapes: egg-shaped, round, and long (resembling summer squash).

Buying tips

When selecting eggplants, look for ones with shiny black patent-leather-like skins and bright green stem caps. Press the skin with your thumb; it should feel firm, not spongy. Usually, large eggplants contain many seeds and have rough or thick skins, whereas smaller ones have fewer or smaller edible seeds and tender skins. Wrinkled-skinned and soft eggplants will often have a bitter taste. Avoid those with dark, rough, or spongy spots.

Eggplants are available year-round, but peak in late summer. A two-pound plant serves four to six people.

How do I use it?

Eggplant can be fried, boiled, baked, or sauteed. Try stuffing one with vegetables as you might stuff a large zucchini. Some compare the taste of eggplant to oysters.

When frying slices of eggplant, place slightly salted $1/4$-inch to $1/2$-inch thick slices on a tray for 30 to 60 minutes to expose them to air. This will remove any acrid flavor and excess moisture, but it also reduces the nutrient content, especially of vitamins C and B-complex. Dip them in eggs and bread crumbs for a coating, then fry them in olive oil. Eggplant can also be fried for fritters or chips.

One of the more popular ways to serve this vegetable is in eggplant parmigiana—fried slices of eggplant layered with tomato sauce, mozzarella, and Parmesan cheese, then baked for 20 to 30 minutes at 350°F.

Europeans use eggplant for a number of dishes, including Turkey's imam bayeldi—eggplant simmered in olive oil for several hours; France's ratatouille—a stew of onions, garlic, zucchini, spices, and chopped eggplant; and Italy's caponata—pickled eggplant.

Have you ever had eggplant dip? Blend left-over cooked eggplant, add lemon juice and seasonings, and eat it with crackers or raw vegetables.

How nutritious is it?

Eggplant offers small amounts of protein; vitamins A, B-complex, and C; potassium, phosphorus, and calcium. It is a good source of fiber and is low in calories.

Although eggplant is sometimes eaten as a main course, it should have cheese, seafood, or other vegetables added to provide more nutrition.

✦ Nutritive Value: Appendix, 391, 498.

How do I store it?

Refrigerate eggplant. It will keep up to one week if it is wrapped in plastic or stored in a covered container. Use it as soon as possible. Cooked eggplant will be usable for three or four days if it is refrigerated and tightly covered.

Where does it come from?

Eggplant originated in China and India and has been used extensively in the Middle East-Mediterranean region.

Most of the eggplant produced in the United States is from Florida. During the winter and spring, eggplant is imported from Mexico.

Garlic

What is it?

Someone somewhere pegged garlic as the "atomic bomb of the vegetable world" because of its strong aroma. Now scientists have developed garlic with patented odor control.

A garlic head consists of from eight to forty cloves attached to a root base, each clove covered with white or purplish skin, which is in turn surrounded by a papery white covering.

A large type of garlic called *Tahiti* or *elephant garlic* has five or six huge, pullet-egg-size cloves per bulb. It is less strong than regular garlic. One elephant garlic clove is equivalent in size to eighteen regular cloves.

Buying tips

Select garlic with firm, filled-out bulbs and clean skins. Avoid soft, moldy, or shriveled bulbs. Sprouted cloves are okay to use but they can become soft and rubbery. Garlic is available all year and is in greatest supply during the summer.

How do I use it?

If you want garlic to impart the strongest flavor, peel and mash it just before using rather than chopping, slicing, or mincing it. Cloves are easier to peel when you hit them with a knife handle to break the skin. To mince garlic, first cut the clove from stem end to the bottom, then slice it horizontally. Saute or fry garlic only until tender, as the pieces will taste bitter if they are allowed to brown. Add garlic to soup or sauce just prior to serving, so the flavor does not dissipate with the heat.

To enhance the flavor of salads, rub the inside of the salad bowl with raw garlic before adding greens. Make garlic-flavored French bread by melting 1/2 cup butter, adding 4 minced cloves, and allowing both to gently simmer before spreading the mixture on pieces of bread. Broil or bake the bread until toasted.

Cooked or baked unpeeled garlic cloves have a sweet, nutlike flavor and will not give the eater garlic breath.

How nutritious is it?

Garlic is generally consumed in such small portions that its nutritive value is insignificant. There are no outstanding amounts of any vitamin or mineral in garlic.

Garlic has long been used medicinally for colds and as a purgative. It has recently been cited as a possible aid for heart conditions, as the allicin (an amino acid in garlic oil) was shown to reduce cholesterol levels. It is also speculated to have antibiotic properties.

✦ Nutritive Value: Appendix, 499.

How do I store it?

Keep garlic in a cool, dry place. If you refrigerate it, store it in a tightly closed glass jar to prevent its odor from penetrating other foods. A hanging braid of garlic will last several years in a root cellar or other cool place.

Where does it come from?

Most of the garlic sold in North America is imported from Italy, Spain, Mexico, or Peru, although a small amount is produced in California and Louisiana. Much garlic is added to processed foods, such as ketchup and sausages, or is sold as garlic powder.

GREENS

Greens are the leaves of various plants that can be eaten raw in salads or sandwiches, steamed for a side dish, or cooked and chopped or pureed for soups and casseroles.

Greens should be crisp, fresh looking, and of good color. Avoid ragged, wilted, yellowing, or excessively dirty leaves and those with signs of excessive insect damage. All of the common greens are available year-round. One pound of greens will serve two or three people.

Because sand tends to stick to the leaves, wash them in lukewarm water. Be sure to shake off as much water as possible before using greens for salads.

Greens are excellent sources of vitamins A and C, iron, calcium, magnesium, and potassium. They will stay fresh for at least a week—some types up to three weeks—when stored in a plastic bag in your refrigerator.

Arugula

Funny how a plant can be considered both a pesky weed and a gourmet's delight. Arugula, or *rocket cress,* holds this dichotomous distinction—wild and unwanted in country croplands, tangy and arrogant in urban salads.

Arugula looks and tastes similar to watercress. It is sold in bunches and is generally available from spring to autumn. Allow one bunch for two salad servings, unless you plan to mix this peppery plant with other greens.

Use arugula in salads, omelettes, burritos, and sandwiches. Try it minced and blended with butter, cream cheese, tahini, or tofu for a vegetable dip or spread.

To prepare arugula, snap or cut off the roots and any discolored leaves. Slosh it in a bowl of water to loosen any sand or mud, then drain in a colander or on a towel.

Arugula provides calcium, potassium, phosphorus, and vitamin C. It does not store well, so refrigerate it until ready to serve and use it within a few days after picking or purchasing.

Chard

Chard is an offshoot of the beet family that was developed from wild leafy strains of beets found in the Mediterranean region. Sometimes called *Swiss chard,* this vegetable was so dubbed because of a Swiss botanist who, in the sixteenth century, described yellow chard.

Chard can grow to two feet high and produces large, crinkly leaves with thick stems. Yellowish or green chard is popular, and a red *rhubarb chard* is sometimes available.

Like beet tops and spinach, chard leaves can be eaten as a salad green or cooked as a side dish. Its stem or stalk can be prepared as you would celery. About one pound of chard serves two to three people. It is on the market from mid-summer to fall.

Nutritionally, chard is very similar to beet tops. Raw chard contains vitamin E.

Store chard in a plastic bag in your refrigerator, where it will keep for about two days. It can also be frozen for up to one year: blanch it in boiling water for a few minutes, then freeze it in pint- or quart-size containers. Use frozen chard in soups or casseroles.

Collards, Kale, Mustard

These three leafy greens in the genus *Brassica* (cabbage) are somewhat similar in taste and appearance.

Collards are a nonheading cabbage, sometimes called *black cabbage,* with broad, smooth, dark green leaves and fairly long stems. The name is derived from *coleworts,* an old English term for plants in the genus *Brassica.* Collards are often used for animal feed as well as for human consumption.

Kale could be considered collards with curls, as the leaves are quite frilly. Two types are sold: Blue, which has bluish green leaves; and Scotch, which has bright green, very curly leaves. It has a robust flavor.

Mustard greens can be large, green, smooth but toothed leaves with white mid-ribs, or bright green with yellow-tinged, curly-edged leaves. The flavor of mustard greens is mildly pungent. Wild mustard is considered a weed but the leaves can be eaten as you would eat cultivated mustard. The seeds of a certain variety of mustard are used in pickling and are ground and mixed with vinegar and spices to make the condiment known as mustard.

✦ Nutritive Value: Appendix, 382, 383, 394, 395, 406.

Dandelion

This plant gets its name from the French *dent de lion*—lion's tooth. The jagged-leaved perennial grows nearly everywhere and is usually considered a weed. The new dandelion leaves that appear in early spring are mild, but they turn bitter as they grow larger.

Cultivated dandelion leaves have been bred to taste mild; they grow larger than wild plants. Reportedly, those that are still attached to the roots are juicier and will keep longer than leaves that have been separated from the roots.

Dandelion roots are also edible: Simply peel and eat them, or slice them into soups or salads. Sometimes they are dried, roasted, and ground for use as a coffee substitute.

Eat dandelion leaves in salad or soups. The bright yellow flowers can be used to make dandelion wine.

✦ Nutritive Value: Appendix, 390.

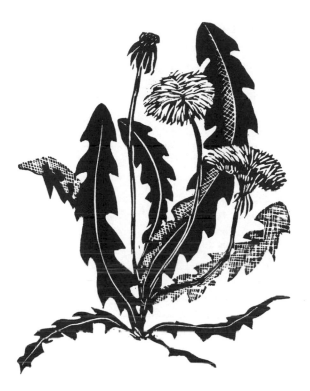

Endive, Escarole, Belgian Endive

Three greens in the chicory family may be mistaken or misnamed. So, to set the record straight, *endive* (also called *curly endive* or *chicory endive*) is the frizzy-leaved member of the family. Its leaves have a dark green exterior and yellowish interior. *Escarole* is the bushy but smooth-leaved variety with twelve- to fifteen-inch heads. Both endive and escarole are fairly bitter and are best added in small portions to milder salad greens.

Belgian endive looks like a fat whitish cigar. It is preferred by gourmet cooks for eloquent entrees. Because of its usually select clientele and long distance to markets—most is air-freighted to North America from Belgium—it is quite expensive. Belgian endive can be sliced raw for salads, braised and served with poultry, or served as a hot vegetable.

✦ Nutritive Value: Appendix, 392.

Watercress

Unlike other greens, the round, peppery leaves of watercress grow in running water, especially brooks and springs. Watercress is also grown commercially in shallow artificial pools. It is related to mustard and nasturtium. You will find it sold in bunches. One bunch serves four people.

As a salad green, watercress should be used as an accompaniment to lettuce or other mild-tasting leaves. When steamed, it loses much of its bite and tastes quite unique. Try it in soups or in an avocado sandwich.

KOHLRABI

The Germans named this vegetable *cabbage turnip* (*kohl* = cabbage; *rabi* = turnip). It resembles both in appearance and taste.

Kohlrabi is popular in northern Europe but is relatively uncommon in North America. It can be light green or purple skinned.

Small kohlrabi bulbs—about the size of a large egg—are preferred; big ones are usually tough or woody. You can eat them raw, or peeled and sliced into rounds or sticks for a mild, crunchy snack or appetizer. Try grating them into salads, or cook them like other vegetables. The tops can be used as a green.

Kohlrabi bulbs provide vitamin C and calcium in notable amounts. The tops are high in vitamin A.

Store kohlrabi in your refrigerator and use it within a week.

✦ Nutritive Value: Appendix, 396, 500.

LETTUCE

What is it?

What vegetable do you think of when salad is mentioned? Lettuce, undoubtedly.

Lettuce is in the plant family that includes daisies and thistles. There are five basic types of lettuce, each with a number of varieties. Most types are available all year.

- Head (Crisphead, Iceberg)—The most popular type in North America. It may also be referred to as *cabbage head lettuce.* The name "iceberg" apparently resulted from the commercial practice in past years of shipping lettuce in ice-covered rail cars to maintain crispness during long travels. Refrigeration and select breeding have enabled growers to produce head lettuce that is specifically destined for long-distance markets. We each eat, on the average, twenty-five heads of this type of lettuce every year.

  Head lettuce should be firm, green, springy, and have no rust. Light heads usually taste sweet and the leaves are easily separated. Hard, heavy, white head lettuce is overmature. A test of freshness is to smell the bottom (if the head is not wrapped); it should smell sweet. Brown or black butt ends indicate age, although the ends are often trimmed by retailers when discoloration occurs.

- Cos or Romaine—A long, tall, firm-leaf variety with crisp, bright green outside leaves and golden inside leaves. The taste is less bitter than head lettuce.

- Butterhead—Also referred to by the varieties: Boston, popular in that city; and Bibb, named after Major John Bibb, who developed it. The tender leaves are rounded and have a medium-green color. They grow bunched up similar to the petals of a rose. The taste is mild and delicate.

- Leaf—Frequently grown in home gardens, this type of lettuce has leaves attached to other leaves by a small core. Most varieties have curly leaves—green or red in color—but flat-leaved varieties are known. Some varieties of leaf lettuce are quite delicate and do not store well or ship well. One variety, a common type called *corn salad* or *lamb's lettuce,* grows in bunches.

- Stem—Called *celtuce,* it is a cross between celery and lettuce and tastes like both. The raw leaves are considered to be unpalatable, but they can be cooked as greens. The stems can be eaten raw, although they are more often boiled, sauteed, or stir-fried.

How do I use it?

Lettuce adds a crispy texture to sandwiches and tacos, and it generally makes the salad. Always wash lettuce well by rinsing or sloshing it in water to remove any sand that may be tucked inside the leaves. Shake off as much excess water as possible.

Head lettuce can be cored easily by whacking it stem side down on a counter, then twisting out the core. This will enable a more thorough washing.

When making salad, allow 2 loose cups of lettuce per serving—less if other vegetables are added. Do not overtoss, as lettuce leaves bruise easily. For extra crispy lettuce, place it in your freezer for about 2 minutes, but not much longer! Don't throw away the nutrient-rich outside dark leaves (unless they are wilted)—add them to the salad.

Leftover or limp lettuce can be cooked for 5 minutes and pureed in a blender, then added to soup stock to make cream of lettuce soup. If nothing else, save it for your (or a neighbor's) rabbits.

How nutritious is it?

Lettuce provides small amounts of potassium, phosphorus, calcium, and B-complex vitamins. Comparatively, leaf and romaine lettuce have about twice as much vitamin A as butterhead, and butterhead has more than twice as much vitamin A as head lettuce. All types have some fiber and are low in calories.

✦ Nutritive Value: Appendix, 397–402.

How do I store it?

Lettuce should not be stored near apples, bananas, pears, tomatoes, or other ethylene gas-producing foods, as the gas will cause russet spots or deterioration.

Head lettuce will keep for about two weeks under refrigeration. Other types of lettuce will stay crisp for about a week if refrigerated in a tightly closed plastic bag or covered container.

Where does it come from?

Lettuce has been grown for thousands of years and was popular during Roman times. (The name *romaine* is derived from Roman.) Its use has grown considerably, at least in the United States, where per capita consumption doubled from the 1940s to the 1970s. Much of this increase is attributed to wider availability and better storage and transportation conditions. About seven billion pounds are grown annually in the United States, mostly in California and Arizona.

MUSHROOMS

What are they?

Mushrooms aren't really vegetables. Rather, they are fungi, some types of which are edible, others poisonous (toadstools) or hallucinogenic (psilosybe).

The most commonly available species of mushroom, *Agaricus campestris*, is a direct descendant of the field mushroom. It can be pearly white, tan, or brown and ranges in size from one to four inches high. It is sold fresh and in cans.

Other edible mushrooms available in stores and markets are:

- Chanterelle—The queen of wild mushrooms, this golden-orange or white funnel-shaped fungus is sought after by many foragers. This very flavorful and versatile mushroom is favored for soups and sautes. Commercially available chanterelles are usually quite expensive. They are available in autumn.

WILD MUSHROOMS

Edible wild mushrooms, such as puffballs, morels, and inky caps, are a gourmet's delight—but only if they are the edible types. Because there are many look-alikes, wild mushroom hunting and eating should be undertaken with caution. Poisonous mushrooms can cause serious illness and death. To be sure you pick the edible ones, consult a mushroom handbook or go hunting with a knowledgeable and trusted partner.

- Crimini—A brown, full-flavored, gilled mushroom that looks like its white cousin *(A. campestris)* and can be used in the same way.
- Enoki—A thin, creamy-white mushroom with a tiny cap and long stem, often used in Asian soups and stir-fried dishes.
- Matsutake—Also called *Japanese pine mushroom,* is a large white or brownish fungus found in Pacific Northwest woods in autumn. Foragers may confuse it for one of the poisonous amanitas, but its flavor and texture are not mistaken.
- Morel—A large, wrinkly, tannish brown or black mushroom with indentations in the caps, cherished by wild mushroom pickers for its delectable flavor. Morels are available in spring in some regions of the United States. They require unique soil conditions found in certain woodlands, such as under old apple and elm trees.
- Oyster—A soft, smooth, almost frilly mushroom that is good in soups and casseroles. Oyster mushrooms are cream colored or light brown. This shelf mushroom grows on logs and tree stumps. Wild oysters are available from spring through autumn. A smaller, more delicate wild cousin called *angel's wings* can be found in autumn.
- Portabello—A big, brown, meaty, gilled mushroom that loves to be sauteed as an entree unto itself.
- Shiitake—A brown shelf mushroom that grows on logs and is popular in Japan. It is quite aromatic and chewy, and it is often used in Asian cooking. Shiitakes are harvested from the wild as well as grown commercially. Shiitake-growing kits are also available for home production.

Mushrooms need no light to grow—only a constantly cool 56°F and a moist atmosphere, as well as rich, composted soil. They reproduce by spores rather than by seeds, and they literally grow overnight, doubling in size within twenty-four hours.

Buying tips

Fresh mushrooms have closed caps and are firm. In a few days, or more accurately, with moisture loss, the caps open to reveal the separating gills, or "veil." Some people prefer mushrooms with open caps, claiming they have more flavor than those with closed caps.

Mushrooms exposed to room temperature or a dry atmosphere will turn dark brown, dehydrate, and become spongy, wrinkly, slimy, and tough. Size is not a determining factor in the age of mushrooms, as they are mature when they are picked and will not ripen any further. One pound will serve 3 or 4 people and is equivalent to 36 to 46 small mushrooms, 25 to 30 medium, or 12 to 15 large mushrooms. They are available all year.

How do I use them?

When preparing mushrooms, rinse them under cold water and rub off any dirt with your fingers or a dampened towel. Trim a small amount off the stem ends, but do not discard stems or peel the caps, as all of the mushroom is usable. You can now slice or chop them and use them raw in salads or sauteed for gravy, omelettes, casseroles, or soups. Do not wash mushrooms until you plan to use them, and never soak mushrooms, as this will cause a loss of nutrients.

Small mushrooms (sometimes called *buttons*) can be blanched by dipping them in boiling water for 1 minute, then quickly cooling them in cold water for 3 minutes. You can also batter-fry mushrooms to serve as appetizers.

When sauteing mushrooms, do not cover the pan, because mushrooms release a considerable amount of water and the moisture should evaporate. They cook quickly—in 10 minutes or less. If they are fried or sauteed too long, they will become black and mushy. Mushrooms can discolor aluminum, so use stainless steel or cast iron pans.

How nutritious are they?

Mushrooms are, surprisingly, over 90 percent water. They provide some protein, phosphorus, potassium, calcium, iron, and other trace minerals. Raw mushrooms are high in biotin, one of the B-complex vitamins.

✦ Nutritive Value: Appendix, 403–405.

How do I store them?

Fresh mushrooms will keep for about a week if they are refrigerated in a moisture-proof container.

You can easily dry mushrooms: String them with a needle and thread, then place them in sunlight for six to eight hours. About 1 pound of fresh mushrooms yields 3 ounces dry mushrooms. Store them in tightly closed glass jars in a cool place, where they will keep for up to a year. Reconstitute dry mushrooms by soaking them in hot water, saving the water for soups or other foods. Use reconstituted mushrooms in stuffing, omelettes, casseroles, and soups, but not as a side dish.

Freezing mushrooms is also possible. Either slice and saute them, or scald them whole, with 1 tablespoon of lemon juice per quart of cooking water. Scald them for 4 minutes, drain, then pack into freezer containers.

Where do they come from?

Mushrooms are ancient foods that have for centuries been linked with magic and myth. Many of the commercially available mushrooms sold in North America are from Ontario and Pennsylvania, where they are grown in abandoned underground mines—ideal growing environments for mushrooms. Commercial mushroom houses have no windows and are air-conditioned. Other states that produce mushrooms include California, Washington, Oregon, Michigan, New York, and Delaware.

OKRA

Okra is a green fingerlike pod of a plant related to cotton. This unique vegetable is native to Africa and is popular in the southern United States, where much of it is grown. Its nickname, *gumbo,* is derived from the African term *quingumbo.*

Young okra pods are selected for eating, as they are tender and have small seeds. Small, two- to four-inch pods are graded Extra Fancy, while medium-size pods are graded as Fancy. Large pods are often hard or tough, but they can be dried and ground into a protein-rich flour. Okra is available all year, especially in the South, and peaks from July to October. One pound (22 to 28 small pods) serves 4 people.

Okra seeds are pressed for edible oil in some parts of the world. They can also be roasted and ground for use as a coffee substitute.

Okra is generally cooked for soups and stews. It has a mucilaginous, or thickening, property. It can be coated with cornmeal and deep-fat fried.

Sliced raw okra adds attractive stars to salads. Okra is also processed for commercial vegetable soups, such as chicken and gumbo soup. It is sometimes used to thicken ketchup.

Okra contains vitamins A, B-complex, and C. It is a good source of calcium and contains phosphorus, potassium, and other trace minerals. The fat content is minimal.

Fresh okra does not store well and should be used within three to five days. Keep pods wrapped in a plastic bag in your refrigerator. Blanch and freeze them for long-term storage.

✦ Nutritive Value: Appendix, 407.

ONIONS

Take your pick—there are a number of onion varieties and types to satisfy almost any eater:

Dry Onions

- Bermuda-Granex-Grano—Also known simply as Bermuda or Granex-Grano, these onions are flattened or top-shaped and have a mild flavor. They are early season onions—March to June—but do not store well.

- Globe (also called Creole)—Round to oval, strong-flavored onions used primarily for cooking. Most globe onions are yellow skinned, although white-skinned varieties are sometimes available. They are on the market most of the year. The yellow-skinned varieties are good keepers.

- Red Italian—Flat, red-skinned onions that are often sliced for hamburgers. They are available all year.

- Shallots—Actually a garlic cross, they have clustered, rounded bulbs and a mild, sweet flavor that won't linger on your breath. Shallots are available fresh or dried.

- Spanish (or Sweet Spanish)—Large, round, usually yellow-skinned onions that are favored for slicing into salads but can also be used in cooking. Spanish onions are sold from September to March and can be stored for several months. Some sweet onions are named after the areas in which they are grown, such as Vidalia (Georgia) and Walla Walla (Washington).

Fresh Onions

- Chives—Small, narrow tops but no bulbs to speak of. The tops are snipped and used as a culinary herb, either fresh or dried.

- Green (scallions)—Young, small-bulbed onions used mostly for their tops. White varieties are most often grown for green onions. They are quite perishable and are available year-round, especially in summer.

- Leeks—A separate species of onion, although they look similar to green onions. Leeks have wide, flat tops and just a bulge for bulbs. They are very mild and sweet and are available year-round.

- Pearl (or Canada)—Small white bulbs, used for boiling, pickling, and cocktails. They are on the market all year.

Buying tips

Dry onions should have papery, crackly skins, should be firm, and should have little or no neck. Avoid soft or moldy onions. Onions with green sprouts can still be eaten or even planted; most likely they were in storage too long or stored where the temperature was too high. Dry onions are available in three basic sizes: small (1 to 2¼ inches in diameter); medium (1½ to 2 or 3¼ inches in diameter); and large or jumbo (over 3 inches in diameter).

Fresh green onions are usually sold in bunches. They should have bright green, vibrant tops and bulbs without insect damage or bruises. Yellowed, brown, or wilted tops indicate age or prolonged storage.

The serving portions of onions is a matter of

personal discretion, but a fair estimate is one pound dry or two bunches fresh per four servings.

How do I use them?

Onions can accompany nearly any food—except sweeteners or fruits—and can be prepared in dozens of ways: chopped or sliced raw for salads and sandwiches, sauteed, fried, boiled, baked, and steamed. Chopped onion tops or scallions are flavorful additions to soups, salads, omelettes, and casseroles.

A number of suggestions have been offered regarding how to prevent the tears caused when onions are peeled or chopped. One way is to peel them under running tap water. Another way is to eat some cheese or bite on a crust of bread while peeling or chopping onions. Refrigerated onions tend not to release tear-producing vapors as much as those stored at room temperature. Peeling is simplified by first soaking onions in hot water to soften the skins. A special kitchen utensil—a jar with a blade attached to a springed handle—makes chopping a breeze but cleanup a bit messy, as the onion pieces stick to the glass.

Onions will become tender by frying or sauteing them for 10 minutes. Boiling takes 10 to 35 minutes, depending on what size the onions are and whether you slice them or leave them whole. You can steam whole or halved onions in 10 to 15 minutes.

Do you like sweet-tasting onions? Bake them, unpeeled, for $1^1/2$ hours at 350°F. To hasten baking, first boil the onions until partially cooked, then bake for 30 to 40 minutes on a cookie sheet or pie pan. Cutting an **X** in the top will allow steam to escape.

How nutritious are they?

Onions contain vitamins A, B-complex, C, calcium, magnesium, potassium, and traces of other minerals. Onion tops are very high in vitamin A. Onions are about 90 percent water.

✦ Nutritive Value: Appendix, 408–412.

How do I store them?

Dry onions should be stored in a cool, dry place, such as in a basket or net sack, and hung in a root cellar, basement, or porch. They can also be refrigerated in a tightly closed plastic bag—away from foods that can absorb odors—where they will keep for several months. Do not store onions near or with potatoes because the tubers give off moisture, and that could cause onions to sprout or rot.

Fresh onions stay fresh for only about a week. Store them in a plastic bag in your refrigerator.

For longer storage and convenience, try dehydrating or freezing onions. Dehydrated and frozen onions have less flavor, so you will need to add more of them than if you used fresh onions.

To dehydrate onions, peel and slice them very thinly (to a thickness of $1/8$-inch), and place the slices on trays in the sun for 2 or 3 days, then in a 175°F oven for about 10 minutes. If you use a food dehydrator, it will take several hours at 130 to 140°F. Store dehydrated onions in a tightly capped jar.

To freeze onions, chop them and spread the pieces on a cookie sheet. Put them in the freezer until stiff. Pack them loosely in a jar or freezer container. Scoop out pieces as needed.

Where do they come from?

Onions probably originated in Middle Asia or India. They have been grown and eaten since recorded history.

Wild onions were found growing in North America. The Native Americans of the Great Lakes region called them *she-khe-ony*, from which the city of Chicago reportedly got its name.

Most commercial onions sold in the United States are from California, Oregon, New York, Colorado, and Idaho, with a total annual crop of five billion pounds.

PARSLEY

Parsley, a member of the carrot family, is typically used as a culinary herb. It is available in two forms: *curly leaf* and *flat leaf* (Italian). Curly leaf parsley is the most popular, while Italian parsley is said to have more flavor.

A less popular but zesty-tasting type of parsley is *cilantro,* also called Mexican or Chinese parsley. Cilantro is the leaf of coriander, the seeds of which are used as a spice.

Even less common than cilantro is Hamburg parsley, also called *parsley root*. It resembles parsnips and tastes similar to celeriac. It is often used to flavor soups.

Look for clean, dark green parsley with no signs of yellowing or wilting. It is available all year and is in greatest supply from October to December.

Use fresh parsley in salads, in soups, and as a garnish. It is a natural breath freshener: eat a sprig of it to rid the mouth of the taste of garlic or onions.

Dried parsley, or parsley flakes, can be made by spreading fresh parsley on a cheesecloth-covered tray and putting it in a closet or on a high shelf for a few days. When the parsley is dry and brittle, crumble it and pack it into jars.

♦ Nutritive Value: Appendix, 413, 414.

PARSNIPS

This vegetable looks like a big white carrot. The two plants are related—both parsnips and carrots are members of the Umbelliferae family. The leaves of parsnips resemble those of celery, another cousin.

Parsnips are a cold-climate food and actually become sweeter if they are frozen in the ground. The starch will convert to sugar at low temperatures. Parsnips that are freshly dug in the summer are rather bland tasting.

Look for firm parsnips with no double roots or knobs. Small or medium-size ones are tender, whereas large parsnips tend to have hard, woody cores. Avoid shriveled, soft, or insect-damaged parsnips. Waxed ones must be peeled. One pound of parsnips serves two or three people. They are available year-round, with peak supplies in fall and winter.

To prepare parsnips, scrub them well and remove tops and rootlets. Boil them whole for 20 minutes, or sliced for 5 minutes. You can also bake them in a covered casserole dish for 20 to 30 minutes, or slice and saute them in butter until tender but not mushy. If you prefer eating peeled parsnips, it is easier to peel them if they are cooked and then briefly dipped in cold water. This will prevent them from becoming discolored.

Parsnips offer small amounts of vitamins A and C, calcium, potassium, and phosphorus. They are high in fiber.

Refrigerate unwashed raw parsnips in a plastic bag, where they will keep for two to three weeks.

♦ Nutritive Value: Appendix, 415.

PEAS

There seems to be widespread agreement (or lament) that fresh-from-the-garden peas are the sweetest, best-tasting peas available—but only available to gardeners! Fresh peas have steadily declined in importance as a produce item, since 95 percent of the United States' annual production of peas is now frozen or canned.

When or if you can find fresh peas in the pod, look for small, shiny, velvety pods that squeak when they are pressed or rubbed together. Dull, wilted, or limp pods indicate prolonged storage—peas lose moisture and sweetness very rapidly after picking. Yellow, bulging, or hard peas are old and usually starchy.

Cook shelled peas from the pod in as little water as possible, and only until tender. The French method of cooking peas is to line a pot with lettuce, then add peas and cover with another layer of wet lettuce. Don't add salt to the cooking water, as it will cause peas to become tough.

A type of pea often used in Chinese cooking is called the *snow pea* or *sugar pea*. The pod is tender and edible, and it is picked when it is flat rather than when the peas are filled out. Snow peas, when stir-fried, will become tender in only two minutes.

Although pea pods from common garden peas are usually discarded, they can be juiced raw or steamed and eaten as one would eat globe artichokes—pulled between the teeth to remove the flesh.

Fresh raw peas provide vitamins A, B-complex, C, and E, and copper, iron, phosphorus, and potassium. They are very high in protein for a vegetable and provide a good amount of carbohydrates. Cooked and canned peas have the same nutrients as raw peas, except canned peas have reduced amounts of vitamin C and are usually high in sodium.

Refrigerate fresh peas. Do not shell them until you are ready to use them.

♦ Nutritive Value: Appendix, 416–418.

PEPPERS

What are they?

Mild to hot . . . green, red, yellow . . . fresh, dried, canned, bottled . . . these are just some of the words used to describe peppers.

Peppers are fruits of a plant that is related to tomatoes and eggplant. They are hollow and contain a number of flat, yellowish seeds.

Mild Peppers

The most popular type of pepper used in North America is the *green sweet bell pepper.* It is four to five inches long, two and one-half to four inches in diameter, and is squared or tapered. If it is allowed to fully ripen, it will become bright red. The taste is mild and subtly sweet.

Pieces of red bell peppers are sometimes stuffed into green olives. They are then called *pimientos.*

Firm, bright-skinned bell peppers are best. Avoid any with soft spots, shriveling, thin skins, or pale color. Bell peppers are available all year and are in greatest supply during summer months.

Another large green pepper, often elongated, is the *poblano* pepper. It is often used to make a Mexican dish called chile rellenos, a poblano pepper stuffed with cheese, covered with a special sauce or batter, and fried or baked.

The *banana pepper,* also a mild type, is five to six inches long, two inches in diameter, and yellow to orange-red in color. This pepper is more commonly found in home gardens than on the market.

Hot Peppers

At least fifteen different types of chili peppers are found in Mexican dishes. Some have multiple names.

Jalapeño (pronounced *ha-la-**pay**-nyo*), serrano, and poblano peppers are green, one to two inches long, and quite hot. They are sold fresh and are sometimes canned or bottled.

Reddish brown chili peppers are usually dried. They include the round cherry or Cascabel pepper and the following triangle-shaped ones: Ancho, Chipotle, Guijillo, Mulato, and Pasilla. The Japanese ha-paka pepper is also very hot and usually sold dry. A yellow wax pepper (also called Carribi or Guero) is so hot your eyes may water when you cut it.

How do I use them?

Mild green or red bell peppers can be chopped, grated, or sliced for salads, sandwiches, casseroles, pizza, and egg dishes. Because of their unique shape, you can stuff them with a cheese, rice, and sunflower seed mixture, or any other stuffing. For speedier cooking, boil them whole for a minute, remove top and seeds, then drain them upside down, stuff them, and bake.

Chili peppers should be used sparingly if you are not accustomed to them. Use them to season soups,

---

SEASONINGS FROM PEPPERS

Peppers are often used to add flavor to foods, rather than as foods themselves. These include:

Cayenne—Another red pepper that is often ground into a powder. It is more pungent than chili powder and its color is a fiery orange-red.

Chili powder—Reddish brown seasoning made from ground chili peppers. It is mild to hot in flavor.

Hot sauce—Pureed hot peppers, either red or green types, or a blend of both red and green peppers, sometimes with vinegar.

Paprika—Mostly used as a garnish or condiment, paprika is mild red Hungarian peppers ground into a powder.

Salsa—Hot peppers mixed with chopped onions, cilantro, tomatoes, and other seasonings.

Tabasco—A bright red pepper, one to one and one-half inches long and tapered at the end. Although it is sometimes sold fresh or bottled, much of the tabasco pepper crop is made into Tabasco® sauce.

casseroles, or sauces. Experiment with the different types to learn their pungency and to develop a taste or tolerance for them. Avoid touching your eyes, nose, or lips with your hands after you've handled chilies, as severe burning will result. Wash your hands in hot soapy water to remove the volatile oil.

Fresh chili peppers should be minced as small as possible, so the eater does not get an overwhelmingly hot bite.

Dried chilies can be reconstituted by first washing them well in cold water, removing stems and seeds, tearing or crushing them into small pieces, then soaking in hot water for an hour—1 cup water per 6 chilies. You can then puree them with the soaking water or with beans or other ingredients in a blender or through a sieve. Pureed chilies will be more evenly distributed throughout the foods than chopped or minced chilies would be.

Specialty food markets often offer a stunning array of prepared chili sauces from all over the world. Experiment with the Asian, Latin American, and Caribbean products to find the sauces just right for your culinary needs.

Some of the more unusual prepared foods, available primarily in the southwestern United States, are chili jelly and chili honey. These taste bud-titillating spreads provide a hot-sweet zing to toast and crackers. Green chili pepper-flavored beer is made by some microbreweries and is great with Mexican foods.

How nutritious are they?

Green bell peppers provide a good amount of vitamin C, vitamin A, potassium, and calcium. Red bell peppers are substantially higher in vitamins A and C than green ones.

Hot chili peppers, because they are eaten in small quantities, do not contribute a significant amount of nutrients. Red hot chilies are exceptionally high in vitamin A.

✦ Nutritive Value: Appendix, 419–421.

How do I store them?

Keep peppers in your refrigerator, where they will last for about a week.

You can freeze peppers by simply chopping or slicing them, placing the pieces on a tray, and freezing them until firm. Transfer the pieces to a plastic bag or freezer container and use them as needed.

To dry bell peppers, chop or slice them to a thickness of about 1/4 inch, then place them in the sun or in a food dehydrator until brittle.

String fresh chili peppers and hang them to dry. They will keep for a year or longer.

Where do they come from?

Peppers are native to Central America, where voyaging Spaniards learned of them and erroneously named them after the spice, peppercorns *(Piper nigrum),* which are ground into white and black pepper. The word *chili* is from a Mexican Indian tribe by the name of Chilli.

Approximately five hundred million pounds of peppers are marketed in the United States every year. They are mostly from Florida, California, and Texas, or are imported from Mexico, primarily during the winter.

PLANTAIN

What looks like a banana but tastes sort of like a potato? It's a fruit of the plant called plantain. A close relative of bananas (sometimes considered a baking variety), plantains are fatter and usually longer than their sweet cousins, and they often wear their thick green or red skins in the markets. Look for plantains with blemish-free skins and no bruises.

Plantains are popular in Africa and Latin America, where cooks make amazingly versatile meals using these starchy vegetable-fruits. They are often sliced and fried but can also be roasted, boiled, steamed, or baked like potatoes. Plantain flour is also used for thickening soups or adding to baked goods, imparting a subtle sweetness.

Because plantains are mostly starch and water, they are a good source of carbohydrates as well as potassium. Plantains also provide vitamins A and C, folic acid, and phosphorus.

Store plantains at room temperature. However, they should be refrigerated after they become soft.

✦ Nutritive Value: Appendix, 220, 221.

POTATOES

What are they?

Potatoes are tubers, the swollen stems of a plant related to tomatoes and peppers. They are unique vegetables: They grow underground and are propagated by budding rather than by seeds.

In the United States, about one hundred pounds of potatoes are eaten by every person every year. There are generally five classifications of potatoes, and each type has a certain use in cooking.

- New—The young, freshly dug potatoes with thin, feathering skins and sweet flavor. New potatoes cook quite rapidly compared to mature potatoes. They are on the market from January to September, and they can be stored for only one or two weeks.

Mature potatoes are those that have been cured and have developed thick skins. Due to moisture loss, they will absorb more water or oil during cooking. These include:

- Round red—Skins are reddish, netted, or russeted; insides are white and firm. Round red potatoes are recommended for roasting, boiling, and slicing for potato salad. Occasionally they are artificially colored or waxed. The package or label will state if coloring or wax has been added.
- Round white—Tannish-colored skins, usually smooth and sometimes shiny; the inside texture is firm.
- Long white—Like round whites, the skins are tannish and smooth and the insides are firm. Their shape is cylindrical or elongated.

    Both long white and round white potatoes are all-purpose cooking, baking, and frying types.
- Russets—Brown, spotty, or russeted skins, usually cylindrical in shape. The insides are mealy—a desired trait for baking. The Russet Burbank variety is the most popular potato for growing in the gardens and for eating.

Buying tips

The best way to buy potatoes is to pick them out yourself from a bin or bulk display so you can examine each one for possible defects. Netted or paper bags often obscure the contents.

Buy only as many potatoes as you can use within a few weeks, unless you have proper storage facilities. That twenty-pound bag is not a bargain if half the potatoes rot!

Look for clean, firm, well-shaped "spuds" with few eyes and no knobs. (Knobs usually result in excess waste.) Avoid cracked or bruised skins, excessive sprout growth, and potatoes that smell moldy or musty. Potatoes with green skins or spots indicate exposure to light during storage or growth. They contain solanine and are toxic and bitter, so avoid them or cut off the green areas before cooking.

In the United States, potatoes are sometimes inspected and graded by the Department of Agriculture according to appearance and size. *U.S. Extra No. 1 potatoes* are premium grade and often cost more than other grades. No sprouts and only slight defects are allowed. They are a minimum of two and a half inches in diameter and must be packed in uniform-size lots. *U.S. No. 1 potatoes* have few defects and are the most common grade available. The minimum size is one and three-quarters inches in diameter.

Grade labeling is not required, so many potatoes may not be marked.

How do I use them?

Nearly everybody has a preferred method of preparing and eating potatoes: baked, boiled, fried, mashed, as chips or tater tots, or even raw.

- Baking—By far the easiest way to prepare potatoes. Simply scrub them to remove dirt, cut off any eyes, spots, or bruises, then pierce them with a fork to allow steam to escape and prevent explosion during baking. Bake for 45 minutes at 450°F, or 1 hour at 400°F, or 1 hour and 15 minutes at 350°F.

    Coat the jackets with butter or oil to keep them tender. Wrapping potatoes in aluminum foil will also keep them tender, but technically this steams them instead of baking them. For speedier baking, insert a clean long nail, knitting needle, or skewer through the center of the potato. The metal will cause the heat to be more evenly distributed through the potato. Another trick is to first parboil the potatoes for 5 minutes, drain, and dry them. This will reduce baking time by half.

- Boiling—Scrub potatoes, remove defects, and cut large ones in half or quarters. Use cold water, about an inch deep in the pan, and cook for 20 to 40 minutes or until tender. Save the cooking water for soup stock, gravy, or liquid for baked goods. To keep the insides white, add a teaspoon of vinegar, lemon juice, or milk to the cooking water. Reportedly, a dash of sugar in the water will help retain the vitamin C present in potatoes.
- Frying—Shred or thinly slice either raw or cooked potatoes and fry them, covered, in butter or vegetable oil over low heat until tender, 10 to 15 minutes. Increase heat and remove cover. Stir until brown and crispy, about 10 minutes.
- Mashing—After boiling or steaming potatoes until tender, mash them with a mashing utensil or a large fork until crumbly. Add milk, butter and/or egg yolk, then blend or whip until fluffy. If you will not be serving the mashed potatoes immediately, keep them moist by placing them in the top of a double boiler or on a steamer tray.
- Steaming—Place scrubbed and cut potatoes in a steamer and cook, covered, with only a small amount of water for 10 to 20 minutes.

Potatoes can thicken soups: Just grate 3 tablespoons of raw potato per cup of soup and heat the soup for about 15 minutes or until it thickens. If by chance you put too much salt in your soup or sauce, drop in pieces of raw potato and boil the soup or sauce until the salt is absorbed by the potato. Remember to remove the potato pieces before serving.

How nutritious are they?

Potatoes provide protein in small amounts, vitamins C and B-complex, potassium, calcium, and iron. Most of the nutrients are in or near the potato skins, so don't peel or discard them.

Potatoes are low in calories, unless butter, gravy, sour cream or other fats are added. French fries, potato chips, and hash browns are very high in fat and are often heavily salted. An estimated 50 percent of the vitamin C is lost when potatoes are processed.

✦ Nutritive Value: Appendix, 422–428.

How do I store them?

Potatoes like a cool, dry, and dark room for long-term storage, in the 45 to 55°F range. Light (either sunlight or from artificial sources) can cause potatoes to turn green. After several months of storage, potatoes begin to sprout, unless they have been treated with a sprout inhibitor. Sprouted potatoes become shriveled and soft, hence unusable.

Do not refrigerate potatoes, as temperatures below 38°F can convert the starch to sugar and would make the potatoes sweet tasting.

You can successfully freeze mashed potatoes, but raw or boiled ones would become grainy or mushy if they were frozen. Store leftover baked or boiled potatoes in a covered container in your refrigerator and use them within three or four days.

Where do they come from?

Although they originated in the Andes Mountains region of South America, potatoes crossed the Atlantic to Europe before landing in North America in the early 1700s. The name potato is a corruption of *batata,* a West Indian word for the sweet potato. The French call the potato *pomme de terre*—apple of the earth. Likewise, the German term for potato is *Erdapful.* Mexicans refer to them as *papas.*

Potatoes are grown in nearly every province and state in North America. Canada produces five and a half billion pounds a year. The United States averages over thirty-five billion pounds of potatoes annually. Idaho, Washington, Maine, and Oregon lead in the production of potatoes.

Sweet Potatoes
What are they?

Sweet potatoes are plump, smooth-skinned tubers of a plant in the morning glory family. They are sometimes called yams, but true yams are of a different genus of plants that grow in Africa. Blacks in the South referred to sweet potatoes as *nyamis* because of their similarity to the African plant, and the word yams stuck.

There are two types of sweet potatoes: *firm fleshed* and *soft fleshed. Firm-fleshed* ones are mealy or dry and yellowish when cooked, and they are not very sweet. This type is sometimes called Jersey because it was once the main type grown in New Jersey.

Soft-fleshed sweet potatoes are moist, orange, quite sweet when cooked, and are usually fatter or rounder than the firm-fleshed type. Soft-fleshed sweet potatoes are often referred to as yams, while the firm-fleshed type is referred to as sweet potato. The terms *yam* and *sweet potatoes,* however, are interchangeable for most purposes.

Buying tips

Fresh sweet potatoes are sold uncured and cured. *Uncured* ones are those sold right after harvesting. *Cured sweet potatoes* are stored for ten days or longer at 85°F. This converts some of the starch to sugar and allows the potatoes to be stored for several months thereafter without deterioration.

Look for clean, smooth-skinned sweet potatoes with no major bruises or harvesting scars. Avoid those that are displayed on refrigerated racks, as cold temperatures can damage the tubers. They bruise easily, so handle them gently. One pound (fresh or canned) equals 3 medium-size yams or 2 cups cooked and mashed. They are usually available year-round.

How do I use them?

Sweet potatoes are amazingly versatile and colorful additions to meals. You can boil, bake or french fry them as you would other potatoes. Add them to baked goods such as cakes cookies, muffins, or pies. Blend them with fruit juices to make an interesting beverage. They are quite tasty when sliced and fried with tempura batter.

To cook sweet potatoes, wash and scrub them but do not peel. Peeling causes an 8 to 13 percent waste as well as loss of nutrients, flavor, sweetness, and color. Boil in water for 20 to 35 minutes, depending on the size. Cut large ones in half for speedier cooking.

You can bake them, jackets oiled, for 1 to 1¹/₂

hours at 350°F, or for 15 minutes at 400°F, then 45 to 60 more minutes at 375°F. Puncture the skin with a fork to allow steam to escape and to prevent them from exploding.

Cooked and mashed sweet potatoes can replace up to one-fourth of the wheat flour in breads. When serving them as a side dish, add milk or fruit juice to the mashed yams for extra flavor.

How nutritious are they?

Sweet potatoes are rich in carotene and thus in vitamin A. Also present are vitamin C, calcium, potassium, carbohydrates, and fiber. Soft-fleshed (deeper orange) sweet potatoes are higher in vitamin A than firm-fleshed (yellow) ones.

✦ Nutritive Value: Appendix, 442–446.

How do I store them?

Keep sweet potatoes in a cool area (55°F) but do not refrigerate them. They can be stored at room temperature for up to two weeks.

Cooked, mashed yams freeze well. Just pack them into containers and use as needed.

Where do they come from?

Sweet potatoes are native to the West Indies and southern United States, where they were called *batatas.* Today, most of the sweet potatoes grown in the United States are from North Carolina, Louisiana, California, and states in the Southeast; about 1.2 billion pounds are grown annually.

Jicama

Jicama (pronounced **hee**-*ka-ma*) is a tuber in the morning glory family. It grows in Central America, where it is used extensively. It is a cousin of the sweet potato.

This large, brown, turniplike tuber has two forms: *agua* (watery juice) and *leche* (milky juice). Both types are thirst quenching and taste similar to water chestnuts, for which jicama can be substituted.

Eat jicama slices as a raw vegetable or cooked like potatoes. One pound yields four servings. Store it in your refrigerator for up to two weeks.

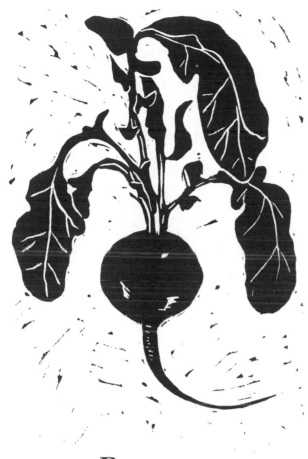

RADISHES

An early spring vegetable, but one that is on the market all year, is the radish. This cousin of mustard is usually red and round, and it has a mild bite. Also available are long red, long white, round white, and long black radishes. Each size and color of radish has its own degree of hotness.

One particular variety, *daikon,* is eight to ten inches long, white, and quite hot. This Japanese radish is generally grated for relish and salads, sliced for soup and stir-fried vegetables, or pickled whole. Another type, called *horseradish* or *German mustard,* is often ground and made into a pungent condiment.

Cherry-type *red radishes* should be firm, crisp, and have no insect or worm damage. Avoid spongy or woody ones. Large radishes are often pithy inside.

Use radishes as an appetizer, in salads, or cooked for soups and sauteed vegetable dishes. The tops, if they are present, are fine to cook as greens, although they may be a bit fuzzy or prickly.

Nutritionally, radishes offer small amounts of vitamin C, potassium, and other trace minerals. They are about 94 percent water.

Radishes keep best if the tops are removed. Refrigerate and use them within a week.

Radishes are native to China and have long been used in the cuisine of developed nations, including ancient Greece and Egypt. Today, four hundred million pounds of radishes are sold in the United States every year. They are grown commercially in California, Florida, Ohio, and Illinois, among other states.

✦ Nutritive Value: Appendix, 431.

RUTABAGAS

Rutabagas have smooth, tannish yellow skins with purple-crowned roots and bluish green, smooth leaves. They are thought to be a cross between turnips and cabbage.

The rutabagas available in grocery stores are often waxed to prevent moisture and weight loss, and they are usually sold without the leaves. Large rutabagas may be woody or fibrous, so select those of small to medium size.

Rutabagas cook in 5 to 15 minutes, depending on the size of the pieces. They must be peeled: first cut off the crown, then slice the vegetable into circles and peel the skin from each circle.

Besides serving them as a side dish, rutabagas can be mashed and added to pies, casseroles, and soups. Use them raw in salads or for hors d'oeuvres, cut into cubes, curls, sticks, or triangles. Try french frying rutabagas to arouse the curiosity of your friends and family.

Rutabagas are nutritionally similar to turnips, but they also have vitamin A and a good amount of calcium and vitamin C.

Store rutabagas in your refrigerator, where they will keep for a month or longer. Diced pieces ($1/2$-inch cubes) can be frozen without blanching.

✦ Nutritive Value: Appendix, 501.

SPINACH

Spinach is the most popular green for cooking, but it is also good raw in salads. The spinach variety that is sold fresh is *savoy*; it has wrinkled leaves. *Flat-leaved spinach* is generally frozen or canned.

Several other greens similar to spinach are Chinese spinach and tampala, used in Asia; Good King Henry (also called goosefoot or wild spinach); and New Zealand spinach, a triangle-leaved, sprawling plant that originated in New Zealand but is not in the same botanical family as common spinach.

When buying fresh spinach, look for crisp, springy, bright leaves and short stems. Avoid those with wilted, torn, or yellowed leaves, long stems, seed shoots, and excessively dirty roots. Spinach is available all year. One pound yields 4 cups raw or 1¹/₂ cups cooked, enough for 2 to 3 servings.

Spinach cooks in a very short time—5 to 8 minutes. To prepare it, rinse it several times in lukewarm (not cold) water to remove sand, then drain or shake off the water and steam the spinach, using only the water that clings to the leaves. Do not overcook spinach, or it will result in a mushy mess. Cooked and pureed spinach is excellent for soups, quiche, and homemade pasta.

Spinach is exceptionally high in vitamins A and C, calcium, and iron. However, it also contains oxalic acid, which can prevent calcium absorption. The iron in spinach is a type that is not readily assimilated by the body.

Spinach will keep for only two to four days, so refrigerate it in a plastic bag and use it as soon as possible. It can be frozen for long-term storage by blanching it in boiling water for about a minute and packing it into freezer containers.

✦ Nutritive Value: Appendix, 435–439.

SEA VEGETABLES (SEAWEEDS)

What are they?

Sea vegetables (seaweeds or algae) are the plants of the sea. They grow in a wide variety of sizes, shapes, and colors, ranging from microscopic to those that are hundreds of feet long; from flat and round to feathery and elongated; and from blues to browns. Unlike plants of the land, sea vegetables do not have flowers, tubers, or fruits—only fronds (leaves) and stems.

Most seaweeds are inedible, but some are quite palatable. The Japanese have been consuming sea vegetables for more than three hundred years and have over twenty different kinds in their cuisine. People in the British Isles and on the coast of New England have also incorporated sea vegetables into their diets. Today, many North Americans are learning to use seaweeds as vegetables and as food supplements.

Seaweeds grow wild in the ocean. Some cause surface waters to be green and slimy, or red as in the Red Sea. Others are farmed as agricultural products—the seeds are planted in empty clam shells and are shortly thereafter transplanted to large nets that are lowered into offshore waters. When mature, the plants are harvested with the use of large machines similar to hay reapers, then they are placed on racks or bamboo mats and dried.

The types of sea vegetables typically available or used in the food industry are:

- Brown—kelp, kombu, wakame (alaria)
- Green—sea lettuce
- Red—agar-agar, dulse, Irish moss (carrageenan), nori (laver)

They are usually sold as dried sheets or strips, powder, or flakes.

Another food that grows in water—but in lakes or ponds rather than the sea—is an algae called spirulina. It is used as a food supplement rather than eaten as a vegetable.

How do I use them?

Sea vegetables can be crushed or chopped and added to soups, casseroles, and salads. They are great with rice and seafood. You can also boil or steam them and eat as cooked green vegetables. Crumble or sprinkle dulse or kombu on pizza to simulate the taste of anchovies.

Be sure to clean and wash seaweed sheets and strips prior to cooking or eating to remove any sand or tiny shells that may cling to the fronds.

Some people, especially Westerners, are not accustomed to eating sea vegetables. To allow the intestinal flora to adjust to the new food, start by eating seaweeds in small portions, then gradually increase the amount you consume.

Sea vegetables are naturally salty—or have salt added—so you can eliminate other salts when you use them in cooking. Try sprinkling powdered kelp as a seasoning instead of salt.

How nutritious are they?

Sea vegetables are high in fiber and complex carbohydrates, so they add bulk to the diet. Most types provide a good amount of protein and are low in fat. Some of them also contain vitamin A, B-complex vitamins, and small quantities of vitamin C.

The real benefit of sea vegetables is their outstanding mineral content. The nutrients in water are absorbed through the seaweed fronds, so iron, calcium, phosphorus, potassium, and iodine are widely abundant in sea vegetables. The sodium content is also high, due to the salty sea water in which the plants grow.

✦ Nutritive Value: Appendix, 433, 434, 502–507.

How do I store them?

Dried sea vegetables will keep indefinitely if they are stored in moisture-proof containers. Powdered sea vegetables will lose some flavor during prolonged storage—which may be desirable because the taste is sometimes strong.

Agar-Agar

Agar-agar, or simply agar, is an extract of red seaweed. After harvesting, the flat, fernlike seaweed is washed and sun bleached. Its mucilage is strained and allowed to harden and dry in the sun. This becomes a papery, whitish clear product and is sold as bars, flakes, or granules. Agar-agar has virtually no taste or smell.

Industrially, agar-agar is used in the manufacture of silk, textiles, and foods such as ice cream, jelly beans, and preserves. In science and research it is used as a medium for growing cultures.

Agar can be used as a jelling agent. Boil 1 bar broken into pieces, or 3 tablespoons flakes, or 2 teaspoons granulated agar-agar with 4 cups liquid (water, fruit juice, or vegetable juice). It is a great substitute for Jello® or other gelatins derived from animal sources. Try agar-agar in jelled salads, light puddings or desserts, and jellies.

Agar-agar is mostly indigestible complex carbohydrates that pass through the body unchanged. It adds bulk and is considered a laxative.

The word *agar* comes from a Malayan term for alga. It is sometimes called *kanten*. Agar-agar has been commercially harvested in Japan since 1769. The Japanese had a monopoly on sales up to the mid-1940s. Agar-agar is now grown in California as well.

Algin

Algin, alginate, and *sodium alginate* are names of extracts from kelp that are frequently used in the food industry.

Algin is found in the cell walls of kelp. Alginate is the salt of algin, and sodium alginate is one of the four salts present. (The other three salts are ammonium alginate, calcium alginate, and potassium alginate.) Alginate acts as a gelatinizing and stabilizing agent in ice cream, yogurt, and other processed dairy foods; frozen desserts; and candy. Sausage casings are sometimes made of it, and it is occasionally used to thicken custards and puddings.

Scientific research during the 1960s found that alginate was able to absorb and eliminate strontium-90 from the body. Strontium-90 is a deadly radioactive isotope created by nuclear fission. It can concentrate in bones and body tissues. Alginate, however, is not utilized by the body and passes unchanged through the intestines.

Dulse

Dulse is a red seaweed with flat, fan-shaped fronds. It has been dubbed the "beef jerky of the sea" because of its chewy, stringy texture and salty taste. Dried dulse can be eaten raw; chopped or crumbled for salads, soups, and vegetable dishes; or twisted on a tong and roasted.

The use of dulse as a food dates back to the eighteenth century in the British Isles, where it was commonly eaten with fish, potatoes, and butter. Dulse grows in the North Atlantic Ocean near Maine, Scotland, and Wales.

Hijiki

Hijiki (also spelled *hiziki*) is a black, stringy sea vegetable that is often sauteed with vegetables or crumbled into soups and salads. It has a milder sea taste than dulse, kombu, or nori, and it blends well with many foods. Dried hijiki should be soaked in warm water for 30 minutes and carefully lifted out so that any sand or shells that have come loose stay at the bottom of the pan. The soaking process causes hijiki to quadruple in size.

Hijiki grows and is harvested off the coast of Japan.

Irish Moss

This red seaweed is also fernlike and flat. It is inedible when raw but can be cut up and added to soups or stews.

Most of the Irish moss sold or gathered is used as a thickening agent. Its jellylike substance, called carrageenan (also spelled caragreen), is popular in desserts, puddings, yogurt, sour cream, and other dairy products.

Unlike agar-agar, carrageenan will jell in cool (not boiling) water. Nutritionally, however, they are quite similar—they provide bulk but offer few nutrients.

Irish moss grows off the coast of Ireland, hence the name, but much of what is harvested comes from the Atlantic coast of Canada and the northeastern United States.

Kelp

Kelp is the fastest growing plant on land or in the sea. It can grow two feet a day and reach lengths of over one hundred feet.

After harvesting and drying, kelp that is to be sold for human consumption is usually powdered and put in capsules or sold as a mineral supplement or seasoning. Add powdered kelp to the salt shaker; mix it with beverages; or add it to casseroles, soups, crackers, or baked goods to give these foods a subtle sea flavor.

Kelp is farmed commercially in southern California and grows along the east and west coasts of the United States.

Kombu

Kombu, also called *tangle* and *sea cabbage,* is a brown seaweed that has been eaten by people in Russia, Wales, and Iceland for several hundred years. It is sometimes used as a chewing tobacco substitute. You can eat it as a raw vegetable or cook it with carrots, beets, and tomato sauce.

To make instant soup or stock, soak a strip of kombu in 3 cups water for 6 hours or overnight, then heat until the water boils. Remove kombu, and save the liquid stock in a jar in your refrigerator. Cleaned and dried kombu can be chopped and fried in oil with onions, peppers, and other vegetables, or it can be shredded and powdered for use as a seasoning.

This robust-flavored seaweed grows in the Arctic Ocean and off the coasts of Hawaii, Japan, the United States, and Europe.

Nori

Nori, or *laver,* is classified as a red seaweed; although it is bright lavender in water, it dries to a dark purple or black color, and turns green upon cooking or toasting. It is a thin, rubbery plant with a hearty sea taste.

Nori is widely used in Japan for sushi—rice, fish, and vegetables wrapped in the seaweed for a meal in a pouch. Nori sheets can be chopped or broken and added to soups and salads. To make a seasoning or garnish, toast nori and crumble it into or onto casseroles. Make sea bread by boiling 1 cup of nori in 2 cups water until it becomes jellylike. Cover it with oatmeal and fry it until brown.

Nori can be found off the coasts of Hawaii, Japan, Europe, and California.

Sea Lettuce

Sea lettuce is a bright green, ribbed plant that resembles leaf lettuce. It has a mild flavor and is good as a fresh, finely chopped salad green when it is picked at an early stage. Older fronds may be dried and added to soups.

Sea lettuce grows close to shore and is found along the west coast of the United States, Japan, and Hawaii.

Spirulina

Spirulina maxima is a blue-green microalga, or vegetable plankton, that grows in alkaline waters throughout the world. The plant grows in single cells that resemble filaments—tiny spiral wires—to about one millimeter in length.

Anabaena is also available. It is a blue-green microalga similar to spirulina, but it grows in fresh water.

Although spirulina is relatively new to North Americans, Aztecs ate it as a staple food, mixed with maize. They called it tecuilatl. Natives of the Sahara dry it with grains, vegetables, and seasonings to form dihé, practically a meal in itself.

Much of the spirulina on the market is sold in tablet or capsule form, often combined with other food supplements such as food yeast, comfrey, ginseng powder, and bee pollen. It is quite expensive.

This so-called miracle food is high in protein, vitamin A, B12 (the vitamin previously thought to be found only in animal products), calcium, phosphorus, iron, magnesium, and potassium. The protein makes up 60 to 70 percent of the product—30 to 40 percent of which is usable. It is low in fat and calories.

There have been reports of spirulina being imported to the United States that was contaminated with rodent hairs and insect parts. Most of it is imported, although a spirulina farm has been set up in California.

Wakame

Wakame, sometimes referred to as *alaria* or *fingers,* is a brown seaweed that grows sporophylls—fingerlike protrusions—that reportedly taste like peanuts.

To use wakame, soak it for 15 to 30 minutes, then strain it, saving the water for soup stock. It will swell to five times its dry size. Wakame can also be eaten as a fresh vegetable. Dice it (fresh or reconstituted) into 1/2-inch pieces and use it in salads, soups, or rice dishes.

Wakame grows in the northern coastal waters of Japan, Alaska, and the British Isles.

SQUASH

What is it?
There are two types of squash: the soft-skinned or summer varieties, and the mature, hard-skinned winter squash.

Summer Squash
The young, immature berries of certain varieties of squash used to be available only in summer, hence the name. They include:

- Caserta or Cocozelle—Like zucchini, these types of squash are dark green, although caserta is light-green striped and cocozelle is yellow striped. Both are best when they are six to eight inches long.
- Chayote—A green or white pear-shaped squash with deep, lengthwise furrows and slightly wrinkled skin. It is three to eight inches in length, and has a large soft inedible seed pit and solid flesh that tastes like a cross between cucumber and apple. Chayote is native to Mexico and Central America, where it is popular as a vegetable side dish, in salads, and pickled as a relish. It can also be added to soups and casseroles or served raw with salsa or other dips.
- Crookneck—One might easily think of a goose when observing crookneck squash. The best size for this type is eight to ten inches long. But, like zucchini, if it is allowed to keep growing, it may reach unwieldy dimensions.

- Scallop or Patty Pan—Light green to white colored, this rounded squash has scalloped edges and slightly bumpy skin. Pick ones that are four inches across or smaller.
- Straightneck—This summer squash is basically the same as crookneck, except for the shape of the stem end.
- Zucchini—By far the most popular summer squash, zucchini is a variety that was developed in Italy from cocozelle squash (also called vegetable marrow). It has dark green with yellow-striped or mottled skin and white flesh. Most commercial zucchini is four to nine inches long, although the prolific plant can produce zucchini the size of baseball bats. Its versatility is nearly unrivaled by any other vegetable. You can eat it raw in salads, marinate it, panfry or stir-fry it, stuff and bake it, puree it for soups or sauces, pickle it, and even make marmalade with it.

Buying tips

Summer squash is most tender when it is picked fairly small, in sizes noted above. Test it for tenderness by poking a fingernail into the skin; it should penetrate easily. Excessively large or mature summer squash has hard skin, dry or fibrous flesh, and hardened seeds. Smaller ones have soft-shelled, edible seeds—fewer seeds than large squash. Some types, such as zucchini, are on the market all year. One pound generally serves two to three people.

How do I use it?

Slice raw summer squash for salads, sandwiches, and appetizers. Chop and puree it for relishes and sauces. It is attractive and tasty in stir-fried vegetable dishes, and it can be dipped in tempura batter (or breaded) and fried. Try it in casseroles, omelettes, and shish kebabs.

How nutritious is it?

Nutritionally, summer squash has fair amounts of vitamins A and C, potassium, and calcium. It is mostly water (94 percent) and is very low in calories.

✦ Nutritive Value: Appendix, 440.

How do I store it?

Use summer squash as soon as possible. To store it, wrap it in a plastic bag and refrigerate it for three to five days. Cooked summer squash can be frozen.

You can also dry raw, thinly sliced squash in a food dehydrator for several hours or until leathery, then store the slices in a tightly closed jar. Used dried squash slices in soups or omelettes.

Winter Squash

By far the best-known type of winter squash is pumpkin. Other common types are acorn, banana, buttercup, butternut, hubbard, and warren turban. Mature squash is typically harvested in autumn and will, upon proper curing and handling, keep well into the winter months.

- Acorn—As the name suggests, this squash is shaped like an acorn (the seed of oak trees). It is sometimes called *table queen.* The skin color is dark gray and changes to green with an orange spot as it matures. It is ribbed, and is usually five to eight inches long and about five inches across the stem end.
- Banana—A large, elongated squash that, like a real banana, turns from green to yellowish brown (or orange). Banana squash is about nineteen to twenty-four inches long and about six inches in diameter.
- Buttercup—Also called *turban* because of the turban-shaped blossom end. It is about eight inches across the top and five inches long. The skin is dark green, with a light green or bluish turban. The bright orange flesh is usually quite sweet.
- Butternut—This squash does not resemble a real butternut; it is more bell shaped, or at least bottom heavy. The color of its very hard skin is pale orangish brown. Its size is usually nine to twelve inches long and three to five inches across. The seeds are concentrated in the bulbous blossom end, while firm yellowish flesh fills up the stem end.
- Delicata—An elongated yellowish orange or green and tan-striped squash with tender yellow flesh. It may also be called *Bohemian squash* or *sweet po-*

tato squash. The taste is similar to corn, although slightly sweet. To prepare, cut it in rings or chunks and bake it or steam it for 20 minutes. Delicata can be stuffed with apples, croutons, or mushroom and rice mixtures for casseroles.

- Golden nugget—A small round squash with an orange hard-ridged skin (like a small pumpkin). The flesh has a full squash flavor and is slightly sweet. This squash should be baked in halves or quarters. Bake, covered, for 20 to 25 minutes at 350° F.

- Hokkaido—A pumpkinlike squash named after a Japanese island. The skin may be bluish green or orange, with a smooth surface. The flesh is very sweet. Use it as you would acorn or buttercup squash.

- Hubbard—Named after Elizabeth Hubbard of Massachusetts, this large winter squash may remind you of Thanksgiving. The dark green or reddish orange pebbly skin and its large size—it looks sort of like an overgrown, swelled crookneck squash—make hubbard squash unmistakable. It can weigh up to thirty pounds and is usually baked.

- Kabocha—Another Japanese variety, kabocha squash is ball shaped and has a greenish gray skin. The flesh is sweet and rich tasting. It is excellent baked with butter and served as a side dish, or stuffed with vegetables for a main course. Use it as a substitute for sweet potatoes.

- Pumpkin—The Greek word for a large melon is *pepon,* and through French and English translations the word became *pumpkin.* Its fame is primarily due to its role as Halloween jack-o'-lanterns, but few would argue the popularity of pumpkin pie or pumpkin bread, pumpkin butter, pumpkin bars—even pumpkin ice cream!

  Fresh pumpkins are typically large—one to twenty-five pounds—and available from September to December. Most pumpkins are, of course, sold in October. A 5 pound pumpkin will yield 4½ cups of cooked and mashed pumpkin flesh.

- Spaghetti—A yellow-skinned, roundish or elongated squash (actually an edible gourd). When it is baked for 1½ hours at moderate heat, it results in stringy flesh that resembles spaghetti noodles. It can be served with butter and cheese or tomato sauce. A three-pound squash serves four people.

- Warren turban—A larger variation of buttercup, usually eight to ten inches long and twelve to fifteen inches across. The skin is bright orange-red and is sometimes striped and pebbly. It has a light blue turban.

Buying tips

Look for winter squash with clean, hard skins and no soft spots, decay, cracks, or bore holes. They should feel heavy for their size. Acorn, buttercup, and hubbard squash usually have yellowish orange "ground spots" that are considered to be indicators of maturity.

When you purchase cut portions of squash, such as a half of hubbard squash, look for white, clean seeds. The flesh should smell squashy, not moldy or peppery. Generally, 1 pound of raw squash will yield 1 cup cooked and mashed. Most types are available in fall and winter. Acorn and butternut squash are often available year-round.

How do I use it?

Winter squash is boiled or baked and eaten out of its skin, or it is mashed and added to other foods. To cook squash, wash and cut it in half, quarter it, or cut into several pieces. Remove the seeds, and boil or steam the flesh for 10 to 20 minutes or until tender. The pieces are easier to peel after cooking, but you must wait for them to cool off. Then the flesh usually slips right off the shell. It can now be mashed or pureed in a blender and added to baked goods (pies, cakes, cookies, casseroles, and so forth) or frozen for later use.

Acorn, buttercup, and hubbard squash are great to bake. Bake them whole for 1 to 1½ hours at 350°F. You can also cut them in half or into pieces, or cut off the top to make a cap. Scoop out the seeds and stringy pulp, then bake the pieces as is or stuffed with apples, sunflower seeds or nuts, rice and vegetables, or other foods.

Do you like pumpkin seeds? Try making your own. Roast the squash seeds on a cookie sheet for 5 to 10 minutes or until they begin to pop (not brown). Then remove them from the oven and let them cool. Eat them as a snack as you would sunflower seeds in the shell, or grind them in a blender and press the meal through a sieve to make pumpkin seed butter.

How nutritious is it?

Winter squash is an excellent source of both vitamin A and potassium. It provides notable amounts of vitamin C, calcium, and fiber, and it is fair in protein and carbohydrates.

✦ Nutritive Value: Appendix, 429, 430, 441.

How do I store it?

Freshly harvested winter squash will keep for about a month at room temperature. For long-term storage, it must be cured by holding it at 85°F for ten days, then storing it in a cool, dry place. It will keep for about three months.

It is important to handle squash gently because it bruises easily. Bruised areas will become soft and rotten. Do not refrigerate it or keep it below 50°F. Squash can get chill damage, and that affects the flavor.

TOMATOES

What are they?

The debate about whether tomatoes are a fruit or vegetable can be easily resolved: they are both. Botanically, they are fruits, the parts of a flowering plant that contain seeds. But then, so are peas, peppers, and pumpkins. Tomatoes are generally prepared as a vegetable—in sauces, ketchup, soups, or salads.

In the tomato (or Solanaceae) family you will also find potatoes, eggplant, peppers, tobacco, and deadly nightshade. Of tomatoes alone, some five hundred varieties are available, and thousands are known. They can be white, green, striped; square, bell, or vase shaped. The red, round varieties are the most popular, though, especially beefsteak and cherry tomatoes.

Many commercial tomatoes are picked and shipped at a mature green or pink stage, then they are ripened artificially in ethylene gas chambers. Some are ripened slowly in warm rooms out of di-

CANNED TOMATO PRODUCTS

We each eat, on the average, between fifty and sixty pounds of tomatoes per year—up from twenty to thirty pounds per person at the turn of the century. Most of this increase can be attributed to the wide availability of processed tomatoes.

According to the United States Food and Drug Administration, the following standards must apply to canned tomato products:

Tomatoes — Mature tomatoes, peeled and cored. Citric acid, calcium salts (which keep tomatoes firm), spices, salt, and flavoring may be added. Canned tomatoes are 5 to 6 percent solids. Solids are the amount of residue left if all of the water were evaporated.

Tomato juice—Liquid extracted from tomatoes, plus salt. It is 5 to 6 percent solids.

Tomato paste—Extracted liquid and pulp of tomatoes, which is concentrated to no less than 24 percent solids; baking soda, spices, salt, and flavoring may be added.

Tomato puree—Extracted liquid and pulp of tomatoes, which may or may not be concentrated. Salt is sometimes added. It is not less than 8 percent nor more than 24 percent solids (usually in the 10 to 12 percent range).

Tomato sauce—Extracted liquid and pulp of tomatoes, plus spices, sweetener, salt, vinegar, onion, or garlic. No standards exist for percent of solids, although the range is usually 10 to 12 percent.

rect sunlight; these are called *vine-ripened* tomatoes. Also available are greenhouse tomatoes and hydroponically grown tomatoes, which are usually "perfect" in shape and color and have the stem cap attached. Locally grown tomatoes are usually picked when red ripe.

SUBSTITUTING TOMATO PRODUCTS

You can substitute canned tomato products in some recipes, with certain alterations:

- 2 cups canned tomatoes, *or*
    1 pound fresh, simmered and seasoned
        For 1 cup tomato sauce

- ½ cup tomato sauce plus ½ cup water or other liquid, *or*
    ¼ cup tomato paste plus ¾ cup water or other liquid
        For 1 cup tomato juice

- 1 cup tomato sauce
    For 1 cup tomato puree (but reduce or don't add seasoning and salt)

- 1 cup tomato puree
    For 1 cup tomato sauce (but add seasonings)

- 1 cup tomato puree
    For ½ cup tomato paste (but subtract ½ cup liquid and reduce the amount of seasoning and salt)

Buying tips

As with other fresh vegetables, look for unpackaged tomatoes so you can examine them for bruises, dark or moldy spots, cracks, or other blemishes. Choose firm, well-shaped ones with a tomatoey aroma. The best time to buy tomatoes is in the late summer when there are peak supplies. Tomatoes available in winter and spring are imported from Mexico or are greenhouse grown. Greenhouse tomatoes are usually offered at higher prices than others.

How do I use them?

Round or beefsteak tomatoes are good for slicing, stewing, cooking, and canning. Green beefsteak tomatoes can be pickled, or fried as you would eggplant. Never eat raw green tomatoes, as they contain a toxin known as solanine.

Cherry tomatoes are usually reserved for salads and vegetable trays, or they are used as garnishes on casseroles. Italian (plum or pear-shaped) tomatoes are often made into paste because they are fleshy and have few seeds. Bell tomatoes are less common and resemble bell peppers. They are good for stuffing, as the centers are less pulpy than other types.

For maximum flavor, serve raw tomatoes at room temperature. More juice is retained if you slice tomatoes vertically, stem side up, rather than across the middle.

Tomatoes for home canning should have a pH of 4.6 or less; this indicates an acid content sufficient to prevent the growth of harmful bacteria. So-called low-acid tomatoes—usually yellow or orangish when fully ripe—are actually more acidic then red ones. Overripe tomatoes, however, have a lower acid content (higher pH) and are not recommended for canning.

How nutritious are they?

Tomatoes are well known for their high vitamin C content. Those that are picked while green or that were treated with ethylene gas have about one-third less vitamin C than tomatoes that were allowed to become red on the vine. Tomatoes used for commercial processing are usually picked when red ripe, so they may have more nutrients than tomatoes that are shipped green and sold as "fresh" tomatoes. "Low-acid" tomatoes are usually a bit higher in vitamin C than red tomatoes.

Vitamins A and B-complex, and the minerals potassium, magnesium, phosphorus, and calcium are present in tomatoes. Raw sauce, puree, and paste have proportionally less water and more nutrients by weight. Canned tomato products are often high in sodium because of the salt used in processing, although sodium-free products are readily available in most grocery stores.

✦ Nutritive Value: Appendix, 447–452.

How do I store them?

Green or pink (unripe) tomatoes will ripen at room temperature in a few days. Put them stem side down on a window sill or in a bag. Enclosing a banana or apple in the bag will hasten ripening, as these fruits give off ethylene gas.

Refrigeration is not recommended for tomatoes because cool temperatures (below 55°F) can adversely affect their taste. If you store them in your refrigerator, take them out an hour or so before serving.

Fresh whole tomatoes will normally keep for a week or two. One long-term storage technique is to put alternating layers of coarse salt and tomatoes in a wooden barrel, repeating the layers until the barrel is full. Space the tomatoes on the same layer an inch apart.

It is normally recommended, however, that tomatoes be stored or placed no more than two layers deep to prevent squishing. Stem caps should be removed so that holes are not poked into other tomatoes.

You can also freeze cooked or raw tomatoes. Frozen raw ones cannot be used for slicing, however, as they become mushy when they are frozen. Frozen whole tomatoes should be used within six weeks. Frozen pureed tomatoes will keep for up to one year. Use them for sauce and in soups, casseroles, or omelettes.

Where do they come from?

The origin of tomatoes has been traced to the Andes Mountains of Peru. The name, however, is from the Mexican (Mayan) term *xtomatl*.

The United States' annual commercial production of tomatoes is over two billion pounds. Another seven hundred to eight hundred million pounds are imported to the U.S. from Mexico every year. About 85 percent of the tomatoes sold domestically are grown in California. Three-fourths of these are processed into sauce, paste, and other products.

TURNIPS

Turnips are plants in the *Brassica* (cabbage) family that have white, purple-crowned skins, round or top-shaped roots, and thin, green, hairy leaves. They are cousins of rutabagas.

Look for firm, fairly small (two to three inches in diameter) turnip roots with no insect damage or major blemish. Large roots are often pithy, fibrous, or woody. Turnips are available year-round and are in peak supply October through March.

Cook turnip roots in boiling water for 10 to 20 minutes if they are sliced or diced, and for 30 minutes if they are whole. Turnips are good in soups and casseroles as well as for eating as a side dish. You can also make turnip kraut (like cabbage sauerkraut).

Turnip roots offer vitamin C, potassium, calcium, and small amounts of other minerals. They will keep for at least three weeks under refrigeration.

Like other green leafy vegetables, turnip leaves (also referred to as *turnip tops* or *turnips greens*) should be crisp, fresh, and have no insect damage. Avoid yellowed or limp tops.

Use turnip leaves as you would spinach, in salads, soups, or casseroles, raw or cooked. Turnip leaves are the highest-ranked vegetable in terms of nutrition. They are very high in vitamins A and C and calcium, and they contain potassium, magnesium, and B-complex vitamins.

Turnip leaves will stay fresh for less than a week. Refrigerate them in a closed plastic bag.

Turnips probably originated in Russia or Scandinavia, and they have been a staple food in the diets of northern Europeans for a long time. They are popular in the southern United States.

✦ Nutritive Value: Appendix, 453–455.

Other Foods

Carob

What is it?

A chocolate substitute? That is what carob has come to be known as, although it rightly deserves credit on its own.

The carob plant is an evergreen tree with dark green, glossy leaves and small, clustered, red flowers. Long brown pods form on the tree, which hold five to fifteen seeds within sweet pulp. These seeds are the source of *locust bean gum* (carob gum), an additive used in ice cream, cheeses, and confections to improve the texture by thickening and stabilizing the food.

After being sun dried, the seeds are removed and the pulp of the carob pods is ground into *carob powder* (also called *carob flour*). To make carob syrup, the powder is dissolved in water and boiled until it is the consistency of honey.

Carob confections have become quite popular in the natural foods industry. Some manufacturers mix carob with sweeteners, fat, and other ingredients to make carob chips, which are often used to replace chocolate chips. The same mixtures are used for carob candies; as coatings for nuts, seeds, or raisins; and for blocks of carob for baking or cooking purposes. Also available are powdered carob mixes that can be added to milk or other beverages.

How do I use it?

Carob is a naturally sweet addition to baked goods. Its taste is not as rich as chocolate or cocoa.

Carob powder can be used to supplement or replace sweeteners and chocolate in brownies and puddings. Some people prefer to combine carob and chocolate rather than using either one separately.

Use carob one-for-one as a cocoa substitute, but reduce the amount of sweeteners in the recipe by about one-fourth. Try adding carob powder to the dough of dark breads, such as pumpernickel or Russian rye, for extra color and flavor.

Carob powder is less soluble than cocoa, and it is gritty—that is, all the particles of carob powder do not dissolve, and sediments may remain in beverages or other foods. This problem can be minimized by making a smooth paste of carob powder and warm water before adding it to the other ingredients in a recipe.

How nutritious is it?

Carob is high in carbohydrates. It also contains calcium, phosphorus, and a trace of iron. The protein and fat levels are low.

In comparison to chocolate, carob has a very low fat content, no caffeine, and is less allergenic. It does, however, contain a notable level of tannin, as do cocoa, coffee, and teas. Tannin is an astringent that can bind elements together to form indigestible compounds when combined with protein.

✦ Nutritive Value: Appendix, 290.

How do I store it?

Store carob in a closed container in a dry place. Excess moisture will cause the powder to form lumps, making it harder to dissolve. If this happens, break or crush the lumps in a separate bowl before adding the carob to your recipe.

Where does it come from?

Carob originated in the Mediterranean region, from where most of it still comes. The trees grow to fifty feet and, after they reach maturity, they produce over one hundred pounds of pods each year. They thrive on dry soils and reportedly never need fertilizer or spraying against pests and diseases. The pods, however, may be fumigated after harvesting. Much of the carob that is harvested is fed to horses, mules, and pigs.

Legend has it that Saint John the Baptist once survived in the wilderness by eating locust beans (carob pods) and wild honey, hence carob's nickname of Saint John's bread. He might really have been eating the insects called locusts, though, since they have some resemblance to carob pods.

The seeds of the carob bean are very uniform in size, and it is thought that they were used as the standard carat weight for early goldsmiths.

CHOCOLATE/COCOA

What are they?

"Food of the gods" is what the Aztecs called cacao, or cocoa. The enticing taste of this food has been cherished for centuries in Mexico and the West Indies, and today it is one of the most popular ingredients in candies and baked goods.

The cacao tree is a tropical plant that grows to thirty feet and bears fruit from age four through forty years. The ripe pods are seven to twelve inches in length and dark red, brownish, or purple in color. Inside the tough, thick rind is a mass of slippery, whitish pulp that holds the cacao beans. About forty of these almond-size seeds are in each pod. They are very bitter and have no chocolate taste at this stage. Ten pods will yield approximately one pound of dry cacao.

After hand-picked harvesting, the pods are cut open to remove the pulp and bean seeds. The beans are placed in fermentation tanks to cure, during which time they become reddish and less bitter. Then the beans are cleaned, sorted, roasted, and cracked to remove their hard shells. These cocoa nibs are then ground into a thick, oily paste called chocolate liquor and blended according to the desired specifications of chocolate and cocoa manufacturers.

How are they made?

The types of cocoa products available are made as follows:

- Cocoa butter—Chocolate liquor is placed in a hydraulic press to extract this yellowish white oil. Although most of the cocoa butter obtained is used in the cosmetics industry, a portion of that procured is added to some chocolate products.
- Cocoa powder—The drier portion that remains after pressing cocoa butter from the chocolate liquor. This pressed cake is pulverized, sifted, and sold to be used in candies, syrups, and beverages.
- Dutch cocoa—Cocoa powder that has been processed with alkali (usually potassium carbonate) to neutralize the natural acids and to enhance the color of the cocoa powder. The name was given to this process because Dutch people developed it. Labels of foods containing this product may state "cocoa, processed with alkali."
- Imitation chocolate—A cheaper product being used in many foods that formerly contained pure chocolate. Rather than cocoa butter, imitation chocolate has vegetable fat added, such as coconut oil, palm oil, or palm kernel oil. This costs less and at times is more suitable for the food being made, due to the different melting points of cocoa butter and other fats. For example, the substituted fat may have a higher melting point, which is better for candy coatings so the confections won't melt in your hands. Products that contain imitation chocolate are often labeled "chocolate flavored" or "chocolatey."
- Milk chocolate—Sweet chocolate is mixed with dry milk solids, or sometimes milk or cream. It is also referred to as Swiss chocolate (it was developed in Switzerland) and is a favored coating and base for candy.
- Plain or bitter (dark) chocolate—The chocolate liquor is poured into molds and refrigerated to harden. The resulting unsweetened squares are sold for use in baking and cooking.
- Sweet or semisweet chocolate—Plain chocolate is mixed with cocoa butter and sugar, then poured into square and rectangular molds or dripped to form chocolate chips.

- White chocolate—Cocoa butter is sweetened with sugar or the meal of sweet chestnuts.

How do I use them?

Chocolate and cocoa are used predominantly in candies, cookies, cakes, ice cream, and beverages. They are invariably sweetened with some form of sugar to mask the natural bitterness. Cocoa powder is generally sweetened with an equal amount of sugar.

If you use chocolate squares or chocolate chips for recipes that require melting, be sure to melt them slowly over very low heat or in the top of a double boiler to prevent scorching and thickening. Grate or chop the squares first to speed up the process. Unless the directions state otherwise, do not add water or milk to the melting chocolate, as this would cause it to become hard rather than more liquid. If you want a thinner paste, melt vegetable shortening or cocoa butter with chocolate.

To make cocoa syrup, boil cocoa powder with water instead of milk to bring out the flavor. Chocolate cakes are reportedly brighter in color if cocoa powder is added to the batter before shortening or other fats.

You can substitute chocolate and cocoa products:

- 2 ounces (2 squares) plain chocolate = 6 tablespoons cocoa powder + 2 tablespoons fat or oil

and

- 1 ounce (1 square) plain chocolate + 7 tablespoons sugar and 2 tablespoons fat = 1 cup (6 ounces) chocolate chips

How nutritious are they?

Chocolate is about 50 percent fat, most of which is saturated. The fat content of cocoa ranges from 8 to 25 percent fat, depending on how much cocoa butter was extracted. Both chocolate and cocoa have 10 to 20 percent protein, carbohydrates, and negligible amounts of B-complex vitamins and vitamin A.

The minerals found in cacao products are magnesium, copper, potassium, phosphorus, iron, and calcium. Cocoa processed with alkali is often high in sodium.

The stimulants caffeine and theobromine are present in chocolate and cocoa. Also present are tannic acid, which can stunt growth in laboratory animals, and oxalic acid, which can block calcium absorption.

✦ Nutritive Value: Appendix, 327, 328, 460.

How do I store them?

Chocolate stored in a cool, dry place (50–60°F) will remain usable for 12 months. Storage beyond a year may result in a rancid or wormy product. Do not refrigerate, as moisture may collect in the container or package and affect the texture. Hot weather or excessive heat (over 75°F) will cause the cocoa butter to float to the top of chocolate squares or chocolate chips, and this makes the surface of the chocolate grey or white.

Keep cocoa powder in a cool, dry area in a tightly closed container. Too much moisture may cause lumping or mold growth, and cocoa stored beyond 6 months might lose flavor or become discolored and musty.

Where does it come from?

Although cacao was originally found in Latin America, most of the world's supply now comes from western African countries.

The Aztecs relied on cacao beans as their money. Spanish explorer brought cacao back to Europe, where English-speaking Europeans corrupted the name to cocoa.

EGGS

What are they?

Eggs are the round or oval-shaped reproductive cells of birds and reptiles. The eggs sold to North American consumers are from chickens; but duck, turkey, quail, turtle, and even ostrich and iguana eggs are eaten in other parts of the world. Consumers in the United States each eat an average of 235 eggs every year.

Hens (female chickens) and the eggs they lay are sometimes referred to by the environment from which they come. *Free-range* hens are those that are kept outside most of the year and scratch around

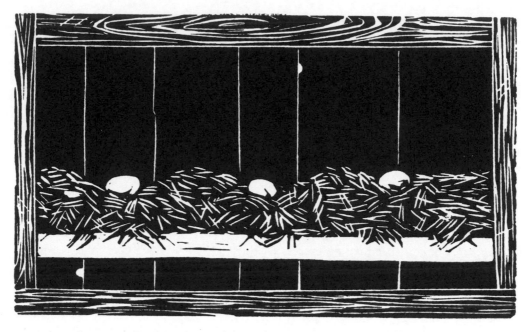

for insects and seeds to eat. *Fertile* eggs are those laid by hens that have been associating with roosters (male chickens). *Battery* hens are birds that are penned up in cages and fed grains and often growth hormones to stimulate egg laying, as well as antibiotics because the immobile birds frequently become sick. Most eggs sold in supermarkets are from battery hens. You can find free-range and fertile eggs in some food co-ops and natural foods stores.

Buying tips

Eggs are graded according to how they look when held in front of a bright light (a process known as candling). Those with small air cells, centered yolks, no cracks in the shell or dark spots in the yolk, and apparently thick whites are given a high grade (AA or A). Likewise, those with large air cells, off-centered yolks, cracked shells, and blood or meat spots are given a lower grade (B or C). There is no qualitative or nutritional difference between brown- and white-shelled eggs.

Several sizes of eggs are sold: jumbo, extra large, large, medium, small, and pullet or peewee. For price comparison, small eggs are economical if they cost one-fourth less than large eggs, and medium eggs are a good buy if they are at least seven cents per dozen less than large eggs.

How do I use them?

Eggs should always be cooked or fried over low heat, as the protein can become tough and plastic from high heat.

Hard-cooked eggs are preferable to hard-boiled eggs, as boiling may result in tough egg whites. Use eggs that are a few days old for best results. Cover eggs with water and heat until the water starts to boil. Then either cover and remove pan from heat and leave eggs in the pan for 20 minutes, or reduce heat so the water in the pan simmers but does not keep boiling, and leave eggs in the pan for 10 minutes. When time is up, rinse eggs under cold water and serve, or store in the refrigerator. (Mark the shells so the cooked eggs don't get confused with raw eggs.) For soft-cooked eggs, keep them in heated water for 1 to 3 minutes, then rinse under cold water. To prevent cracking of the shell during cooking, poke the large end of the egg with a pin, or add salt to the cooking water.

Do you know how to tell if an egg is hard-cooked or raw? Try spinning the egg—raw eggs wobble, while cooked ones spin around.

A test for determining if an egg is fresh or old and possibly rotten is to place it in a bowl of cool, salted water. The fresh egg will sink or stand on end, while the old or bad egg will float or bob in the water. To avoid the possibility of mixing spoiled eggs with other foods, crack and separate eggs one at a time into a different cup or bowl and add them to the other ingredients one at a time.

When a recipe calls for separating egg whites and yolks, try pouring eggs into a narrow-holed funnel. The whites should flow through while the yolks stay in the funnel.

Egg whites are easier to whip at room temperature, so remember to take eggs out of the refrigerator 30 to 45 minutes before using. Be sure to use clean, oil-free utensils and remove all traces of yolk in the whites before whipping. This can be done by dipping a wadded corner of paper towel into the whites, which will absorb the yolk but not the whites.

How nutritious are they?

Eggs contain all the amino acids necessary for complete protein synthesis in the body. Egg whites are mostly water and protein. Yolks contain protein as well as iron, phosphorus, potassium, and calcium. Vitamins A, D, and B-complex are present.

The fat in egg yolks is roughly one-third saturated and two-thirds unsaturated or polyunsaturated. The cholesterol level in eggs is very high and is the subject of much controversy regarding its possible effects on heart disease. Some nutritionists and doctors believe cholesterol is a major contributor to hardening of the arteries, but others in the medical profession claim a high level of cholesterol consumption has little effect on the net amount of cholesterol in the blood plasma. There is no conclusive evidence for either theory, although a substantial amount of research supports the claim that high cholesterol intake is hard on the heart.

✦ Nutritive Value: Appendix, 92–98.

How do I store them?

Keep raw eggs refrigerated, preferably covered in cartons to prolong freshness, and use them within a week. They will keep better if the shells are not washed, as washing can promote germ penetration.

Separated egg whites can be stored up to a week in a covered container, or frozen for up to six months. They freeze well in ice-cube trays, one per cube. Thaw them in the refrigerator before using.

EGG SUBSTITUTES

The cholesterol controversy of the last thirty years has prompted the manufacture and sale of egg substitutes that have little or no cholesterol. The imitation products are usually mixtures of egg white, nonfat dry milk powder, corn oil, vegetable lecithin, synthetic vitamins, and artificial flavor and color additives.

Egg substitutes can be used for baking and scrambling but not for poaching or cooking. They have been recommended for people on cholesterol-free diets, but they are not advised for people who are to abstain from all egg products, since the imitation food contains egg whites.

Leftover yolks will keep for two or three days if stored under cold water in a closed container in the refrigerator. Discard water before using the yolks.

LECITHIN

What is it?

Lecithin is a substance found in virtually all living organisms. Chemically, it is a mixture of diglycerides in stearic, palmitic, and oleic fatty acids joined with the choline ester of phosphoric acid. It is known as a *phosphatide* or *phospholipid* and is also referred to as *phosphatidyl choline*. Lecithin is sold as a goopy brownish liquid or solid yellow pellets.

Commercial lecithin is derived from egg yolks or soybeans, particularly from soybean oil during the refining process (see page 34, "Fats and Oils"). The human body also synthesizes lecithin.

Most commercial lecithin is used as an additive to stabilize and emulsify processed foods, such as baked goods, chocolate, frozen desserts, margarine, and salad dressings. It is also used in industrial products, such as soap, cosmetics, and paint.

How do I use it?

Lecithin is available in both liquid and granulated form. Liquid lecithin is an excellent substance to keep foods from sticking to pans; aerosol nonstick coatings are made from lecithin. It may also be added to home-baked cakes, cookies, and pie crusts.

Granulated lecithin is sold as a food supplement. It resembles millet seeds, although lecithin is more golden and appears waxy or oily. It has a nutlike flavor. Sprinkle it in beverages, on cereals, or in cake batters and other foods to help keep ingredients from separating.

How nutritious is it?

Lecithin has been promoted as a substance that helps break up cholesterol deposits by preventing fat from sticking to the arteries. It has also been cited as an aid for people with such ailments as neurological disorders, senility, arthritis, and fatty liver problems. Some health professionals claim there is no evidence that extra lecithin in the body, taken as a supplement, helps or hinders such ailments. It is not considered an essential nutrient, nor does it have any recommended dietary allowances.

How do I store it?

Commercial lecithin may contain some oil, so for long-term storage keep it refrigerated to prevent rancidity. It is handy to keep a small bottle of liquid lecithin near the stove to brush on your griddles and pans.

SALT

What is it?

Salt is a mineral found naturally in sea water. As a mineral, it is called *sodium chloride* and contains about 40 percent sodium and 60 percent chloride.

All salt is derived from the sea. Inland salt deposits, such as those found in Utah and elsewhere, are the remains of ancient oceans that dried up.

Salt has been used as a flavor enhancer and food preservative for thousands of years. People in the United States now use about one million tons annually for food preparation or processing, a figure which translates as four to fourteen pounds per person.

To be sold in the United States, food-grade salt must meet certain standards established by the Food and Drug Administration. It must be at least 97.5 percent sodium chloride. Another 2 percent can be anticaking agents that prevent the salt from lumping (keep it free flowing), such as silicon dioxide, yellow prussiate of soda (sodium ferrocyanide), green ferric ammonium citrate, or magnesium carbonate.

Iodized salt contains no more than .01 percent potassium iodide. Iodine is needed for proper thyroid functioning and was not widely present in the diets of most North Americans during the early 1900s. Iodized salt was considered necessary to prevent goiters. Iodine is now plentiful in the diets of people in the United States.

How is it made?

The salt that is processed for human consumption is obtained by several methods. In *solar evaporation,* sea water is pumped into large ponds and allowed to dry to a salt concentration of 3 percent; the water is supersaturated to 25 percent salt. At this point the water is drained and the salt crystals are harvested. The salt may also be dried in kilns at 300 to 400°F to kill any bacteria that might be present. Solar evaporation of salt takes five years. Only about 5 percent of the table salt sold in Canada and the United States is solar evaporated.

In a process known as *shaft mining,* a narrow passage, or shaft, is dug to the layer of earth where rock salt is deposited. This salt is then mined and crushed to different grades of coarseness. Most rock salt is used industrially, such as for highway and street de-icing, rather than for food purposes.

Finally, in *solution mining,* a well is drilled to the salt bed layer in the earth, and water is piped in to dissolve the salt, which forms a brine. This brine is piped to the surface, heated to precipitate impurities, filtered, and evaporated by steam heating. The resulting crystals are most commonly used for food-grade salt.

How do I use it?

Salt is an excellent natural preservative because it inhibits bacteria and mold growth in canned and pickled products, meats, and cheeses. It can control the rate of yeast development in breads, and it helps to stabilize colors, flavors, and textures of vegetables.

Unfortunately, we know how to use salt too well. Salt is present in just about every processed food on the market. For example, one large dill pickle contains nearly 5 grams of salt—over 1,900 milligrams of sodium—while a large raw cucumber contains only about 6 milligrams of naturally occurring sodium. Snack foods such as potato chips and pretzels are typically high in salt, but so are canned vegetables, dry cereals, packaged dry soups, and processed meats.

Besides all the salt found in processed foods, we add it to our cooking water for vegetables, to doughs and batters for baked goods, and to foods at the dinner table. Our taste buds soon forget how foods really taste if they don't taste salty.

The United States Dietary Goals, established by the Senate Select Committee on Nutrition, recommend that our consumption of salt and other sodium products be reduced from the present daily average of about 15 grams to 5 grams of salt—or about 1 teaspoon of salt—per day. We can try to do this by avoiding foods that are high in salt, by not adding extra salt to cooked foods, by experimenting with herbs and spices to enhance the taste of vegetables and meats, and by eating fresh raw fruits and vegetables.

If by chance you put too much salt in soup, stew, or chili, you can cut a raw potato into a few pieces and add them to the broth. The potato pieces will draw out the salt. Remove the pieces before serving.

How nutritious is it?

Salt contributes sodium, a mineral necessary for proper regulation of body fluids, for converting carbohydrates to fat, for ridding the body of carbon dioxide, and for heart and muscle contractions. Not enough sodium in the diet can result in symptoms similar to a heat stroke (usually caused by excessive sweating, which reduces the salt in the body). The symptoms include faintness, nausea, vomiting, weakness, and muscle cramps.

Too much sodium, on the other hand, may result in water-weight gain because salt can cause water retention and can make you thirsty. Swelling of the face, ankles, or hands may occur, or you may be short of breath when relaxing or upon slight exertion.

Excessive sodium consumption can also contribute to hypertension. Sodium constricts the small blood vessels, forcing the heart to pump harder and thus increasing blood pressure and the risk of heart disease. An estimated 25 million people in the United States have hypertension.

The chloride in salt is needed by the body to produce hydrochloric acid, the main digestive juice in the stomach, as well as to balance the body's acid/alkaline level and to stimulate the liver.

About .05 to 1 percent of food-grade salt consists of trace minerals (calcium, potassium, and magnesium), but in levels insignificant for nutritional purposes.

✦ Nutritive Value: Appendix, 461.

How do I store it?

Salt that contains anticaking additives (magnesium carbonate, et al.) will stay free-flowing indefinitely. If the salt does not have anticaking agents, add a few grains of rice to your shaker to absorb excess moisture. Keep larger quantities of salt in a tightly closed container and in a very dry place to prevent lumps.

Where does it come from?

Most food-grade salt sold in the United States comes from New York, Michigan, Ohio, Kansas, Utah, and California. Some is imported from France.

Many cities were built near salt beds or deposits, including Syracuse (New York), Detroit, and of course, Salt Lake City, Utah. Salt was used as payment for labor in ancient Greek and Roman civilizations, hence the word *salary*.

VINEGAR

What is it?

Vinegar is a liquid derived from fermented foods and is used primarily for pickles and salad dressings. Although vinegar can occur naturally, that which is sold commercially is processed to enhance the natural fermentation of sugars and to regulate the growth of bacteria.

The sources of fermentable sugar are grape wine for wine vinegar, apples for cider vinegar, grains or potatoes for malt vinegar, and molasses for sugar vinegar. The fermentable sugar is called the mash.

How is it made?

The traditional method of vinegar processing is the Orleans method. First, wine or apple cider that has turned hard is allowed to ferment with an equal volume of nonpasteurized vinegar. The liquids are placed in wooden barrels or small, enclosed vats until the proper level of acetic acid is formed (4 grams acetic acid per 100 milliliters). This process is rather slow—it takes four to six months—but the aroma and flavor of the resulting vinegar are considered to be superior to those of the vinegars produced by the quick method. In that method, the fermentation is done in generators that recirculate, pump, filter, and heat the mash until it attains proper acidity. After fermentation, the vinegar is allowed to age for several weeks in tanks or airtight wooden barrels, after which time it is filtered, bottled, and pasteurized.

Vinegar that is produced and sold as is retains its distinct aroma and flavor, and it has an amber color. This type is called *nondistilled vinegar. Distilled vinegar* is made by distilling off the alcohol produced by the fermented mash, and then converting this alcohol to acetic acid by adding special bacteria. Also available is cider-flavored vinegar, which is distilled white vinegar with a small amount of concentrated cider stock and some coloring added.

Gourmet cooks frequently use vinegars that have been flavored with aromatic herbs, such as tarragon, garlic, oregano, basil, thyme, and savory. These herb vinegars enhance salads, seafood, and sauces. You can make them yourself (see above).

Balsamic vinegar, another specialty product, is used to jazz up salads, vegetables, pasta entrees, and other recipes calling for red wine vinegar. It has a strong, sweet-sour flavor, so you need to use only a small amount. Balsamic vinegar is aged for

SEASONED VINEGAR

Seasoned vinegars are easily made by soaking herbs or spices in vinegar until their flavors accentuate that of the vinegar. Basil, tarragon, garlic, or dill, for example, can be used.

To every pint of vinegar, add 1 loosely packed cup of fresh, slightly crushed leaves or sprigs, or 2 teaspoons crumbled dry leaves, or 1 ounce crushed seeds or minced garlic. Allow the vinegar and herbs to blend for 3 to 4 days or until the desired taste of the herbs is attained. The slower the aging process the stronger the vinegar will be. Strain the mixture and seal the vinegar in a tightly capped jar.

ten years in red oak, chestnut, mulberry, and juniper kegs. It is made only in the Modena province of Italy.

How do I use it?

Make your own salad dressing by blending wine vinegar, oil, and herbs—or mix cider vinegar with mayonnaise—and pour it on fresh vegetables. Add sweetener to the vinegar mixture and use it to marinate vegetables or as the sauce for three-bean salad.

Mix 2 teaspoonsful each of cider vinegar and honey in a glass of water for a refreshing thirst quencher in the summer.

Vinegar for pickling should have 4 to 6 percent (40 to 60 grain) acidity. Vinegars with unknown acidity may cloud the liquid or cause improper pickling of the food. For light-colored pickles, use white distilled vinegar. Cider vinegar carries its flavor and color into the pickles, so it is good to use for spicy products or dark relishes but may overpower bland foods and fruits. If your pickling liquid is too tart, add more sugar rather than reducing the vinegar content.

Vinegar is also used to increase the acidity of

foods, such as tomatoes, in preserving and canning, and it thus helps to prevent growth of foodborne bacteria such as botulism. The pH of vinegar ranges from 2.4 to 3.4, which is very acidic. Most foods are in the pH range of 5 to 8, making them slightly acidic to slightly alkaline.

How nutritious is it?

Vinegar is a liquid, so it is mostly water. There are, however, some trace minerals present (calcium, iron, phosphorus, potassium), but in very insignificant amounts.

This low-calorie, low-carbohydrate condiment is excellent for people who are watching their weight and need an alternative to commercial salad dressings that are high in fat.

✦ Nutritive Value: Appendix, 462.

How do I store it?

Vinegar will keep indefinitely if it is stored in an airtight container. Cider vinegar may become cloudy or have dark residue at the bottom of the jar. This sediment is not harmful and can be mixed in or filtered out.

YEAST

What is it?

Yeast is a type of microscopic fungi that grows on plant sugars. The tiny, single-celled plant occurs naturally in honey, soil, tree sap, and on rinds or peelings of fruits such as grapes. It can grow by budding—one cell shooting out a bud as do leaves on tree branches—or sexually by spore formation within a mother cell.

There are about 350 different species of yeast, but the main one used for baking, brewing, and nutritional yeasts is *Saccharomyces*, "sugar fungus." The yeast is grown in factories under carefully controlled conditions to produce pure strains that will respond uniformly to temperature and humidity, unlike wild natural yeasts that might contain impurities or grow sporadically.

The two main functions of commercial yeast are for fermentation and for growing nutrients. Fermenting yeasts include those used in baking and in brewing wine or beer. Nutrient-growing yeasts produce vitamins, enzymes, amino acids, and other microbial nutrients used in scientific research studies as well as for human or animal consumption.

How is it made?

Baking and nutritional yeasts are grown by introducing pure strain cultures of yeast into a sugar medium. Beet or cane molasses is typically used, although the medium can also be starch from potatoes or grains, or whey (the liquid by-product of cheesemaking).

The yeasts grow on the medium and cause it to ferment, and this converts the sugar to alcohol and carbon dioxide. When fermentation ceases, the liquid yeast is washed and concentrated by separators to become yeast cream. After refrigeration, the yeast cream will become one of three types of yeast:

- Active dry—After the removal of excess water, the yeast cake is pressed into thin threads and is dried under controlled temperature and humidity to a moisture content of 5 to 8 percent.
- Compressed—Excess water is pressed out of the yeast cream, resulting in a spongy cake of yeast.

  Compressed and active dry yeasts are refrigerated to prevent further yeast growth during storage. Some active dry yeast is packaged under nitrogen gas into laminated aluminum foil envelopes and does not require refrigeration.
- Nutritional yeast—The yeast cream is pasteurized to stop further yeast growth, dried in huge drums, then ground into textures ranging from flakes to fine powder. It is a pale yellow color and has a distinct but pleasant aroma. Nutritional yeast needs no refrigeration.

Two other types of yeast are available to consumers:

- Brewer's yeast—left over from the beer-brewing process. The original yeast is grown on barley malt, rice, corn or corn syrup, and hops. After brewing, the yeast is removed from the vats, debittered (to get out the hops flavor), and dried into a powder. The resulting product is a "spent" or dead yeast that is quite nutritious. Brewer's yeast is sold as a food supplement, usually in capsules or mixed with other vitamin and mineral supplements.

- "Food" yeast—may be one of several yeast strains: *Torulopsis utilis* (torula yeast) or *Candida utilis*. Torula yeast is a product grown on food-grade ethyl alcohol, which is obtained as a by-product of petroleum refining and paper making. Torula yeast is added to processed foods, such as dessert toppings and pastries, and it is used as a meat substitute in imitation meat products or as a meat extender. Known in the industry as Torutein®, torula yeast is over 50 percent protein—high in the amino acid lysine—and relatively inexpensive to produce. These two factors account for its increased popularity in the food industry. *Candida utilis* may be grown on pine chips and marketed as torula yeast. Its tastes very bitter.

How do I use it?

Baking yeast is used as a leavening agent to make bread dough rise. It also makes the product more digestible and flavorful.

Upon mixing baking yeast with warm (105–115°F) water and a small amount of sweetener, it will again grow and cause the sugar to break down. The resulting carbon dioxide gas forms air bubbles, and this causes the dough to rise.

A ⁵⁄₈-ounce cake of compressed yeast is equivalent to a ¼-ounce envelope *or* 1 scant tablespoon of active dry yeast.

Never use water that is hotter than 140°F, as the yeast will become inactive above that temperature.

Honey, molasses, or sorghum can be used as the sweetener. Don't eat dough that contains baking yeast, because yeast could grow in your stomach and cause intestinal problems.

Nutritional yeast is considered a "dead" yeast and will not work for leavening. It is a food supplement and can be added to baked goods, casseroles, beverages, and snacks. It is great as a seasoning on popcorn and is good mixed with fruit juices.

How nutritious is it?

Nutritional and food yeasts are 40 to 55 percent protein and contain all of the essential amino acids needed for complete protein utilization. They are very high in B-complex vitamins and provide many trace minerals, including iron, phosphorus, and potassium.

✦ Nutritive Value: Appendix, 463, 464, 509.

How do I store it?

Compressed yeast is highly perishable, so keep it refrigerated and use it within six weeks. You can freeze it for longer storage—up to six months—but defrost it at room temperature or in the refrigerator overnight, then use it the next day.

Active dry yeast sold in jars or in bulk at food stores will keep at room temperature for fourteen months if it is tightly sealed. Once opened, however, it should be refrigerated. It will remain active for two years.

Keep nutritional yeast in a tightly closed container. It will last indefinitely.

DIETS

VEGETARIAN DIET

In the last two decades, the vegetarian diet has become widely accepted and more commonly practiced throughout the world. An estimated 5 to 10 percent of the people in the United States consider themselves to be vegetarian. Many more have experimented with a meatless diet, and an ever-increasing number of people are reducing their consumption of red meat. Vegetarian entrees are now offered in many restaurants in North America, particularly in towns and cities that also have natural foods stores or food co-ops.

What is a vegetarian diet?

A vegetarian diet consists of foods from plants generally classified as vegetables (from which the word *vegetarian* derives), as well as fruits, grains, legumes, and nuts. Dairy products and eggs are also consumed by some vegetarians.

Various terms are used to describe people who limit their diets to particular foods:

- Fruitarian—One who eats only plant foods that allow the plants to continue living. These include fruits, berries, nuts, and certain vegetables. Some fruitarians eat only raw food, believing that heat from cooking or baking destroys too many life-giving properties in the foods.
- Lacto-ovo vegetarian—One who eats plant foods as well as dairy products and eggs (*ovo* refers to ovum, or egg).
- Lacto-vegetarian—One who eats plant foods as well as dairy products (*lacto* is a Latin word for milk).
- Vegan—One who eats foods solely of plant origin. No dairy products, eggs, or honey (from bees) are consumed.

Between lacto-ovo vegetarians and meat eaters come *semivegetarians, pisco-vegetarians,* and *protovegetarians.* Semivegetarians are vegetarians usually, although meat is eaten at social gatherings, restaurants, and/or occasionally at home. Pisco-vegetarians are people who generally eat a vegetarian diet but also include fish (Latin: *piscis*) and/or poultry, but no red meat. Finally, protovegetarians are those who are in transition, phasing out or cutting back on animal products.

Why choose a vegetarian diet?

Reasons for eating a vegetarian diet are as varied as the types of vegetarians. They include:

Health—Probably the main rationale for restricting or reducing meat consumption is the belief that one will be healthier by doing so. Red meat consumption has been criticized by health professionals, who claim it contributes to heart disease, cancer, and other ailments. Animal and fish products are also more susceptible to food-poisoning bacteria than are plant foods. In addition, some people are allergic to or have a dietary intolerance for proteins or sugars in animal products, especially milk. Some people are also leery of eating meat because of antibiotics, growth hormones, and the high pesticide residues that may be found in meat.

Economic—Historically, meat and other animal products have been more expensive than plant foods. During the early 1970s some U.S. consumers boycotted meat in an attempt to bring the prices down. People on limited or fixed incomes may be de facto vegetarians because they can't afford meat.

Environmental—The croplands used for growing grains consumed by animals could more efficiently be used to grow food for direct human consumption. As pointed out in Frances Moore Lappé's classic book, *Diet for a Small Planet*, by eating certain plant foods one can obtain complete protein and thus eliminate the need for meat, which would in turn (theoretically) free more land to grow food for people. (See pages 71, 112, and 203 for more information on protein.) This argument is even more poignant when one considers the destruction of tropical rainforests in Central and South America, carried out for the sole purpose of clearing the land to raise cattle that often end up as hamburgers in fast-food restaurants.

Another argument against meat raising is the amount of methane gas produced by belching cows and manure piles. Methane gas is thought to contribute to the greenhouse effect. Agricultural runoff from cattle operations also pollutes streams and results in excessive water weeds and nitrates, thereby affecting fish habitat and contaminating drinking-water supplies.

In some areas, catching or digging fish and shellfish are restricted due to heavy metal concentration or bacterial contamination. In the 1950s, about 1,200 people in Japan were poisoned by seafoods from Minamata Bay because of the high levels of methylmercury, an industrial waste product; this epidemic became known as "Minamata disease." Harvesting of clams, oysters, and other shellfish products in the Puget Sound is regularly curtailed or banned due to excessive undesirable bacteria.

Humanitarian—Animals are living creatures and therefore have a right to keep living instead of being slaughtered and eaten by humans. This respect for life frequently extends to chickens raised three or more to a small cage, dairy cows and calves confined by stanchions and small pens, and other practices considered inhumane by animal-rights activists, who therefore refuse to eat any meat, eggs, or dairy products. Taken to an extreme, some militant vegetarians have scrawled "Meat is Murder" on public structures, modified billboards that advertised steak restaurants, brought cows into McDonald's

establishments, and picketed stores that sell fur coats—all to promote their beliefs (or to polarize the meat-eating public against them, depending on how outrageous their direct-action tactics were).

Religious—Scriptures from the Bible, the Koran, and other holy books are considered God's or Allah's messages to people to not eat animal products. The Seventh Day Adventists are probably the best-known Christian vegetarians, while Moslem, Hindu, Buddhist, Jewish, and other religious groups also have special dietary practices, such as no pork or only kosher foods. Catholics restrict their consumption of meat during Fridays in Lent, often substituting fish instead.

Cultural—Anthropological studies have found tribes and societies throughout the years who apparently ate no meat. (There have, of course, been many records of meat eaters, too.) The traditional diet of India is, for the most part, vegetarian. A few decades ago, culturally-ignorant people used to joke sarcastically that the starving people of Bangladesh should eat their sacred cows—not realizing that the cows were (and still are) a main life-support system, providing considerable amounts of dairy products and dried dung used for heating fuel.

Philosophical—Throughout the years, eminent figures have advocated or practiced vegetarianism. Pythagoras, known as the "father of vegetarianism," is occasionally quoted, as are George Bernard Shaw, Sylvester Graham (the inventor of graham crackers), Henry David Thoreau, and Mohandas Gandhi. Adolf Hitler was also rumored to be a vegetarian, although this has been disputed.

Fashion—Performers such as Michael Jackson, Paul and Linda McCartney, and Madonna are or were vegetarians, so people who want to emulate celebrities may modify their diet accordingly. Occasionally a fad diet will call for a meatless regimen, which will result in temporarily vegetarian weight-loss hopefuls. Some people claim that a vegetarian diet helps people lose weight or stay trim, but that's a matter of opinion.

Political—Events such as labor disputes and subsequent boycotting of a meat-packing company may make people think twice about eating meat. On a broader scale, this may lead them to withhold support for a meat marketer who mistreats its workers, has a history of corporate irresponsibility, or has increased its concentration or attempted monopolization of the meat industry.

Personal—Some people dislike the taste or smell of cooked meat. Others may have never learned to prepare it, or they may simply refuse to eat meat because of unpleasant experiences with animals or from a debilitating illness caused by eating contaminated meat. An outbreak of *E. coli* bacteria at a fast-food burger restaurant in Seattle resulted in several deaths and many illnesses; many people have suffered from milder forms of food poisoning after eating improperly prepared chicken, fish, or other flesh foods.

Whether or not you are—or choose to become—a vegetarian, it is wise to be tolerant of others who, for whatever reason, choose to eat differently than you. Criticism tends to solidify people's beliefs rather than change them; encouragement, example, and explanations allow people to decide what is best for themselves. Eat to your heart's content—literally.

MACROBIOTIC DIET

The word *macrobiotic* means great *(macro)* life *(biotic)*. The word implies an encompassing of all the things around us, although when some people hear or see the word—particularly those who eat standard North American fare—they may think it's a diet with seemingly limited (and rather weird) kinds of foods.

The concept of macrobiotics began in Japan about one hundred years ago, when a Western-trained doctor, Sagen Ishizuka, cured himself of a supposedly incurable disease. He studied ancient medical texts of the Japanese and Chinese that discussed how food caused and cured illnesses. His studies resulted in a book, *Shoku-Yo: A Chemical Nutritional Theory of Long Life* (1897). He became known as "the doctor who cures with food."

George Ohsawa, a student of the Shoku-Yo theory, cured himself of tuberculosis and in 1956 introduced the concept to the West. Ohsawa expanded the theory to include Taoist beliefs and coined the term *macrobiotics: the great art of life.* Michio and

FOODS COMMONLY EATEN IN A MACROBIOTIC DIET

ADUKI BEANS (AZUKI, ADZUKI)—Small red beans about the size of lentils (see page 100).

MISO—A fermented paste made from soybeans and/or grains, used as a condiment and flavoring agent (see pages 105–106).

SEAWEEDS (SEA VEGETABLES)—A variety of plants harvested and eaten fresh, cooked, or dried. These include hijiki, a black, stringy, mild-tasting plant often crushed and added to soups; dulse, a red, chewy, salty seaweed; and wakame, a brown, finger-like plant used in salads and stir-fry dishes (see pages 172–175).

SEA SALT—Salt that remains after sea water has evaporated. It reputedly contains more trace minerals than salt mined and refined from earth deposits (see pages 187–189).

TAMARI (ALSO CALLED SHOYU)—A natural soy sauce used to flavor foods (see pages 106–107).

TOFU—A white, soft cake of curdled soybean milk, used for a variety of preparations (see page 104–105).

UMEBOSHI—A pickled, very salty plum used to season soups and as a condiment (see page 64).

Aveline Kushi further developed and promoted this diet and have taught and published numerous books on the subject.

What is a macrobiotic diet?

At the heart of macrobiotic philosophy is the concept of balance. To maintain balance one must choose elements in life that accommodate change. All elements in life are believed to represent a duality represented by *yin* and *yang* elements: cool/hot, weak/strong, expansive/contractive, acid/alkaline, feminine/masculine, and so forth. The macrobiotic philosophy states that when the forces of yin and yang are at an equilibrium, we are balanced—that is, healthy.

Macrobiotic practice emphasizes the importance of diet in our lives. It recommends organic, locally grown foods eaten in season and with the goal of establishing a balance between yin and yang elements. Foods are generally classified as follows:

- Yin (expansive): vegetables, fruits, beans, and nuts
- Extremely yin: refined sugars, coffee, and drugs
- Yang (contractive): grains, seeds
- Extremely yang: animal products (cheese, fish, meat), salty foods

Balance results when, for example, vegetables (yin) and grains (yang) are eaten together. The more extreme a food is, the more desire there is for a food at the other extreme, such as sweets (cookies, candy, desserts) and meat—typical foods in the diets of most North Americans. Even though these foods balance each other on the yin/yang scale, it is believed that they put more stress on the body and thus may cause or contribute to diseases. A macrobiotic goal is to maintain a steady, moderate balance rather than to swing from one extreme to the other.

Early teachers of macrobiotics were from Japan and ate foods native to their country. These foods—rice, tofu, miso, seaweeds, aduki beans—were therefore considered to be what constituted a macrobiotic diet. But because one of the tenets of macrobiotics is to eat food grown locally and in season, the macrobiotic diet has in the past twenty years expanded to include other grains and beans, more vegetables and fruits, and nuts and seeds native to the country in which the person practicing macrobiotics resides.

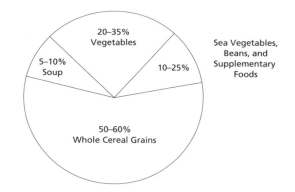

STANDARD MACROBIOTIC DIETARY APPROACH

Macrobiotic dietary recommendations

The following guidelines are adapted from *Macrobiotics—Standard Dietary and Way of Life Suggestions*, an information sheet by the East West Macrobiotic Foundation of Baltimore, Maryland.

1. Whole-cereal grains: 50–60%

    Cooked whole-cereal grains include brown rice, barley, millet, oats, corn, rye, wheat, and buckwheat. Only a small percentage should be noodles, unyeasted breads, and other flour products, as these are considered difficult to digest.

2. Soup: 5–10%

    One or two bowls per day of miso or tamari-broth soup, with some vegetables and seaweed added, is recommended.

3. Vegetables: 20–35%

    Each meal should include vegetables: two-thirds cooked by steaming, baking, or sauteing; one-third boiled or pressed or as raw salad. Recommended vegetables are cabbage, kale, broccoli, cauliflower, collards, pumpkin, watercress, bok choy, greens, carrots, and other local products. Not recommended are plants in the nightshade family (potatoes, yams, tomatoes, eggplant), asparagus, beets, zucchini, or avocado.

4. Beans and Sea Vegetables: 5–15%

    Cooked beans, notably aduki, chickpeas, and lentils are recommended; eat others only occasionally. Eat seaweeds, such as hijiki, kombu, wakame, nori, dulse, and Irish moss, in soups, with vegetables, or as side dishes.

5. Supplementary Foods: 5–10%

    Once or twice a week eat white-meat fish, fruit desserts (locally grown fruit only), roasted seeds for snacking, and foods made with rice syrup or barley malt.

6. Beverages

    Tea is recommended, especially bancha twig tea, roasted grain tea, and dandelion tea.

7. Foods to Avoid

    Avoid meat, eggs, poultry, animal fat, all dairy products, tropical fruits and juices; sodas, coffee, peppermint tea; artificially colored, flavored, sprayed, or treated foods; refined grains; mass-produced (canned, frozen) foods; hot spices; and artificial vinegar.

8. Additional Suggestions

    Use only unrefined sesame oil or corn oil, in moderate amounts. Use sea salt, shoyu, miso, and umeboshi plums. Cook everything. Attend macrobiotic cooking classes.

THE PYRAMID DIET

First there was the Basic Seven—food groups with recommended daily servings for each of the seven categories. Then the United States Department of Agriculture condensed it to the Basic Four. Now there's the Food Guide Pyramid, brought to you by the USDA and the Department of Health and Human Services.

The Basic Seven food groups, as promoted in the 1950s, were as follows:

1. Meat, eggs, dried peas, and beans
2. Dairy products, excluding butter
3. Green leafy and yellow vegetables
4. Citrus fruits, tomatoes, and raw cabbage
5. Potatoes and other vegetables and fruits
6. Breads and cereals
7. Butter and fortified margarine

To simplify this, the Basic Four was devised and popularized in the 1960s:

1. Meat group, including beef, veal, pork, lamb, poultry, fish, and eggs, with alternates such as dry beans and nuts—2 servings per day

2. Milk group, including cheeses, ice cream, and yogurt—2 to 4 cups of milk per day (more for children and teenagers)

3. Vegetable and fruit group—4 or more servings per day

4. Bread and cereals group, with recommendations for whole grain, enriched, or restored products—4 or more servings per day

During the 1970s, a fifth group was added, with words of caution: Fats and sweets—high in calories, low in nutrients.

The diets of many North Americans have changed significantly in the last fifty years. The food made and eaten at home now is often bought pre-processed and packaged for quick preparation. Consumption at fast-food restaurants has soared. Nutritional deficiencies show up as excesses such as obesity, heart disease, and tooth decay, all of which have been on the rise in the last fifty years. To try to reverse our declining standard of dietary living, the USDA formulated the Food Guide Pyramid, a more graphically understandable approach to educating consumers about healthy food choices.

The Food Guide Pyramid, first published in 1992, incorporates the Dietary Guidelines for Americans, which are based on advice from nutrition scientists and are now part of a federal nutrition policy. These guidelines are:

- Eat a variety of foods.
- Maintain healthy weight.
- Choose a diet low in fat, particularly in saturated fat and cholesterol.
- Eat plenty of vegetables, fruits, and grain products.
- Use sugars, salt, sodium, and alcoholic beverages in moderation.

The Dietary Guidelines alert people to the fact that certain foods, even though they are in a basic food group, contain high levels of undesirable substances. Many cheeses, for example, are high in saturated fat. Liver and eggs provide significant amounts of dietary cholesterol. Sweeteners and salt are processed into many commercial products and are therefore less detectable.

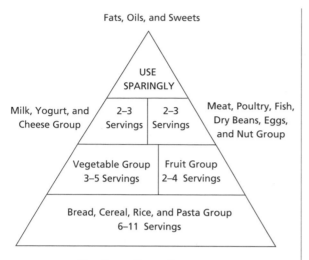

THE FOOD GUIDE PYRAMID

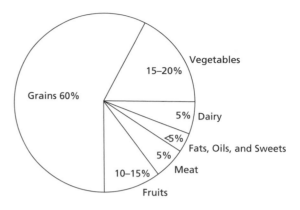

THE FOOD GUIDE PYRAMID, PRESENTED AS A PIE CHART, IS SIMILAR TO THE CHART FOR THE STANDARD MACROBIOTIC DIETARY APPROACH (SEE PAGE 194).

Ironically, the foods to be used sparingly are at the top of the pyramid. Given society's tendency to perceive vertical hierarchy as better, this may have been a dubious choice in graphic design. Nor is there mention of caffeinated beverages, particularly coffee and soda pop, and the effects of caffeine on the body. Some dairy and meat producers (and lobbyists) weren't particularly pleased with the place that their products occupy on the pyramid.

The Dietary Guidelines strongly urge people to limit their total fat consumption to 30 percent of total calories; saturated fats should only make up one-third of that, or 10 percent. The guidelines also suggest limiting intake of dietary cholesterol to 300 milligrams or less per day (one egg yolk contains 213 milligrams); sodium to 3,000 milligrams or less per day; and added sugars to no more than 6 teaspoons a day (if your total caloric intake is 1,600 a day).

In order to determine if you meet, exceed, or fall short on any of the guidelines, record all the foods and beverages you consume, then measure the fat, cholesterol, sodium, and sugar. These mea-

surements should be done over a certain period of time (a week or a month) then averaged and compared. If you find that your diet is deficient or excessive in any foods or nutrients, you can then alter your diet and retest yourself after several months on the new plan.

The Food Guide Pyramid and Dietary Guidelines for Americans will probably be superseded by another system of food groupings and recommendations after more studies in nutrition science and eating habits are conducted. Statistics published by the USDA indicate that per capita consumption of fats and sweeteners continued to increase during the 1980s and early 1990s. By the year 2000, with continued publicity about reducing intake of these substances, we may see some numbers sliding down the pyramid. By 2010, the government may be warning us (too late) about the dangers of genetically engineered or irradiated foods and long-term consumption of growth hormone residues in dairy products. It's up to us as consumers to change our diets for the better, and to keep watch on those who want to alter foods under the guise of scientific advancement.

NUTRIENTS

What are they?

Nutrients are substances or elements that provide nourishment. They are chemicals and compounds that have specialized roles in maintaining and sustaining our health. Nutrients are energy givers, bone builders, blood makers, and waste eliminators, working together to keep us alive.

The four basic elements needed by all plants and animals, including humans, are:

- Air—Clean air fills our lungs and pores with oxygen. The first nutrient a newborn receives is air. In some traditions, air is associated with clarity, the direction north, and winter.
- Light—Sunlight improves the human disposition. In measured doses, it helps maintain healthy skin and regulates our internal and external clocks according to the day/night cycle. The second element received by a newborn is often light. Some traditional societies associate light with new ideas, energy, the direction east, and spring.
- Earth—Soil, dirt . . . the stuff that we walk on, plants grow from, and to which our bodies return. The earth provides us with most of our food. As an element, it is associated with growth, endurance, the direction south, and summer.
- Water—Pure water quenches thirst and keeps our blood flowing. A newborn is usually given mother's milk, a form of water, soon after birth. Water is associated with fluid power, connectedness, the direction west, and autumn.

From a whole-life perspective, these four elements are essential nutrients. At the present time, air and light are still "free" elements. Water, however, has become a marketable item, along with substances from the earth. Nutrition classes and textbooks typically give the most attention to the earth element—that is, individual vitamins, minerals, fats, proteins, and carbohydrates that can be isolated or synthesized from plants and animal substances.

Many other essential nutrients, are as yet immeasurable by scientific instruments or have not been assigned Recommended Daily Allowances. These include: physical activity and exercise, touch, friendship, laughter, affection, sexual pleasure, psycho-spiritual connectedness, solitude, communing with nature, having fun, and a myriad of interpersonal "vitamins and minerals." While we can't currently buy a supplement to heal a broken heart or resolve a conflict with a co-worker or family member, we can at least be aware of physical, social, and emotional nutrients we personally need. For example, it is good to try to alleviate stress by maintaining a healthy diet of nutrition-rich foods and taking care of the body in relaxing ways, such as by receiving massages, as well as to endeavor to change the situations or attitudes that perpetuate undesirable or destructive stress. Popping B-complex vitamin pills may reduce irritability, thus enabling us to better cope with stress. Taking a vacation would probably help, too, as would earning a living by doing something we enjoy rather than despise.

Assessing nutritional needs

Nutritionists and dieticians currently use certain techniques to determine the adequacy of individual and institutional diets. The most common assessment method is recording the food intake of an individual, measuring the composition of that food in terms of calories, protein, minerals, and vitamin content, and then comparing the measurements to the Recommended Dietary Allowances. The RDAs, established in 1941 by the Food and Nutrition Board of the National Research Council–National Academy of Sciences, are based on age, sex, weight, and activity level. The RDAs have been revised several times in the last thirty years.

Some nutritionists or health practitioners assess trace minerals by hair analysis. A small quantity of hair is cut from the back of the neck and sent to a laboratory that analyzes the levels of both desirable and potentially toxic minerals. It is believed that mineral deficiencies or excesses show up in the hair and would therefore be present throughout the body.

Nutrient levels (or secretions) may also be determined by urine and fecal analysis and by blood samples. Cholesterol, in particular, is measured from serums in blood.

Other less popular and sometimes controversial methods are employed to determine the adequacy of an individual's diet or overall health. Iridology, muscle testing, blood-type categorizing, and comparing physical traits or characteristics with an established norm are some of the methods. The self-reporting of a person seeking medical assistance can often provide clues about their nutritional status. For example, someone who complains of kidney pains may be eating too much fat or salt or not drinking adequate amounts of water.

You can try to assess your own nutritional and health status by paying attention to the following factors:

- Energy level—Do you generally feel alert and spunky, or are you chronically exhausted?
- Skin condition—Does your complexion glow and show good color, or is it dull, blotchy, scaly, or prone to rashes and acne?
- Hair condition—Is your hair shiny, vibrant, and bouncy, or is it dull, oily or brittle, full of split ends or excessive dandruff?
- Tongue condition—Is your tongue pink with uniformly textured taste buds, or is it cracked, coated, spotted, pale, or dark red?
- Taste and smell—Do you detect the full flavors and aromas of foods and beverages, or does everything seem bland?
- Eye condition—Do your eyes sparkle or shine or are they dry and dull? Do you have perpetual shadows under your eyes or excessively baggy eyelids?
- Fingernails and toenails—Are they strong and pliable, with no irregular spots on or underneath them, or are they excessively soft, brittle, or chipped?
- Motor functioning—Are you agile, mobile, and coordinated, or do you frequently lose your balance, stumble, or bump into things?
- Vocal tone—Is your voice generally cheerful, upbeat, or neutral, or do you mumble, grumble, or growl?
- Attitude—Are you usually happy, encouraging, or tolerant, or do you complain about anything and everything?
- Frequency of colds, flu, headaches, and stomach upsets—When your body is not well, it's trying to tell you something. Instead of masking the symptoms with medications, listen to the symptoms and their implicit messages.

Adequate nutrition is not simply a matter of isolating particular nutrients and determining if you meet or exceed the suggested dietary intake levels. It's a whole body/mind experience that needs to be considered within the context of overall health and lifestyle. It may help to understand how each of the individual nutrients contribute to our well-being by picturing the nutrients as little people holding hands in a circle around us, smiling and harmoniously singing our favorite songs. Give them thanks—they like attention, too.

WATER

Water is our most important nutrient. Without it we would die in a matter of days.

The life-sustaining properties of water are equal to that of air. Water is often taken for granted, but due to its major presence—both the human body and planet Earth are about 70 percent water—it should not be overlooked as a vital element nor take a back seat to such micronutrients as vitamins B-

SUBSTANCES AND FACTORS THAT DEPLETE NUTRIENTS

Depleter	Nutrients Affected
Air pollution	All vitamins
Alcoholic beverages	Vitamins A, B-complex, C, D, E, K, choline, magnesium, pangamic acid
Antacids	Vitamin B_1 (thiamine), iron, phosphorus, protein
Antibiotics (penicillin, etc.)	Vitamin B-complex
Antihistamines	Vitamin C
Arsenic, arsenicals	PABA, vitamin A, selenium
Aspirin	Vitamin C, folic acid
Barbiturates	Vitamin C
Caffeine (coffee, some soft drinks)	Vitamin B_1 (thiamine), biotin, inositol, pangamic acid, potassium, zinc. Blocks assimilation of calcium and iron.
Calcium (high intake)	Magnesium, zinc
Carbon monoxide	Vitamin C
Chlorine (from municipal water)	Vitamin E
Cold water	Vitamin A
Cortisone	Vitamins A and C, potassium
Diuretics	Potassium, sodium, zinc
Contraceptives, oral	Vitamins B-complex and C, folic acid, copper, magnesium, zinc
Exercise:	
lack of	Calcium
overexertion	Vitamin A
Fish/shellfish, raw	Vitamin B_1 (thiamine)
Flour, refined	Vitamin B-complex
Fluoride (from municipal water)	Vitamin C
Laxatives	Vitamins B_{12}, D, and E, potassium
Menstruation	Vitamin B_{12}, calcium, iron, magnesium
Mineral oil	Vitamins A and D
Nitrates/nitrites	Vitamins A, C, E
Oxalic acid (in beet greens, chard, chocolate, rhubarb, and spinach)	Calcium, magnesium
Perspiration (excess of)	Sodium
Phytic acid (in grain fibers)	Calcium, magnesium, phosphorus, zinc
Radiation, X-rays	Vitamins B_6 and F
Salt (high intake)	Potassium
Sodium bicarbonate (baking soda)	Vitamin B_2 (riboflavin)
Stress (all types)	All vitamins, zinc
Sugar	Vitamin B-complex, calcium
Sulfa drugs	Folic acid, PABA
Tannic acid (from tea and chocolate)	Vitamin B-complex, calcium
Tetracycline	Vitamin C, calcium, iron, magnesium
Tobacco (inhalation of smoke)	Vitamins B-complex and C, folic acid, calcium, phosphorus
Water (excess consumption)	Vitamins B-complex and C, sodium

(Adapted from Vita Chart, Bronx, NY, and *The Vitamin Robbers* by Earl Mindell, R.Ph., Ph.D., and William H. Lee, R.Ph., Ph.D., New Canaan, CT: Keats Publishing Inc., 1983.)

complex and C, which are themselves water-soluble substances.

Water facilitates major bodily functions, including alleviating thirst; regulating body temperature; eliminating waste via kidneys, bowel, liver, lungs, and skin; supplying and transporting nutrients; maintaining the health of cells and skin; and mediating metabolic biochemical reactions, such as the production of energy and the maintainenance of the acid/alkaline balance.

The amount of water each person needs varies, just like food intake, activity level, exposure to heat and dry air, and sleep requirements vary. It is often recommended, however, that we drink eight ten-ounce glasses of liquid every day. The eight-glass-a-day guide is based on an estimated daily water loss by an average, healthy adult of 80 ounces (2,500 milliliters) through urination, defecation, respiration, and perspiration.

Because we take in varying amounts of water from foods and the body's own chemical reactions, we may find that eight glasses of liquid a day is inadequate and leads to over- or underhydration. The first sign of excessive water intake is excessive urination, which is not damaging to the kidneys unless one consumes about twenty glasses per day. The first sign of dehydration is weakness and lethargy. You can also determine the status of your body hydration by pinching a fold of skin on the back of your hand. A fold that does not readily return to normal indicates dehydration. One indicator of inadequate fluid intake (or mineral leaching) is excessively dark urine; another is body odor. Sore muscles may also be due to an insufficient consumption of water.

To estimate your water requirements, calculate your total fluid intake for one day. Drink from premeasured containers, and include fresh foods that are predominantly water, such as fruit and vegetables (many are 90 percent water), fish (approximately 80 percent water), and bread (approximately 30 percent water). Remember that cooked whole grains such as rice contain about twice as much water as the dry grains. Then, measure and/or guesstimate the amount of excreted body fluid from urine, bowel movements, and perspiration.

It takes about twenty minutes for a human body to absorb eight ounces of fluid. If you are trying to increase your fluid intake to assist in normalizing bowel patterns, solubilizing kidney stones, detoxifying, or any other reason, it is best to sip liquids throughout the day rather than chugging a large quantity at one sitting. Carry a water bottle with you, or have a water bottle in each place where you regularly spend time, such as certain rooms in your home or in your car, office or workplace, or school. Guzzling fluids tends to add too much air to the digestive tract and can cause belching and other discomforts. Medical centers and other health-care institutions often recommend drinking liquids through a straw to minimize air ingestion.

Some people question if drinking fluids with meals is healthful. They may experience digestive upsets or may believe it dilutes their digestive juices. Both of these are valid personal concerns but have not been scientifically substantiated. Since individual variation seems to be the rule rather than the exception, consider the following:

- Observe your bodily reactions to eating with and without drinking water or other beverages.

- Vary your fluid intake according to meal composition. Sipping tea or soup may actually enhance digestion.

- Choose beverages that combine well with other foods. Milk, for instance, is high in protein and is therefore not necessary with a protein-rich meal. Fruit juices are high in sugar, which may cause fermentation and incomplete digestion, which leads to flatulence. Consider diluting fruit and vegetable juices by 30 to 50 percent.

- Try thinking not about what you need to do after lunch but instead about the gift of the food in front of you, and how it is contributing to your well-being. People who do not chew their food completely may have a tendency to wash it down with whatever beverage is handy. Eating and drinking in an unhurried, relaxed manner aids in digestion and reduces stress.

WATER ADDITIVES

Chlorine

Throughout history, people have become ill or died from drinking contaminated drinking water. Cholera epidemics are still a concern in some countries, as they were in the United States and Europe during the mid- to late-1800s. Consequently, municipalities began to add chlorine to public water supplies as a precautionary measure to kill disease-producing bacteria. Thereafter, the rates of sickness and death from gastrointestinal diseases fell dramatically.

Unfortunately, chlorine can react with organic matter to produce cancer-causing compounds called trihalomethanes. Some municipal water departments monitor their supplies to assure that the level of such hazardous compounds are below maximum contaminant levels set by a state or local government board of health. The health effects from cumulative concentrations of chlorine are also suspected to contribute to high blood pressure.

Since chlorine is a gas, it can be cleared from your tap water at the drinking glass level. One method is to simply allow an uncovered container of water to sit overnight. Since temperature affects the rate and quantity of gas-off, do not place the container in the refrigerator. A more effective process is to boil your water. This will drive off most of the chlorine, as well as sterilize the water of bacteria, when boiled for at least 20 minutes. Boiling also helps remove volatile organic chemicals such as gasoline that may be present in minute amounts.

Fluoride

This naturally occurring mineral is present in soil, sea water, plants, and the living tissue of bones and teeth. It is dissolved by water and found in virtually all drinking water supplies at some level. Fluoride-rich water was discovered to be an effective barrier to tooth decay, as people in areas with naturally high levels of the mineral (such as Naples, Italy, and Colorado Springs, Colorado) showed substantially fewer cavities than the rest of the population. These discoveries in the early 1900s led to widespread support by dentists and other health professionals for adding fluoride to municipal water supplies.

Various studies have shown a 40 to 65 percent decrease in tooth decay where cities have added fluoride to the water (usually added to achieve a level of .6 to 1.5 parts per million). This resulted in a substantial cost benefit to the consumer, as far less was spent on the municipal fluoridation systems than on dentists' bills.

Excessive fluoride, however, actually weakens tooth and bone structure and may cause numerous other health problems. In areas where aluminum is refined, people have been poisoned by fluoride emissions from the aluminum smelters. (The fluoride that is a by-product of the aluminum industry is sold to municipal fluoridation systems.)

Caustic Soda (Lye, Soda Ash) and Lime

Some municipal water departments add trace levels of these chemicals in an effort to keep water pipes clear. The levels are measured in parts per billion and therefore are not considered a health hazard. Lime is derived from limestone, not the fruit lime, and may be added to balance the acid/alkaline level of the water or to reduce leaching of toxic metals that may be present in old pipes, such as lead or cadmium.

BOTTLED WATER

Bottled water sales have more than tripled since the 1970s. Bottled water was the fastest growing beverage category in the United States during the mid-1980s, exceeding imported and domestic beers, wines and wine coolers, and regular soft drinks.

More than seven hundred brands of bottled water are on the market. These include uncarbonated drinking waters, which make up about 90 percent of the sales, and carbonated sparkling waters, which constitute the other 10 percent of all bottled water sales.

Many people buy bottled water assuming that it is better (i.e., more healthful) than tap water. While bottled water is generally better tasting than tap water, the bacteria and potential contaminants may not be reduced. Bottled water companies often reprocess water from municipal systems by running the water through charcoal, limestone, and mechanical filters. They may also pass the water through an ozone column to kill bacteria and through a polypropylene filter to remove sediment or particles. The treated or *purified water* may indeed be superior to tap water at this point, but it is bottled in containers that may not be clean, have residues from cleansing agents, or transmit noxious gases. In California, bottled water plants were cited with problems such as "off" taste and odor (musty, like gasoline); contamination by algae, dead flies, and beetles; excessive levels of phenol, nitrates, pesticide residues, and bacteria; improper sanitizing of dispensers; and phony or incomplete test records. These problems were in part due to the reuse of five-gallon water bottles, which can serve as storage containers for other liquids in a household, as well as provide an environment for trapping insects or fostering the growth of bacteria and algae. If you buy bottled water in returnable containers, always return clean bottles to the stores or delivery person.

Sparkling water is water that has had carbon bubbled into it. This effervescence is often enhanced by fruit flavors, such as lemon, lime, and berry extracts. While there are naturally carbonated waters in some places, most of the bottled "fizzy" water available in stores is charged, just like other soda pop. But no caffeine, sweeteners, or artificial color are added to most sparkling waters. You pay for the shapely bottles and transportation, especially for fancy water from Europe.

Distilled water has been heated until steam forms, then the droplets are collected and bottled. It has negligible to no levels of minerals, which is why it's recommended for use in car radiators and clothes irons. Some health professionals recommend drinking distilled water while others advise against it, claiming it may leach minerals from the body.

Mineral water is water that contains dissolved minerals. Essentially all water that isn't distilled is mineral water. Some locales, such as California and countries in Europe, have regulations on what constitutes mineral water. Water is rated as hard or soft, depending on the level of minerals. The harder the water, the higher the mineral content. Soft water is often preferred for washing, as it leaves fewer residues on clothes and skin and encourages soap to foam. Water can be softened by adding special salts to change the ratio of sodium, calcium, and magnesium ions.

Artesian water is tapped from underground aquifers or wells. It may be filtered, bottled, and sold as mineral or spring water, although *spring water* technically springs from the earth by its own pressure or through rock fissures. Sparkling spring water is naturally carbonated.

Whatever water you drink, think about where it came from and where it goes. The hydrologic cycle includes us, and if we contaminate our water before or after we consume it, what goes around will return to us in some way.

CARBOHYDRATES

Carbohydrates are organically derived compounds made up of carbon plus hydrates such as water or other hydrogen and oxygen combinations. Simply put, "carbs" are sugars and starches that are widely prevalent in all plants—fruits, grains, legumes, nuts and seeds, and vegetables—and, to a lesser extent, animal products.

Most of us eat 200 to 300 grams of carbohydrates every day. A deficiency of carbohydrates, through high-fat diets or prolonged fasting, can cause ketosis, the breakdown of tissue protein, and dehydration. A daily diet of 50 to 100 grams of carbohydrate will prevent ketosis.

Carbohydrates also provide dietary fibers that absorb liquid and help move food through the digestive tract. Stools that float are thought to indicate adequate levels of fiber in the diet. Lack of fiber results in constipation and may lead to hemorrhoids, bowel diseases, and cancer, as well as tooth decay, ulcers, gallstones, and atherosclerosis. Too much fiber, however, particularly phytic acid from bran or whole grains, may cause the minerals calcium, iron, and zinc to be bound and thus unabsorbable. Some plant fibers may also irritate the colon walls or prompt diarrhealike symptoms.

For further discussion of carbohydrates, see "Sweeteners," pages 128–130.

FATS (LIPIDS)

Fats are discussed in "Fats and Oils," pages 20–35.

PROTEIN

What is it?

People often consider protein a nutrient of prime importance. Not surprisingly, the word protein is derived from the Greek words *proto* (first), or *proteios* (of first quality). Protein may also have been named for Proteus, the Greek sea god who could change shape to suit the occasion, the same of which can be said about this nutrient.

An estimated one-fifth of our total body weight, or one-half of our dry weight (if water is removed) is protein. Of the dry weight, about one-third of the body's protein is in the muscles, one-fifth in bone and cartilage, and one-tenth in skin; the rest is in blood, body fluids, and tissue.

Protein is unique among the three macronutrients (protein, carbohydrates, and fats) in that its chemical structure includes carbon, hydrogen, and oxygen, *plus* nitrogen. Nitrogen is the key element in determining the crude protein content of foods, calculated by multiplying the number of nitrogen atoms by 6.25 (that figure is based on an average nitrogen content in protein of 16 percent).

Protein is also distinguished by its origin. Plant proteins are found in the seeds and leaves of many plants, notably grains, legumes, and nuts. These proteins are from 73 to 90 percent digestible. Animal proteins are found in the eggs, milk, and flesh of poultry, livestock, and fish. Other than eggs and dairy products, this book does not elaborate on animal products. Animal proteins are 90 to 95 percent digestible.

Protein is really an umbrella term for twenty-two organic compounds called amino acids, most of which have unusual names ending with *-ine*. The biochemical makeup of the human body gives us the ability to synthesize thirteen of these amino acids;

those thirteen are consequently considered nonessential to our diets. Eight amino acids must be obtained from dietary sources, however, and are therefore called *essential amino acids*. Two amino acids, arginine and histidine, are considered essential for infants and/or children or animals but are not required for adults. All the amino acids are thought to be needed in the body at the same time and in the right amounts for proper protein formation.

ESSENTIAL AMINO ACIDS	NONESSENTIAL AMINO ACIDS
Arginine	Alanine
Histidine	Asparagine
Isoleucine	Aspartic Acid
Leucine	Cysteine
Lysine	Cystine
Methionine	Glutamic Acid
Phenylalanine	Glutamine
Threonine	Glycine
Tryptophan	Hydroxyproline
Valine	Proline
	Serine
	Tyrosine

How does my body use it?

Protein synthesis involves a series of digestion and absorption processes. Food that contains protein starts breaking down in the stomach, where it mixes with hydrochloric acid, pepsin, and the enzyme protease. The protein's amino acids are linked together as peptides; the digestive acids and enzymes go about dissolving those links. The separated amino acids eventually leave the intestine and enter the liver and bloodstream.

An estimated 75 percent of ingested amino acids go into making tissue proteins, protein hormones, and enzymes. Some amino acids are recycled by the liver from old or worn-out tissue proteins. The half-life of liver proteins is thought to be ten days; the half-life of muscle proteins, however, is 180 days (about half a year). Even though our daily dietary protein intake may be forty to sixty grams, our bodies each make up to three hundred grams of protein in a day.

The main role of protein in the body is to build and maintain body tissues. It also regulates water and acid/alkalinity levels. Protein plays a big part in the production of antibodies, enzymes, and hormones. Women who nurse their babies need additional protein, as human milk contains about twelve grams of protein per liter.

If the body has a greater need for carbohydrates than is available from food, or if more protein is consumed than is required by the body, the protein will be used to make energy instead of tissue.

Protein absorption may be blocked by antacids such as alkaline tablets, baking soda, or powders that become fizzy in liquid.

How much do I need to consume?

The Recommended Daily Allowances for protein are based on age, height, and weight. Generally, infants need 13 to 14 grams, children need 16 to 23 grams, women (from age 11 and up) need 44 to 50 grams, men (from age 11 and up) need 45 to 63 grams, pregnant women need 54 to 60 grams, and lactating women need 56 to 65 grams. One way to calculate protein need is to divide body weight in pounds by 2.2 (to obtain weight in kilograms), then multiply that number by .8 (gram of protein per kilogram needed). Example: 150 pounds ÷ 2.2 = 68 x .8 = 54 grams.

The quantity of one's protein intake is in some respects less of a concern than the quality. Animal products generally contain higher amounts or better ratios of essential amino acids and are therefore considered to be high-quality protein sources, the egg being close to ideal. Many animal products are also high in saturated fats, and other environmental and health factors may outweigh any benefits of relying on animal products for protein. Plants are often deficient in certain amino acids and are therefore considered lower quality protein sources. But by combining foods, the amino acids can be complemented, thereby creating high-quality protein. Examples of such protein complementarity are eating the following foods together:

Grains with dairy products
Grains with egg
Grains with legumes
Grains with nuts or seeds and with dairy or egg
Legumes with dairy products
Legumes with egg
Legumes with nuts or seeds
Nuts or seeds with dairy
Nuts or seeds with egg
(See also Protein Complementarity, pages 71, 112.)

Protein deficiency is generally not a problem in North America, where the estimated available protein is more than 100 grams per person per day. In other parts of the world, infants and toddlers suffer from kwashiorkor, a disease recognized by a greatly bloated stomach, brittle hair, diarrhea, and stunted growth. Marasmus, or dying-away disease, also affects children in poor countries and is a combination of protein and calorie deficiencies. The body literally starves and becomes a pile of bones with dry, baggy skin and large, sunken eyes.

Certain amino acids may be deficient or completely lacking in the diet, resulting in a nonfunctional protein. The hereditary disease sickle cell anemia, for example, is characterized by blood cells that have a faulty protein.

Excessive protein intake, on the other hand, may compromise good health. Some animal products are high in cholesterol and saturated fat, substances that have been linked to heart disease, whereas plant proteins can reduce blood serum cholesterol levels. Animal products also have a poor phosphorus-to-calcium ratio. A 1:1 ratio is considered desirable; cheese has a ratio of .65:1, cow's milk is .77:1, sunflower seeds are 1.67:1, egg is 3.86:1, whole wheat bread is 4.21:1, sirloin steak is 13.08:1; chicken is 16.67:1. A long-term phosphorus/calcium imbalance may lead to secondary hyperparathyroidism, which may be a major factor in osteoporosis and myopia.

VITAMIN A

What is it?

Vitamin A is a substance formed in human and animal bodies after ingesting plants that contain *carotene*. It is actually the name for several compounds with similar chemical structures. These compounds are technically known as:

Retinol, also referred to as an *ester, retinyl palmitate,* and as vitamin A₁. Retinol is found in butterfat, egg yolks, animal livers, and oils and fats of ocean fish. It is considered an active form of vitamin A.

Dehydroretinol, also referred to as vitamin A₂, is found in freshwater fish and the birds that eat them. Its biological value is about 40 percent as active as retinol, so less attention is given to it in the scientific community.

Provitamin A are certain carotenes that can be converted by the body into vitamin A. Four carotenoids that show provitamin A activity are alpha-, beta-, and gamma-carotenes and cryptoxanthine. Beta-carotene is especially noteworthy, as it provides much of the vitamin A humans need. It is found in green, yellow, and orange-colored vegetables and some yellow, orange, and red fruits. Cryptoxanthine is a carotenoid found in corn.

The term *carotene* is derived from carrots, one of the best sources of carotenes. Carotenes are sometimes referred to as precursors (preceders) of vitamin A.

How does my body use it?

Vitamin A is a fat soluble nutrient, so fat, bile and antioxidants need to be present in the small intestine in order for it to be absorbed by the body.

Vitamin A aids in the development of all the cells in the body, particularly skin, bones, teeth, hair, and tissues. This membrane-active substance is often acclaimed for its role in preventing night blindness and other visual impairments, as well as inflammations of the eyes, such as xerosis (dry eyes) and xerophthalmia, a condition of lusterless or cloudy eyes that, if not treated, leads to total blindness. The "A" in vitamin A is for antinightblindness.

Vitamin A is also necessary for reproduction, as it assists in hormonal functioning. Evidence suggests that vitamin A helps prevent skin cancers and cancer of membranous parts of the body, such as the mouth, hollow organs, and internal passages.

Vitamin A is primarily stored in the liver but is also stored in the kidneys, body fat, and lungs. Adults generally have vitamin A reserves to last four months to a year. Young children, however, have no reserves and are more likely to show signs of deficiency. They may also be susceptible to intestinal parasites, par-ticularly in the tropics, a situation which further compromises absorption of vitamin A and other nutrients.

How much do I need to consume?

The current Recommended Daily Allowances for vitamin A are 2,000 to 3,300 International Units (IU) (400 to 700 retinol equivalents (RE)) for infants and children; 5,000 IU (1,000 RE) for males age 11 and up; 4,000 IU (800 RE) for females age 11 and up; plus 1,000 IU (200 RE) and 2,000 IU (400 RE) for pregnant and lactating women, respectively (based on an average of 1 RE = 5 IU).

Translating food into numbers, a 7-inch raw carrot provides about 20,000 IU (2,000 RE) of vitamin A. A 3-ounce serving of beef liver provides 45,000 IU (13,500 RE). A pat of butter or margarine has about 150 IU (38 RE). Eating as little as a half-cup of green or yellow vegetables per day may easily satisfy your RDA. The darker or richer the color, the more carotenes will usually be present.

Signs of deficiency in vitamin A intake or absorption include stunted growth and bone development, crooked teeth and soft tooth enamel, sinus problems, scaly or dry and rough skin, acne and other blemishes, allergies, and susceptibility to infections.

Ironically, an excess of vitamin A (in retinol form, not from carotenes) can cause symptoms similar to a deficiency condition. Blurred vision, skin irritations, and hair loss can be caused by too much vitamin A. Other signs of toxicity include nausea or vomiting; ankle swelling; fatigue or drowsiness, weight loss; cracking or bleeding lips; and enlargement of spleen, liver, or lymph nodes. Hypervitaminosis A results from ingestion of more than 50,000 IU per day over a long period of time. It is often caused by consuming polar bear liver, which has up to 18,000 IU per gram, or by consuming or injecting the vitamin in high dosages.

Please note that eating large quantities of carotene-rich foods won't cause hypervitaminosis A, but it may cause your skin to turn yellow or orange (if you are of a race with light skin color). Also note that 15 to 35 percent less vitamin A may be available from cooked vegetables than from those same foods when eaten raw. Long-term storage and exposure to ultraviolet light can also destroy carotenoids.

The availability of vitamin A in the body is also affected by other substances and conditions. Many nutrients work together to maintain bodily health; vitamin A needs the vitamins B-complex, C, D, and E, and the minerals calcium, phosphorus, and zinc to be fully functional in the body. Substances that limit vitamin A's availability include coffee, alcohol, mineral oil (blocks absorption), cortisone, laxatives, and an excess of iron. Even cold weather and strenuous physical workouts can reduce absorption of vitamin A.

FOODS THAT PROVIDE CAROTENE VITAMIN A
(MORE THAN 2,000 IU PER SERVING)

    Apricots
    Beet greens
    Broccoli
    Cantaloupe
    Carrots
    Chard
    Chinese cabbage
    Collards
    Dandelion greens
    Endive
    Escarole
    Kale
    Mangos
    Mustard greens
    Nectarines
    Papaya
    Peppers—red and chili
    Pumpkin
    Spinach
    Spirulina
    Squash (winter)
    Sweet potatoes
    Turnip greens
    Watercress

FOODS THAT PROVIDE RETINOL VITAMIN A

    Butter
    Cheese
    Chicken
    Cod liver oil
    Cream
    Eggs

    Fish
    Liver
    Milk (with fat present or fortified)
    Yogurt

B-COMPLEX VITAMINS

What are they?

This group of water-soluble vitamins includes twelve distinct nutrients with similar chemical structures and functions. They are often found together in nature.

As with vitamin C, the other water-soluble vitamin, the discovery and understanding of B-complex vitamins were linked to the study of a disease frequently found in malnourished sailors. Whereas ascorbic acid (vitamin C) was found to cure scurvy, a concentrate originally named water-soluble B was found to prevent beriberi (B stood for beriberi). After initial research by Dr. Elmer V. McCullum at the University of Wisconsin in 1916, scientists learned that vitamin B was actually not one but several substances, now known as the B-complex.

The nine official and three related nutrients that make up the vitamin B-complex are:

B_1—Thiamine
B_2—Riboflavin
B_3—Niacin
B_6—Pyridoxine, pyridoxal, pyridoxamine
B_{12}—Cobalamin
B_{15}—Pangamic acid
Biotin
Choline
Folic acid
Inositol
Pantothenic acid
Para-aminobenzoic acid (PABA)

All these nutrients will be discussed in the following pages.

How does my body use them?

Each of the B-complex vitamins performs special functions in the body, either alone or with other substances. Many of them are present in the same foods, notably whole grains, brewer's yeast, nuts and seeds, eggs, fish, liver, molasses, and some fruits and vegetables. They are all water soluble and excreted by the kidneys in urine. Few are stored by the body, so they need to be consumed on a regular basis, preferably daily.

B-complex vitamins are important for metabolizing carbohydrates, fat, and protein. They enhance appetite, energy, and muscle tone. They can help minimize stressful situations and reduce irritability. B-complex vitamins are beneficial for the brain, eyes, gastrointestinal tract, glands, hair, kidneys, liver, nervous system, and skin. Many of the B-complex nutrients work most efficiently in the presence of other B-vitamins and vitamin C.

Substances that deplete or reduce absorption of B-complex vitamins include alcohol, coffee, drugs (antibiotics, aspirin, diuretics, laxatives, oral contraceptives, sleeping pills, sulfa drugs), excessive sugar, and tobacco. B-vitamins are also made less available by heat (overcooking and high temperatures), refining (particularly grains), and prolonged storage.

How much do I need to consume?

Each nutrient in the B-complex family has a different Recommended Daily Allowance. There is no known toxicity of any of these nutrients except niacin, which if ingested as nicotinic acid at rates of two to three grams per day can cause vascular dilation, liver damage, and other problems.

As mentioned above, a deficiency of B-complex vitamins, notably a lack of thiamine, can cause beriberi. Beriberi can take several forms, all of which debilitate the body's nervous system and cardiac and neurological functioning. Most cases of beriberi are due to a diet of polished rice (rice that has had the outer layers removed).

B-complex deficiencies may also result in appetite loss, bad breath, depression, a dark tongue, fatigue, gastrointestinal disturbances, hair loss, insomnia, irritability, nervousness, and tender muscles.

Lack of B-complex vitamins is a worldwide phenomenon usually caused by limited or restricted diets, often of overrefined foods. Some researchers have postulated that crime and mental illness rates could be reduced if diets contained more nutrient-rich foods and less B-vitamin-depleted (refined) or -depleting (sugar) foods. Because B-complex vitamins play pivotal roles in our thinking and feeling, we can liken an absence of B to an absence of *being*.

Thiamine (Vitamin B1)

What is it?

Thiamine could be considered a miracle drug in that specific ailments can be cured in a matter of hours after ingestion or administration of this vitamin.

The word thiamine is derived from *thio* (Greek *theio*) for "containing sulfur," and *amine*, for "vitamin." Chemically, it is a white crystalline substance made up of carbon, hydrogen, nitrogen, oxygen, and sulfur. Natural thiamine is found in both its free form and bound form (thiamine pyrophosphate, or TPP, a coenzyme). Thiamine is easily destroyed by moist heat, baking soda, and sulfur dioxide. It is stable in dry heat up to 212°F. Synthetic forms of thiamine, such as thiamine hydrochloride and thiamine mononitrate, are more stable. Thiamine mononitrate is a common additive used to fortify flours and commercial cereal products.

Various studies from the late 1800s to mid-1900s determined the healing power of thiamine in cases of beriberi in humans and of polyneuritis in poultry. Because it was the first B-complex vitamin discovered, thiamine was dubbed vitamin B1.

How does my body use it?

Thiamine is absorbed mainly in the upper small intestine and transported to the liver, where it is changed into the coenzyme thiamine diphosphate. Very little thiamine is stored in the body, so tissues can become depleted within two weeks. The tissues take up what they need, depending on individual metabolism, activity level, and diet. For example, people who consume more carbohydrates than fat or protein, or who use their muscles a lot in work or exercise, need more thiamine. Stress also increases the body's need for thiamine.

Thiamine is needed for proper functioning of peripheral nerves and healthy appetite, mental attitude, and muscle tone. As a coenzyme, it is necessary for carbohydrate metabolism and converting glucose to fats. The body uses only what it needs and excretes any excess through urine. There is no known toxicity of thiamine.

How much do I need to consume?

The Recommended Daily Allowances for thiamine are .3 to .5 milligram for infants, .7 to 1.0 milligram for children ages 1 to 10, 1.0 to 1.5 milligrams for adolescents and adults, and an additional .4 to .5 milligram for pregnant and lactating women.

Thiamine is a rather sensitive nutrient in that many things can destroy it before or after you eat it. Baking causes a loss of 15 to 20 percent; toasting (high-temperature dry heat) takes its toll, and normal cooking depletes about 25 percent. When you discard cooking water or meat drippings you throw away this nutrient. Alkalies such as baking soda and the process of irradiation both destroy thiamine.

Thiamine absorption or availability is blocked by ingesting alcoholic beverages, coffee and tea, and other drinks and foods containing caffeine or tannic acid; excess iron and/or sugar; mineral oil; antacids; barbiturates; and diuretics. Abuse of alcohol and subsequent reduction of thiamine may result in deficiencies in motor and eye movements, distortions in perception of reality, and permanent memory impairment.

Other signs of thiamine deficiency are irritability, fatigue, weakness, confusion, short attention span, memory loss, appetite loss, weight loss, indigestion, severe constipation, intestinal inflammation, and numbness or tenderness in the muscles. The measured level of thiamine deficiency is below .2 to .3 milligram per 1,000 calories.

Severe thiamine shortage, usually caused by monodiets of refined rice or unenriched white flour products, results in beriberi. Three forms of beriberi are known. Wet beriberi is characterized by the wasting of tissue. Early signs are numb toes and feet, stiff ankles, and sore leg muscles, which eventually escalate to include nerve degeneration and reduced muscle coordination in the rest of the body. Dry beriberi is characterized by edema, the excess fluid in body tissues, particularly in the legs. Heart disorders, anorexia (appetite loss), and breathlessness are additional symptoms of dry beriberi. Infantile beriberi is a condition in which the skin turns blue due to a lack of oxygen in the tissues. This disease usually affects infants between two and five months who are breast-fed by mothers with inadequate levels of thiamine in their milk. Early symptoms include soundless or weak cries, or very loud, piercing cries, appetite loss, and rapid pulse. Sudden death occurs in advanced stages.

FOODS HIGH IN THIAMINE

Beans (legumes)
Cereals (fortified)
Grains (whole)
Ham
Nuts—almonds, cashews, peanuts, pecans
Organ meats
Peas—blackeyed, green, split
Pork
Spirulina
Vegetables—asparagus, avocado, broccoli,
    collards
Wheat germ

Riboflavin (Vitamin B$_2$)

What is it?

Riboflavin is a pigment found in essentially all living plant and animal cells. The yellowish substance was found in milk in 1879 and named *flavin,* from the Latin word *flavus* (yellow).

Scientists researching what up to 1928 had been called Vitamin B$_1$, the antiberiberi nutrient, started finding that a growth-promoting, heat-stable substance remained after thiamine (vitamin B$_1$) was destroyed by the heat. Some called the substance vitamin G; others named it B$_2$. In 1935, Karrer, a Nobel prize-winning Swiss chemist, gave the nutrient its present name, from ribitol, due to the chemical resemblance to the sugar ribose, and flavin.

Riboflavin is water soluble and, when isolated and dispersed in water, emits a fluorescent yellowish green color. In crystalline form it is a bitter, orangish yellow, odorless substance. It is more stable than thiamine in heat, acid, and water but highly sensitive to ultraviolet light and alkalies, which can kill it.

How does my body use it?

Riboflavin is absorbed in the upper small intestine by a process known as passive diffusion, a kind of time-release or take-what-you-need absorption process. Phosphorus must be present for the vitamin to enter the intestinal wall and be transported by the blood to the body tissues or to be converted to an enzyme in the flavoprotein group. Those enzymes are vital for metabolizing the "big" nutrients (fats or lipids, proteins, and carbohydrates).

Riboflavin has a reputation as being good for the eyes. It also helps form red blood cells and antibodies, and it activates vitamin B_6 (pyridoxine), which then helps to metabolize tryptophan, an amino acid.

Riboflavin is excreted primarily in the urine but also in the feces. Our bodies store very little of this water-soluble nutrient, so it must be consumed on a frequent basis.

How much do I need to consume?

The Recommended Daily Allowances for riboflavin are .4 to .5 milligram for infants, .8 to 1.2 milligrams for children ages 1 to 10, 1.4 to 1.8 milligrams for adolescent and adult men, 1.3 milligrams for females age 11 and up, and an additional .3 to .5 milligram for pregnant and lactating women. The levels at which a riboflavin deficiency is likely are less than .6 milligram per 1,000 kilocalories, or below 1.2 milligrams in body tissue.

Signs of riboflavin deficiency are often physically visible: cracks at the corners of the mouth, chapped and swollen lips, swollen and reddened tongue, bloodshot eyes, and oily or scaly patches of skin, particularly around the nose and scrotum. Blurred vision may also be caused by lack of riboflavin, as may sensitivity to light, tired eyes, anemia, poor digestion, dizziness, fatigue, and slow wound healing. Babies born of riboflavin-deficient mothers may have abnormalities such as short bones and fingers or deformed growth between fingers, toes, or ribs.

There is no known toxicity of riboflavin.

FOODS HIGH IN RIBOFLAVIN

Almonds
Avocados
Bran (wheat)
Cheese
Eggs
Grains (enriched and whole)
Meat
Milk products*
Molasses (blackstrap)
Mushrooms
Organ meats—heart, kidney, liver
Oysters
Vegetables—leafy greens

*Milk stored in glass bottles may have little riboflavin left in it, due to exposure to light.

Niacin (Vitamin B₃)

What is it?

When you think of something being extracted from tobacco, you probably assume it's a cancer-causing substance—certainly not a healthful nutrient. But niacin, first prepared from the nicotine of tobacco, has been a lifesaver.

The word *niacin* is derived from *ni*cotinic *ac*id and the suffix *-in,* which identifies a substance as a pharmaceutical. The nutrient is sometimes referred to as vitamin B₃ or by its two forms, nicotinic acid and niacinamide (or nicotinamide). Despite the names, there is no nicotine in niacin.

The search for a cure for pellagra (an Italian word meaning "rough skin") led scientists and doctors to discover preventive foods before finally isolating niacin as the deficient substance in the diets of people who ate predominantly corn. Pellagra was once widespread in the United States, particularly in the South; 200,000 cases were reported from 1917 to 1918. Corn is low in the amino acid tryptophan, a precursor of niacin, and the niacin in corn is in a bound form. Yeast, beef, milk, and legumes contain tryptophan or niacin but were apparently not part of the diets of people suffering from pellagra. Southerners ate hog products, such as chitterlings and jowls, that do not contain tryptophan or niacin. It wasn't until 1937 that workers at the University of Wisconsin proved niacin could cure the disease.

How does my body use it?

Niacin is absorbed from the small intestine into the bloodstream and transported to the liver, where it is converted to coenzymes. These coenzymes are necessary for cell respiration and release of energy from carbohydrates, fat, and protein. They also synthesize DNA, fatty acids, and protein, with the help of the other B-complex vitamins biotin, pantothenic acid, and B6.

Niacin plays a role in more than fifty metabolic reactions, many of them in conjunction with thiamine, riboflavin, and other nutrients. It is thanks to niacin that cholesterol is reduced, steroids are formed, and sex hormones are produced.

Like other B-complex vitamins, niacin is water soluble and is excreted in the urine or feces. It is more stable in heat, however. Alcoholic beverages can render it unavailable in the body. Coffee, however, actually contains niacin, as much as three milligrams per cup.

How much do I need to consume?

The Recommended Daily Allowances for niacin are 5 to 6 milligrams for infants, 9 to 13 milligrams for children, and 13 to 20 milligrams for men and women from the age 11 and up. These consumptions are based on a caloric intake of 6.6 milligrams per 1,000 kilocalories. The diet of adults should provide no less than 13 milligrams of niacin a day even if total calorie intake is less than 2,000.

Niacin deficiency, as mentioned, can cause pellagra, a disease indicated by the four Ds: dermatitis, diarrhea, dementia, and death. Another D word describes its appearance: dark. A dark (black or very red) tongue and dark skin around the neck ("Casal's necklace") often show up in diseased persons or animals. Once a deadly worldwide disease, pellagra is now found only occasionally, mostly in Africa.

Other signs of niacin deficiency are anorexia (appetite loss), bad breath, canker sores, depression, disorientation, headaches, hallucinations, irritability, memory loss, and nausea.

Niacin is relatively nontoxic; only when large doses are consumed in the form of a supplement (more than 2 grams a day) is there concern that the body may react. Signs of overdose are high blood glucose and blood enzymes, liver damage, peptic ulcer, gastrointestinal irritation, and vascular dilation (itching or flushing of skin).

FOODS HIGH IN NIACIN OR TRYPTOPHAN*

Cheese
Eggs
Fish
Grains (whole or enriched)
Legumes
Meat—beef and lamb
Mushrooms
Nuts
Organ meats, especially liver
Peanuts and peanut butter
Poultry
Seafood

*an amino acid from which niacin can be synthesized in the body

Vitamin B6

What is it?

Vitamin B6 is the name given to a yeast extract produced in 1934 by Dr. Paul Gyorgy, a scientist at the University of Pennsylvania School of Medicine. Subsequent research in Europe and the United States has led to the current understanding of this nutrient, which exists in foods in one of three forms: pyridoxine, pyridoxal, and pyridoxamine. Those names describe the chemical structure, with *pyrid* referring to its pyridine ring of five carbon atoms and one nitrogen atom, and the remaining parts of the words referring to an oxygen component. They are all white crystalline substances.

Vitamin B6 is found in many foods. It is water soluble as well as soluble in alcohol and acetone. The three forms have varying stability, with pyridoxine being less stable in alkaline solutions but more heat tolerant than pyridoxal and pyridoxamine. Radiation (light, ultraviolet light) destroys Vitamin B6.

How does my body use it?

Vitamin B6 is rapidly absorbed in the upper small intestine and enters the body through the portal vein. It concentrates in the liver and other tissues and is excreted in urine.

Vitamin B6 is converted to coenzymes, such as pyridoxal phosphate, needed for protein metabolism and the building and removal of amino acids or substances in amino acids (e.g., sulfur from sulfur-containing amino acids). These coenzymes work with folic acid to enhance metabolism or function of choline and some amino acids. They also help in conversion of tryptophan to niacin; a test for B6 deficiency is measuring the level of xanthurenic acid (a substance that indicates faulty tryptophan metabolism) in urine.

Pyridoxal phosphate, a type of vitamin B6, is needed for the body to synthesize dopamine, gamma-amino butyric acid, and serotonin, three neurotransmitters (nervous system messengers).

The coenzyme of pyridoxine, with the enzyme phosphorylase, converts glycogen to glucose. It is conveniently stored in the muscle to be ready to provide energy. Vitamin B6 is also needed for the body to utilize vitamin B12, for proper function of the body's immune response system, and for synthesis of the nucleic acids DNA and RNA.

Vitamin B6 is more efficiently metabolized when other nutrients are present in adequate amounts. These include linoleic acid (an amino acid), magnesium, potassium, sodium, and other B-complex vitamins (thiamine, riboflavin, and pantothenic acid).

Substances that reduce absorption or availability of vitamin B6 include alcoholic beverages, coffee and other beverages and foods that contain caffeine, tobacco, amphetamines, penicillamine, reserpine, chlorpromazine, oral contraceptives, and postmenopausal drugs, including estrogen.

Pyridoxine has been used to treat carpal tunnel syndrome and is thought to increase our ability to recall dreams after we wake up.

How much do I need to consume?

The Recommended Daily Allowances for vitamin B6 are .3 to .6 milligram for infants, 1.0 to 1.4 milligrams for children, 1.7 to 2.0 milligrams for adolescent and adult men, and 1.4 to 1.6 milligrams for adolescent and adult women. Pregnant and lactating women need an additional .6 to .8 milligram.

Symptoms of vitamin B6 deficiency include an inability by the body to metabolize protein (amino acids); acne or oily face; sore lips or a smooth, red tongue; appetite and weight loss; hair loss; weakness; anemia; convulsions in infants; dizziness; irritability; nervousness; and depression.

There is no known toxicity of Vitamin B6.

FOODS HIGH IN VITAMIN B6

Avocados
Bananas
Broccoli
Brussels sprouts
Cauliflower
Chicken
Fish
Grains (whole)
Meat and organ meats
Nuts
Peanut butter
Soybeans
Rice (brown)
Wheat germ

Vitamin B12 (Cobalamin)

What is it?

Vitamin B12 is a complex vitamin, not only in terms of its chemical structure but also because of its metabolism and functions in the body.

As a chemical compound, vitamin B12 is known as $C_{63} H_{88} CoN_{14} O_{14} P$; it is the only naturally occurring compound with cobalt and is thus called *cobalamin* (cobalt vitamin). The B12 that is manufactured is contaminated by cyanide and therefore named *cyanocobalamin*. Still other forms are designated with a, b, c: B12a is hydroxocobalamin; B12b is aquacobalamin, and B12c is nitrocobalamin.

Research on this nutrient came about because of attempts to find a cure for pernicious anemia, a deadly disease affecting red blood cells and eventually the whole body. Raw liver was found to alleviate its symptoms, but only in large quantities. After more than twenty years of study at various laboratories, in 1948 scientists at Merck & Company isolated a red crystalline pigment from liver, which they named Vitamin B_{12}. Injections of B_{12} are now the fastest remedy for pernicious anemia.

How does my body use it?

This nutrient is unique in that a substance excreted in the gastrointestinal tract called intrinsic factor must be present for its absorption, which takes about three hours (other B-complex vitamins are absorbed within seconds). Five steps are involved for vitamin B_{12} absorption: (1) release of the vitamin from its source protein; (2) linking with a specific glycoprotein named Castle's intrinsic factor, and secretion into the stomach; (3) forming a complex with calcium and traveling to receptor sites in the upper small intestine; (4) crossing intestinal mucosa, which releases B_{12} from the complex; and (5) transferring to a protein called transcobalamin II which transports it to the bloodstream.

An estimated 30 to 70 percent of ingested B_{12} is absorbed. Injected B_{12}, however, bypasses the digestive process and cuts straight to the chase; people suffering from pernicious anemia usually have a lack of intrinsic factor and therefore do not benefit from dietary B_{12}.

B_{12} also stands out in the vitamin B-complex because it is stored in the body for three to five years, primarily in the liver, whereas the other water-soluble B vitamins are excreted in a matter of days. B_{12} is excreted in the bile and via the kidneys in urine.

Vitamin B_{12}, as mentioned, is crucial for red blood cell formation and cell longevity. It helps maintain a healthy appetite and nervous system. It aids in iron absorption and metabolism of carbohydrates, fat, and protein. Absorption of B_{12} requires the presence of other B-complex vitamins, especially B_6. It is enhanced by adequate levels of vitamin C, calcium, potassium, and sodium, as well as the B-complex vitamins choline, folic acid, and inositol.

Like other water-soluble nutrients, B_{12} absorption or utilization can be compromised by ingesting alcoholic beverages, caffeine-containing substances, laxatives, oral contraceptives, and tobacco.

How much do I need to consume?

The Recommended Daily Allowances for vitamin B_{12} are among the smallest of all nutrients: .3 to .5 microgram for infants, 1.0 to 1.4 micrograms for children, 2 micrograms for adults, and 2.2 to 2.6 micrograms for pregnant and lactating women.

Even with so small a requirement, B_{12} deficiency is not uncommon. Some people have hereditary malabsorption or have antibodies to intrinsic factor. Dietary B_{12} is principally from animal products and to a much lesser extent microbially fermented foods. Strict vegetarians (vegans) who eat no dairy products or eggs are considered to be an at-risk population if they do not supplement their diets with the synthetic form of B_{12} (derived from bacteria and fungi) or the few known plant sources.

Symptoms of vitamin B_{12} deficiency include numbness or tingling, fatigue, speech and walking difficulties, appetite loss, slow reflex response, confusion, disorientation, nervousness, memory loss, delusions, gastrointestinal disturbances, inflamed tongue (glossitis), pale face, and abnormally large red blood cells.

There is no known toxicity of vitamin B_{12}.

FOODS THAT CONTAIN VITAMIN B_{12}

Clams
Dairy products
Eggs
Fish
Liver
Meat
Oysters
Seaweed
Spirulina (blue-green algae)

Pangamic Acid (Vitamin B_{15})

What is it?

This nutrient is not an official vitamin in the United States but is considered a food additive by the Food and Drug Administration. In Russia, however, where more studies on it have taken place, pangamic acid is deemed a necessary nutritional substance.

The name pangamic acid is from *pan,* meaning universal, and *gamic,* referring to seed. And that's where it's found: in seeds throughout the world.

Pangamic acid is usually grouped with B-complex vitamins because it is found with them in nature. The other B vitamins reportedly need to be present for pangamic acid to be absorbed, but how it is metabolized is not fully understood.

How does my body use it?
Pangamic acid is thought to be needed for the functioning of nerves and glands and for the stimulation of oxygen uptake. It has been shown to reduce blood cholesterol levels and to inhibit formation of fatty liver deposits. People suffering from heart conditions (angina pectoris, arteriosclerosis, heart attacks, heart failure), liver disease (hepatitis), and skin problems (scleroderma, eczema, psoriasis) have been treated with pangamic acid.

Pangamic acid, like other water-soluble nutrients, is depleted or inhibited by alcoholic beverages and coffee or other substances that contain caffeine.

How much do I need to consume?
There are currently no Recommended Daily Allowances for pangamic acid, nor are there any known levels of toxicity.

Deficiency symptoms are thought to include fatigue, hypoxia (lack of oxygen in tissues), heart disease, and glandular and nervous disorders.

FOODS THAT CONTAIN PANGAMIC ACID

> Grains (whole)
> Liver
> Rice
> Seeds—apricot kernels, pumpkin, sesame, sunflower
> Yeast (brewer's)

Biotin

What is it?
Biotin is a coenzyme that is present in most foods. Experiments with animals fed with raw egg whites led to the discovery of biotin. A protein in raw egg whites called avidin binds with a life-giving substance (originally found in yeast and boiled duck yolks) that scientists called biotin (*bios* = life). Cooking or heating eggs, however, deactivates avidin, thereby allowing biotin to be absorbed.

Chemically, biotin is an odorless, colorless, sulfur-containing simple monocarboxylic acid. It is hot-water soluble and soluble in acetone, ethanol, and ether. It is also stable in heat and more stable to acids and alkalies than other B-complex vitamins. It is metabolically similar to vitamin B_{12}, folic acid, and pantothenic acid.

How does my body use it?
Like other nutrients, biotin is absorbed in the small intestine. Strangely enough, more biotin is excreted by the body than the amount ingested, indicating that biotin is manufactured or synthesized by our intestinal bacteria. However, this self-synthesized biotin apparently shows up too late in the absorption process, so dietary biotin is thought to be necessary. Some biotin is stored in the kidneys and liver.

Biotin is needed for the metabolism of protein (by incorporating amio acids into protein), fats (synthesizing fatty acids), and carbohydrates (obtaining energy from glucose). It also helps convert folic acid to a biologically active form and can reduce symptoms of zinc deficiency.

As mentioned, biotin is inhibited by raw egg whites, as well as alcohol, coffee, and antibiotics. Other nutrients aid or are needed for absorption of biotin, namely other B-complex vitamins, vitamin C, and sulfur.

How much do I need to consume?
The estimated safe and adequate daily dietary intake rates for biotin are 10 to 15 micrograms for infants, 20 to 30 micrograms for children, and 30 to 100 micrograms for people age 11 and up. The estimated dietary intake of biotin is 100 to 300 micrograms a day in the United States, 50 to 100 micrograms a day in western Europe.

A biotin deficiency is rare. Its occurrence is most likely due to high consumption of raw egg whites or an uncommon hereditary disease known as biotin dependency. Symptoms may include appetite loss, grayish or dry skin, fatigue, nausea, and depression.

There is no known toxicity of biotin.

Foods High in Biotin

- Bran
- Cauliflower
- Cheese
- Chicken
- Chocolate
- Eggs (yolk)
- Grains (whole)
- Milk
- Mushrooms
- Nuts
- Organ meats—kidney, liver
- Peanut butter
- Salmon
- Sardines
- Yeast (brewer's)

Choline

What is it?

The scientific description of choline is $C_5H_{15}NO_2$. It is also known as a phospholipid and as a member of the vitamin B-complex family. This simple molecule, found in lecithin and many other foods, is in its isolated form a bitter, colorless syrup or part of two crystalline salts, choline bitartate and choline chloride.

Discovery of choline dates back to the 1840s when N. T. Gobley isolated lecithin from egg yolk (the Greek word for which is *lekithos*). About one hundred years later other researchers determined that choline, a main constituent of lecithin, acted like a vitamin in the growth and health of test animals.

How does my body use it?

Choline is absorbed by the body in the small intestine; after absorption it works to stop fatty deposits from accumulating in the liver. Buildup of liver fats can disturb many other bodily functions. Choline is also needed for transmitting nerve impulses via the nerve fluid acetylcholine. Those nerve impulses prompt muscles to react according to messages from the brain; a shortage of acetylcholine could result in damaged or paralyzed muscles, such as slipped tendons (perosis).

Choline is also reportedly good for the gallbladder, hair, kidneys, and thymus gland. It may also reduce blood pressure and baldness.

Choline can be and is synthesized in our bodies, but apparently not in large enough amounts or fast enough; and several other nutrients—notably folacin, B_{12}, and the amino acids serine and methionine—need to be present in order for that synthesis to take place.

How much do I need to consume?

There are no Recommended Daily Allowances for choline, in part because little is known of its functions in comparison with other nutrients. There is speculation that a choline deficiency can prompt ulcers, intolerance to fats, and bleeding of the stomach. There are no known levels of toxicity for choline.

Foods Known to Contain Choline*

- Bran—rice and wheat
- Cabbage
- Eggs
- Grains (whole)—barley, corn, oats, sorghum, wheat
- Liver
- Milk—dry skim
- Molasses (blackstrap)
- Potatoes—dehydrated
- Soybeans and soy flour
- Turnip greens
- Yeast—brewer's and torula

*Note: The choline content of many foods has not been assayed.

Folic Acid

What is it?

Folic acid gets its name from foliage—green leaves—in which it is found in abundance. Its role as an essential nutrient was discovered at a hospital in Bombay, India, after Dr. Lucy Wells treated pregnant women suffering from anemia with extracts of yeast that later were shown to contain folic acid.

Several forms of folic acid exist in nature, all named with intriguing words such as hepta pteroyl-glutamate. Pure folic acid is also known as pteroyl-monoglutamic acid.

Folacin is the word used to describe folic acid and the group of related substances. Folacin in foods comes in two forms: readily assimilable free folates (which account for about 25 percent of food intake), and bound folates, also known as polyglutamates, that require more digestive processes. In isolated form, folic acid is a yellow crystalline, light-sensitive substance that is water soluble but unstable in acid and heat (in neutral or alkaline solutions).

How does my body use it?

Other nutrients must be present in the body in order for folic acid to be absorbed. These other nutrients are vitamins B_6, B_{12}, and C. Folic acid is metabolized in different degrees of efficiency, depending on its food source: only 10 percent of the folic acid present in yeast, 31 percent present in orange juice, 80 percent present in eggs and liver, and 82 percent present in bananas is absorbed. Apparently, the higher the glutamate components in folic acid, the lower the absorbability of the foods.

Folates are absorbed in the small intestine, are bound to protein, and are carried via the bloodstream to the liver. There they undergo a chemical change (they become methylated) and then are transported to bone marrow and maturing red blood cells. Folate is excreted in the urine and bile.

Folic acid (as folacin enzymes) is needed for building red blood cells by forming heme, the iron-containing substance in hemoglobin. Folic acid also helps form amino acids necessary for protein metabolism, as well as forming purines and pyramines that are needed for synthesizing RNA and DNA, the nucleic acids that contain genetic codes. Folic acid plays a role in converting ethanolamine, an amino alcohol, to choline, one of the B-complex vitamins the body is able to manufacture.

How much do I need to consume?

The Recommended Daily Allowances for folate are 25 to 35 micrograms for infants, 50 to 100 micro-grams for children, and 150 to 200 micrograms for people ages 11 and up. Pregnant women need 400 micrograms, and lactating women need 260 to 280 micrograms a day.

Folic acid is found in many foods, but the average diet may be deficient because leafy green vegetables and organ meats (the best sources) are not as popular as other foods, and overcooking or discarding cooking water diminishes folic acid.

Signs of folic acid deficiency are similar to those of B_{12}: anemia, irritability, confusion, memory impairment, and gastrointestinal disturbances. Glossitis (smooth red tongue) and graying hair may also be evidence of a folic acid deficiency.

Unfortunately, too much folic acid can mask a deficiency in vitamin B_{12}. Large amounts of folic acid can also reduce the effectiveness of anticonvulsive drugs for epileptics. Doses of 15 milligrams a day are considered nontoxic.

Foods High in Folic Acid

Cantaloupe
Eggs
Fish
Nuts
Oranges and orange juice
Organ meats—kidney, liver
Salmon
Soybeans
Vegetables—leafy greens, broccoli, cabbage, celery, peas, sweet potatoes, tomatoes

INOSITOL

What is it?

"Muscle sugar" was the name first given to this substance, now known by its Greek roots: *inos,* for sinew, combined with the suffix -*ose,* indicating a sugar. The biologically active form is called myo-inositol (*myo* is Greek for muscle), and it is present in nearly all living cells of both plants and animals. Inositol is also synthesized in human cells.

Like choline, inositol is found in phospholipids (compounds of phosphorus, fatty acids, and nitrogen) present in animals, and in phytic acid present in plant cells. Phytic acid usually gets a bad rap

Para-Aminobenzoic Acid (PABA)

Para-aminobenzoic acid, or PABA for short, doesn't get much recognition as a nutritional substance, unless you consider it a skin nutrient for its ability to prevent sunburn. PABA is not an official vitamin, either, although it is sold as a supplement. Actually, PABA is part of the folic acid group, making it sort of a vitamin within a vitamin. Its role in the body is similar to that of folic acid.

PABA once gained undeserved fame as a product that could restore gray hair to its natural color—a claim that was never substantiated.

There are no Recommended Daily Allowances for PABA. Deficiency symptoms are the same as for folic acid. The foods high in PABA are eggs, fish, lecithin, liver, blackstrap molasses, peanuts, rice, soybeans, wheat germ, and brewer's yeast.

Sulfa drugs are chemically very similar to PABA and may therefore crowd out and create a deficiency of PABA. This can be prevented as long as there is more PABA than sulfa drug in the body.

because it binds minerals (calcium, iron, and zinc) and renders them unabsorbable.

When isolated, inositol is a sweet, colorless, water-soluble crystal similar to glucose. It tolerates acids, alkalies, and heat. Although inositol was known of since 1850, it was not designated as a vitamin until 1956.

How does my body use it?

Inositol needs B-complex vitamins, especially choline, as well as B_{12} and linoleic acid (an amino acid), in order to be absorbed by the body.

Inositol helps the heart. With choline, it stops fat from hardening in the arteries. It also aids in the body's production of lecithin and thus reduces cholesterol. Inositol is important for hair growth and brain function. Inositol is stored in the brain and in heart and skeletal muscles.

How much do I need to consume?

No Recommended Daily Allowances have been established for inositol, but the estimated daily intake of people in the United States is 300 to 1,000 milligrams.

Deficiencies of inositol are reportedly similar to those of vitamin B_6, and they may therefore be confused. Symptoms include hair loss (as found

in test animals), constipation, elevated cholesterol, and eczema. Large amounts of coffee or other caffeinated substances deplete inositol, as do alcoholic beverages.

Inositol is considered nontoxic.

Foods High in Inositol

Fruits, especially citrus
Grains (whole)
Legumes
Milk
Molasses (blackstrap)
Nuts
Organ meats—brain, heart, kidney, liver
Peanuts
Vegetables
Yeast

Pantothenic Acid

What is it?

Like some bumper stickers about Pagans proclaim, pantothenic acid is everywhere. The name comes from the Greek *pantothen* ("from all sides"), which is derived in part from Pan, the Greek god of pastures, and/or *pan,* a prefix meaning "all."

This nutrient was first fractionated in 1933 by

R. J. Williams, a scientist at Oregon State University studying the growth and fermentation of yeast cells. Chemically, pantothenic acid is a compound of pantoic acid and beta-alanine, an amino acid. When isolated, it is a water-soluble, viscous, pale yellow oil or, as calcium pantothenate, is an odorless, bitter, white crystalline powder. This is the form that is used commercially as a supplement.

How does my body use it?

Pantothenic acid is absorbed in the small intestine and converted to coenzyme A and acyl carrier protein (ACP). These substances also help synthesize and oxidize fatty acids. Pantothenic acid or coenzyme A also helps metabolize fats, protein, and carbohydrates; synthesize antibodies; and promote utilization of vitamin D. Because it is water soluble, pantothenic acid is excreted in urine. Some is stored in the liver and kidneys for a short time.

Pantothenic acid is thought to prevent or alleviate allergies and, with other B-complex vitamins, can keep stress levels from getting out of control.

How much do I need to consume?

The Recommended Daily Allowances for pantothenic acid are 2 to 3 milligrams for infants, 3 to 5 milligrams for children, and 4 to 7 milligrams for adolescents and adults.

Deficiencies in pantothenic acid are considered uncommon because of its widespread availability in many foods. But because many people eat predominantly highly processed and refined foods, there may be widespread undernourishment of this nutrient. A comparison of potato products, for example, revealed that baked potatoes had 4.4 milligrams, boiled potatoes had 3.8 milligrams, instant mashed potatoes had 2.7 milligrams, homemade mashed potatoes had 2.5 milligrams, potato chips had 1.2 milligrams, and canned potatoes had .8 milligram of pantothenic acid per 1,000 kilocalories.

Signs of deficiency of this nutrient may include fatigue, abdominal pains, appetite loss, burning feet, numbness and tingling in fingers and toes, irritability, depression, respiratory infections, heart and intestinal disorders, insomnia, fainting, and hair loss. Laboratory animals fed a diet without the nutrient

had premature graying of the hair, but this phenomenon apparently does not occur in humans as a result of pantothenic acid deficiency.

There is no known toxicity, although extremely high doses (more than 10 grams a day) may cause water retention or diarrhea.

FOODS HIGH IN PANTOTHENIC ACID

Bran
Cheese, particularly blue
Chicken
Eggs
Fish, especially salmon
Dates
Grains (*except* enriched)—especially oats, rice, and wheat
Legumes—dry beans, peas
Mushrooms
Organ meats, especially liver
Nuts
Vegetables—broccoli, carrots, potatoes, sweet potatoes, tomatoes

VITAMIN C

What is it?

Vitamin C, or ascorbic acid, is a well-known essential nutrient with a long history of significance in preventing and curing the debilitating disease known as scurvy.

Scurvy was known of as far back as 1550 B.C. in Egypt and was a common malady for sailors whose diets usually consisted of dried meat and biscuits. Treatment with lemons, limes, oranges, pine branch soup, sauerkraut, and other foods usually did the trick but was not consistently practiced, so the sailors' disease persisted. In 1795 the British Royal Navy, by governmental decree, started giving each crew member an ounce of lime juice every day, prompting the nickname limeys for the sailors. Vitamin C was isolated in 1932 and given the name ascorbic acid in 1938.

Chemically, ascorbic acid is a simple compound known as $C_6H_8O_6$. It's chemical composition is similar to glucose, a sugar from which synthetic vitamin C is made. The word ascorbic is short for antiscorbutic, or antiscurvy; the C in vitamin C is for citrus, fruits in which vitamin C is found. Ascorbic acid is the least stable of the vitamins, due to its water solubility and sensitivity to alkalies and to oxidation by heat and air.

Two forms of vitamin C are found in nature: a reduced form called L-ascorbic acid, and an oxidized form called L-dehydroascorbic acid. The synthetic form of L-ascorbic acid is apparently utilized by the body with the same efficiency as the natural form. Vitamin C as a powder is white, odorless, and quite dry. It is used in many products, including lozenges, tablets, and instant meal powders.

How does my body use it?

Vitamin C is quickly absorbed from the duodenum (the upper small intestine) into the circulatory system. It is then taken up by the retina, adrenal glands, liver, spleen, kidneys, and other organs. Up to 90 percent of dietary vitamin C is absorbed. Due to its water solubility little vitamin C is stored in the body, so daily intake is necessary. Vitamin C is excreted by the kidneys in urine.

Probably the most important role of vitamin C is the formation of collagen, the substance that binds body cells. It is thought that vitamin C activates an enzyme that effects the conversion of the amino acid proline to hydroxyproline, which makes up much of the protein collagen.

Vitamin C also aids in the metabolism of other amino acids, folic acid, iron, and fats and lipids. Bodies that exhibit stress from injury, burns, shock, cigarette smoke inhalation, extremes in temperature, and toxicity from heavy metals also show an increased need for ascorbic acid. One theory holds that the higher the stress, the greater the need for vitamin C.

Vitamin C has been promoted as a cure or preventive for colds, infections, and fever, although various studies have not proven these claims to be reliable.

How much do I need to consume?

The Recommended Daily Allowances for ascorbic acid are 30 to 35 milligrams for infants, 40 to 45 milligrams for children ages 1 to 10, 50 milligrams for adolescents, 60 milligrams for people age 15 and up, and an additional 20 to 40 milligrams for pregnant and lactating women. Scurvy can be prevented with as little as 10 milligrams of vitamin C a day.

Symptoms of vitamin C deficiency include bleeding gums, tooth decay, nosebleeds, poor digestion, low resistance to infection, shortness of breath, anemia, weak cartilage, and slow wound healing. Acute scurvy is characterized by swollen and ulcerated gums, loose teeth, dark spots and bruises on the body, and weak or malformed bones. Sudden death may result from internal hemorrhage or heart failure.

High levels of vitamin C through supplementation may result in diarrhea, nausea, excess iron absorption, inactivation of vitamin B_{12}, formation of kidney and bladder stones, and destruction of red blood cells. Intake of up to 2 grams per day is considered nontoxic, but doses of more than 8 grams a day—more than one hundred times the Recommended Daily Allowance—are considered detrimental and unwarranted.

The availability of vitamin C in foods depends on several factors, including freshness, preparation, and storage. Vegetables have more vitamin C when picked on sunny days and eaten soon after harvesting than those picked during cloudy or rainy days and/or those that have been refrigerated after harvesting. Boiling vegetables depletes more water-soluble nutrients than steaming or pressure cooking; one study at the University of Minnesota showed vitamin C retention in broccoli to be 33 percent when boiled, 78 percent when steamed, and 88 percent when pressure cooked. Storing vegetables in broad daylight or for prolonged periods renders much of the vitamin C useless—there is usually none left in wilted greens.

In some countries, milk is fortified with vitamin C to insure adequate supplies for children. Unfortified milk is not a significant source of vitamin C.

FOODS HIGH IN VITAMIN C

All fruits and vegetables, particularly:
    Acerola (Barbados) cherry
    Broccoli
    Citrus fruits, especially grapefruit
    Currants, black

Elderberries

Green leafy vegetables

Guavas

Kiwi

Mangos

Melons—cantaloupe, cassava, honeydew, watermelon

Papayas

Peppers—green and red bell

Persimmons

Strawberries

Tomatoes

VITAMIN D

What is it?

Vitamin D is the only vitamin the body can manufacture (other than biotin) and therefore is technically not an essential dietary element. The making of it, however, is dependent on ultraviolet light from the sun, which converts a substance found in our skin (the inactive sterol 7-dehydrocholesterol) to another substance (cholecalciferol, or pre-vitamin D_3), which in turn is transported by a special D-binding protein and converted by the liver to a compound (25-hydroxycholicalciferol) that is then further converted by the kidneys to an active form (1, 25-dihydroxycholicalciferol). This compound works with calcium and phosphorus to be absorbed into bones, muscles, and intestines. The conversion process takes several days.

Vitamin D is also a substance found in some plants and animals, number-labeled according to its antirachitic (antirickets) characteristics. D_2, or ergocalciferol, is derived from plants such as alfalfa, fungi, nettles, plankton, watercress, and yeasts. D_3, or animal-derived cholecalciferol, is found in eggs, fish oils, and organ meats.

The history of the discovery of this nutrient is directly linked to the understanding of a disease known as rickets. Children living in slums in England during the 1600s frequently suffered from this disease, due to industrial smoke and high tenement buildings that blocked the sun's ultraviolet rays, but poor hygiene and home environments were considered the culprits. Cod liver oil was long known as a folk remedy for rickets, but no one knew why. A scientist in England in 1918 thought it was due to vitamin A in the fish oil. Subsequent research at various universities in the United States and Europe eventually shed more light on vitamin D, rickets, and natural forms of the nutrient.

How does my body use it?

After cholecalciferol is ingested or metabolized from sunlight, it is converted to other substances, as described above.

Vitamin D acts both as a vitamin and a hormone. It helps regulate calcium and phosphorus metabolism, which is responsible for bone and teeth formation, as well as resorption of calcium from the kidneys. It also maintains the nervous system and influences citrate metabolism and levels of amino acids in the blood.

Vitamin D metabolism is augmented by vitamin A, calcium, phosphorus, and choline. Absorption may be reduced or blocked by mineral oil, phenobarbital, and laxatives.

How much do I need to consume?

As little as 15 minutes a day of outdoor activities can recharge your skin's vitamin D cells, though direct exposure to ultraviolet radiation is influenced by the degree of atmospheric haze and air pollution which block both ultraviolet radiation and sunlight. Less ultraviolet light and sunlight in general are available in the winter, especially in northern regions.

The Recommended Daily Allowances of dietary vitamin D are 10 micrograms (400 IU) or less, with needs decreasing with age. Because this nutrient is fat soluble, it is stored in the body's adipose tissue as well as in the kidneys, liver, and skeletal muscles, and is not readily eliminated.

Milk is often fortified with vitamin D, a practice that has been credited with reducing the incidence of rickets in children. Rickets results in a variety of physical deformities, including curved spine, arm and leg bones; bow legs; knock-knees; enlarged knee and ankle joints; pot belly; protruding forehead; and beaded ribs.

Vitamin D deficiency may also cause osteomalacia, or bone softening, an ailment found mostly in adults who are bedridden or confined and women who have had multiple, closely-spaced pregnancies. Tetany (twitching and cramping muscles) and celiac disease are also affected by a lack of vitamin D. Signs of deficiency include nervousness, insomnia, diarrhea, a burning sensation in mouth and throat, and myopia.

Because vitamin D is stored in the body, toxic levels can accumulate. It is thought that sunshine-derived and normal dietary consumption of vitamin D will not cause hypervitaminosis D—only prolonged supplementation will lead to a high level of accumulation. Intake of more than 400 IU a day is considered excessive; the toxicity threshold is 500 to 600 micrograms per kilogram of body weight. Toxicity symptoms include excessive thirst, nausea, vomiting, appetite loss, increased urination, diarrhea, dizziness, and in severe cases hypocalcemia (elevated blood levels of calcium).

FOODS HIGH IN VITAMIN D

Egg yolks
Fish liver oils—cod, halibut, and swordfish
Liver (beef)
Milk, especially fortified
Salmon
Tuna

VITAMIN E

What is it?

Vitamin E is the epitome of alphabet soup in terms of biochemistry. To understand its composition and functions requires more energy than most consumers care to devote to the problem, so, although they may already be consuming adequate amounts of vitamin E, they are scared into thinking that they need to buy supplements.

The overall term used to describe vitamin E is *tocopherol,* from the Greek words *tokos,* meaning child or offspring, and *pherein,* to bear or bring forth, plus *-ol,* a suffix referring to alcohol. The substance, found in 1922 by H. M. Evans and K. S. Bishop, scientists at the University of California (who called it Factor X), was shown to be needed for successful reproduction in laboratory rats. It was designated as vitamin E in 1924. In 1936, Evans, and colleagues isolated a crystalline form of vitamin E from wheat germ oil and named it tocopherol.

There are four tocopherols and four tocotrienols that make up vitamin E, all named after Greek letters: alpha (α), beta (β), gamma (δ), and delta (Δ); and zeta (ζ), epsilon (ϵ), eta (η), and theta (θ, also called 8-methyl tocotrienol). Together, they are dubbed *all-rac*-α-tocopherol. Because α-tocopherol is the most biologically active form, it is used as a standard for comparative purposes.

To further complicate a layperson's understanding of this nutrient, it is designated differently in scientific and commercial publications, depending on whether it is naturally derived or synthetically produced and whether it's found as (or made with) an acetate or succinate ester. These esters help stabilize vitamin E; when esters are part of the chemical compound, the spelling of tocopherol becomes tocopheryl.

How does my body use it?

Vitamin E is fat soluble—it's found naturally in fats and oils—so bile, pancreatic juices, and fat are needed for its absorption in the small intestine. Only an estimated 20 to 30 percent of ingested vitamin E is absorbed into the lymph and transported to the bloodstream. It is stored in fatty tissue, muscle, liver, adrenal and pituitary glands, heart, lungs, and reproductive organs. Vitamin E is excreted in the feces.

Absorption of vitamin E is enhanced by adequate levels of vitamins A, B-complex, C, magnesium, manganese, and selenium. Chlorine (from municipal water), laxatives, rancid fats and oils, inorganic iron, mineral oil, and oral contraceptives can deter absorption of vitamin E.

The main attribute of vitamin E is its function as an antioxidant. It joins with enzymes to protect polyunsaturated fats in the body from destruction by oxygen-containing free radicals such as peroxides and superoxides. These substances can damage cells and membranes in the body, particularly in the testes. Vitamin E helps protect lungs from air pollution, prevents tumor growth, and is needed for vitamin A utilization. It also protects breast, eye, liver, calf muscle, and skin tissues.

Vitamin E Supplements

Naturally derived vitamin E is labeled *d*-α-tocopherol and is measured in International Units (IU). It is obtained from vegetable oils such as wheat germ. Synthetic vitamin E is *dl*-α-tocopherol and is usually measured in milligrams rather than IU. It is derived from petroleum or turpentine and is comparatively inexpensive to produce. Synthetic vitamin E attempts to duplicate natural *d*-α-tocopherol, but studies have shown that it is significantly inferior in the human body, in some cases only half as potent as the natural form.

Guide to Vitamin E

Type of vitamin E	Form	International Units in 1 milligram
Natural	*d*-α-tocopherol	1.49
Natural	*d*-α-tocopheryl acetate	1.36
Natural	*d*-α-tocopheryl acid succinate	1.21
Synthetic	*dl*-α-tocopherol	1.10
Synthetic	*dl*-α-tocopheryl acetate	1.00
Synthetic	*dl*-α-tocopheryl acid succinate	0.89

From *Natural Nutritional Foods Association* Vitamin E Report 1980.

Some manufacturers of vitamin E supplements sell products that contain blends of naturally and synthetically derived α-tocopherol but downplay or disregard entirely that their products are partly or mostly synthetic. Furthermore, the substances may be composed of more than just α-tocopherol—they may be mixed with β-, δ-, and Δ-tocopherols, for example. Consumers should look on the labels for the words "100% natural source" or learn more about the reputation of the companies.

As with most supplements, megadosing on vitamin E is not only wasteful but usually unnecessary and possibly expensive. One vitamin E pill provides 200 to 1,000 IU—600 to 3,000 percent of the Recommended Daily Allowance! If your diet is low in foods containing vitamin E (or other essential nutrients for that matter), change it rather than relying on the highly profitable commercial supplements. Certain conditions may warrant supplementation, in which case advice from your health-care provider is recommended.

Vitamin E has also been touted as an antiaging substance and fertility booster. It is thought to prevent or remedy dry or dull hair, miscarriages, muscle wasting or weakness, and gastrointestinal ailments.

How much do I need to consume?

The Recommended Daily Allowances for vitamin E are 3 to 4 milligrams for infants, 6 to 7 milligrams for children, 8 to 10 milligrams for adolescents and adults, and an additional 2 to 3 milligrams or more for pregnant and lactating women.

Vitamin E deficiency is considered rare because of its widespread availability in foods and long-term retention in the body. Premature, formula-fed newborn infants are occasionally deficient in vitamin E, as are people who suffer from a protein-deficiency disease called kwashiorkor. Symptoms of vitamin E deficiency include inability to absorb fat, increased fragility of red blood cells, and increased urinary excretion of creatine (a compound formed in the liver) which indicates muscle damage.

Excessive intake of vitamin E, on the other hand, may result in a variety of clinical disorders and was shown to induce abnormalities in laboratory animals. Some of the reported conditions are dizziness, headache, nausea, and chapped lips (all fairly common health complaints) and hypertension. Among the abnormalities reported were altered immune response, altered hormone metabolism, and increased levels of serum triglycerides and cholesterol among women taking birth control pills.

Vitamin E is found in nuts and seeds, particularly those that are pressed into cooking oils. Certain fish and animal organs also contain vitamin E. Due to commercial processing techniques and storage practices, however, vitamin E is often removed from grains during milling and from oils before bottling (see page 27), or it is destroyed while the oils sit on kitchen shelves. "Recycled" cooking oils (from deep-fat frying) are particularly low in or detrimental to vitamin E, as they have been oxidized through boiling and exposure to light and air. To help retain or minimize loss of vitamin E, buy small amounts of cold-pressed oils and refrigerate them, and also keep nuts in their shells or in the refrigerator.

FOODS HIGH IN VITAMIN E

Almonds and almond oil
Beef brains
Blackberries
Cantaloupe
Cod liver oil
Corn, cornmeal, and corn oil
Cottonseed oil
Currants (black)
Grapefruit
Oats
Olive oil
Peanuts
Safflower oil
Sunflower seeds/Sunflower oil
Tuna (in oil)
Wheat and wheat germ
Wheat germ oil (best source)

VITAMIN K

What is it?

Vitamin K is a name for two naturally occurring compounds and one synthetically derived chemical compound. Named by the Danish scientist Carl Peter Hendrik Dam, who conducted extensive studies on what he termed Koagulation (blood coagulation), vitamin K is now recognized as an essential nutrient.

Vitamin K_1, also called *phylloquinone* or *phytylmenaquinone,* is obtained from green plant foods. Vitamin K_2, also called *menaquinones* or *multiprenylmenaquinones,* is synthesized by microorganisms in the intestines. Vitamin K_3, more commonly referred to as *menadione,* is a synthetic compound sold as a vitamin supplement. It is water soluble and has double or triple the potency of the other two forms of vitamin K.

How does my body use it?

Vitamin K is fat soluble and thereby needs bile and pancreatic juice in order to be metabolized in the intestine. An estimated 10 to 70 percent of vitamin K is absorbed and transported to the lymph system, then to the thoracic duct. There it enters the bloodstream and links up with beta-lipoproteins, then goes to the liver and other tissues where it is stored in small amounts. It is excreted through feces and urine.

Vitamin K is essential to the process of blood coagulation (clotting) in assisting the liver in the synthesis of four proteins: prothrombin (factor II), proconvertin (factor VII), Christmas factor (factor IV), and Stuart power (factor X). Other vitamin K-dependent proteins have been found in the kidneys, bones, and liver, but their functions have yet to be determined.

Vitamin K absorption may be stifled by the presence of mineral oil, a nonabsorbable fat; dicoumarol, a substance found in sweet clover; and warfarin, a rat poison. (The latter two items are noted more in terms of pet and livestock nutrition than for human diets.)

How much do I need to consume?

The Recommended Daily Allowances for vitamin K are 12 to 20 micrograms for infants, 15 to 30 micrograms for children ages 1 to 10, 45 to 65 micrograms for adolescents and teenagers, and 60 to 80 micrograms for adults. Our diets generally supply an estimated 300 to 500 micrograms a day, so deficiencies are thought to be uncommon. Vitamin K deficiency is evidenced by slow blood clotting as well as a hemorrhagic disease of newborns, particularly in breast-fed premature babies (mother's milk has less vitamin K than commercial formulas).

Too much vitamin K is possible not from dietary sources but from consumption of the synthetic form, menadione, at levels of more than 5 milligrams a day, which may cause jaundice. The U.S. Food and Drug Administration bans menadione in food supplements intended for prenatal consumption.

FOODS HIGH IN VITAMIN K₁

Alfalfa leaf
Asparagus
Broccoli
Cabbage
Lettuce
Liver
Spinach
Tea (green)
Turnip greens
Watercress

VITAMIN P (BIOFLAVONOIDS)

What is it?

This vitamin holds the dubious distinction of not being recognized as a true vitamin, yet it is an essential and indispensable constituent of foods, and known deficiency syndromes can be cured as a direct result of its administration.

The substances that fall under the vitamin P category are better known as *bioflavonoids*. These yellow-colored plant pigments get their name from *flavus,* the Latin word for yellow. Although about eight hundred bioflavonoids have been identified in plants (thirty in citrus fruits), some of the most commonly known are:

- Citrin—Found in citrus fruits, it was once called vitamin T.
- Hesperidin—Found in ripe orange peels, orange

blossoms, lemons, citrons, and mandarins. It is used in pharmaceuticals as a therapeutic agent.
- Naringin—Found in grapefruit, it is quite bitter and used as a flavoring agent.
- Rutin—Found originally in the garden plant rue (*ruta graveolens*) and later discovered in buckwheat and tobacco. Rutin tablets are sold as a medicinal aid to treat capillary fragility.

Bioflavonoids are generally present in (and therefore consumed with) foods that contain vitamin C. Their metabolism is also similar to vitamin C, which is in part why they have not been officially granted vitamin status.

How does my body use it?

Bioflavonoids help regulate the permeability of capillaries, the smallest blood vessels in our bodies. Capillary breakage is indicative of scurvy, a disease associated with a deficiency in vitamin C (ascorbic acid). Since bioflavonoids and vitamin C are found together in nature and work together in the body, attributing any specific cures or deficiencies to only one of the substances seems moot. Researchers have found many instances where vitamin C was effective only when combined with bioflavonoids.

Bioflavonoids are absorbed in the upper small intestine and excreted in the urine. They are destroyed by light but are resistant to oxygen, heat, dryness, and some acidity.

Bioflavonoids function as antioxidants to preserve fruits and vegetables and as activators of enzymes. They help bind (chelate) metals and help control bacteria and infections. Bioflavonoids can also stop or inhibit the growth of cancer cells and protect against cell damage by carcinogens.

Bioflavonoids have been used to treat health problems concerning blood, including bleeding gums, hemorrhoids, varicose veins, ulcers, excessive menstrual flow, and thrombosis (clot in a blood vessel).

How much do I need to consume?

No Recommended Daily Allowances for bioflavonoids have been determined. An estimated 1 gram of bioflavonoids is consumed by North Americans every day, about half of which is absorbed.

Signs of bioflavonoid/vitamin C deficiencies include tendencies to bruise or bleed easily, bleeding gums, nosebleeds, and frequent colds.

Bioflavonoids are not toxic.

Commercial bioflavonoid products are often extracted from leftover pulp from squeezing and canning fruits for fruit juice or frozen concentrate. For this reason, it is important to eat fresh fruits rather than rely only on fruit juices to meet nutritional needs.

FOODS HIGH IN BIOFLAVONOIDS

Apricots
Beer
Blackberries
Broccoli
Buckwheat leaves
Cantaloupe
Cherries
Coffee
Currants (black)
Grapefruit*
Grapes
Lemons*
Mandarins*
Onions (red and yellow skins)
Oranges*
Papaya
Peppers
Plums
Rose hips
Tangerines
Tea
Tomatoes
Vinegar
Wine, especially red

*Especially the rind, pulp, and membranes

CALCIUM

What is it?

Calcium is the chief mineral in animal bodies. Our bones and teeth hold 99 percent of the 1,200 grams present (about 2 percent of body weight), with the remaining 1 percent distributed in soft tissues and extracellular fluids.

This silver-white alkaline metal requires the presence of an acidic substance in order to be assimilated by the body, as well as adequate levels of other nutrients mentioned below.

As a dietary element, calcium's role in bone formation has been known since at least 1842, when a French scientist named Chossat demonstrated that pigeons fed only wheat died after ten months but others survived after calcium carbonate was included in their diet.

How does my body use it?

Calcium is needed for formation of bones, teeth, and muscles. It plays a role in blood clotting, permeability of cell membranes, nerve transmission, enzyme activation, and with magnesium in muscle contraction and relaxation, including regular heartbeat.

Calcium absorption takes place in the upper part of the small intestine. Only an estimated 20 to 30 percent of ingested calcium is absorbed by most people; 40 percent or more is absorbed by children and pregnant or lactating women, whose needs are greater. Absorbed calcium enters the bloodstream to replace bone tissue and perform its other functions.

Factors affecting calcium absorption include adequate levels of magnesium, phosphorus, vitamins A, C, and D, iron, and the amino acid lysine. Calcium absorption is also enhanced by exercise, sunlight, and lactose (milk sugar). A decreased level of calcium absorption may be caused by the presence of oxalic and phytic acids, dietary fiber, lack of exercise, imbalance in calcium/phosphorus ratio, vitamin D deficiency, too much saturated fat and sugar, diuretics, phenobarbital, and tetracyclines.

Calcium is excreted by feces as well as urine. Postmenopausal women and elderly men lose calcium and consequently are more susceptible to brittle bones and osteoporosis.

How much do I need to consume?

The Recommended Daily Allowances for calcium are 400 to 600 milligrams for infants, 800 milligrams for children age 1 to 10 and older adults, and 1,200 milligrams for teenagers, young adults, and pregnant and lactating women. If calcium intake is not adequate during pregnancy, the fetus absorbs it from the mother's bones or teeth.

Dairy products are often promoted as excellent sources of calcium, although they are also high in saturated fat (particularly cheese and ice cream). Some calcium may be obtained from drinking water but this is usually not considered a major source of the mineral.

Symptoms of calcium deficiency include fragile bones, muscle cramps, leg and arm numbness, eczema, insomnia, irritability, nervousness, brittle nails, tooth decay, heart palpitations, rickets, and stunted growth. Women who suffer from premenstrual syndrome (PMS) and menstrual cramps can benefit from increased calcium and magnesium intake by consuming a drink made with a tablespoon of blackstrap molasses in a glass of milk or water. Exercise, yoga, and restricted intake of sugar, chocolate, and caffeine products also aid in reducing PMS.

Hypercalcemia, or excessive calcium, is often caused by too much vitamin D and can prevent blood coagulation or result in retarded growth and upset stomach. A calcium/magnesium imbalance (more calcium than magnesium) may result in calcium deposits in the heart, muscles, and kidney and could lead to kidney stones. Bone abnormalities such as osteopetrosis (dense bone) may also result from prolonged excessive calcium intake.

FOODS HIGH IN CALCIUM

(100 milligrams or more per serving)
Beet greens*
Bok choy (Chinese cabbage)
Broccoli
Cheese (all types)
Collard greens
Cottonseed flour
Dandelion greens
Figs, dried
Ice cream
Kale

Milk
Molasses (blackstrap)
Mustard greens
Nuts—almonds, Brazil nuts, filberts
Salmon (with bone)
Sardines
Soybeans and soy flour
Spinach*
Tofu (if made with a calcium coagulant)
Turnip greens
Yogurt

*Also high in oxalic acid, a calcium inhibitor

CHLORIDE

What is it?

In its isolated form, this element is a gas named appropriately for its greenish yellow color. The word is derived from the Greek *chloros*. As a dietary mineral chloride is a compound with sodium in table salt. It is also used as a gas (chlorine) to destroy bacteria in municipal water supplies.

How does my body use it?

Chloride is necessary for forming hydrochloric acid, an acid present in gastric juices that helps the liver eliminate wastes. Chloride also plays a role in the body's acid/alkaline balance.

Chloride is absorbed from the small intestine and distributed to body fluids, primarily extracellular fluids, where much of it is stored. Approximately 100 grams are present in extracellular fluids; chloride is also present in blood (450 to 600 milligrams per 100 milliliters). It is excreted through the kidneys as well as through sweat and feces.

Chlorine in drinking water is a highly reactive substance that can bind with other minerals or chemicals to form harmful substances and destroy intestinal flora and vitamin E.

How much do I need to consume?

Because chloride is a component of salt (sodium chloride), no Recommended Daily Allowance levels have been established. We consume an estimated

3 to 9 grams of salt a day—more than adequate to supply dietary chloride.

Deficiencies of chloride result only from purging, vomiting, diarrhea, stomach pumping, excessive intake of diuretics, and extremely restricted salt intake. Infants with inadequate levels of chloride developed hypovolemia and metabolic alkalosis and have urinary potassium loss. Memory loss, psychomotor impairment, retarded growth, hair and tooth loss, and low muscle tone may also result from chloride deficiency.

No toxicity levels have been determined for chloride, as it is believed that excesses are excreted if kidneys are functioning.

FOODS HIGH IN CHLORIDE

Olives (ripe)
Rye flour
Salt
Seaweeds

CHROMIUM

What is it?

Chromium is a hard shiny metal used for plating automobile trim, bumpers, and other items for which corrosion resistance is desired. Derived from the Greek word *chroma,* meaning "color," chromium is often found in ores with varied color compounds that are used as pigments and dyes.

Dietary chromium has four functions: as an essential element, as a hormone, as a vitamin, and as a poison.

How does my body use it?

Our bodies contain minute amounts of chromium, an estimated 20 parts per billion in blood and 6 milligrams in total body weight. The availability of chromium in the diet is affected by the type of cooking utensils used, its content in soils in which food is grown, extent of processing and refining, and fermentation.

Chromium absorption may be hindered by inadequate protein intake, excessive consumption of processed and refined foods, and high iron levels. It is also reduced by repeated pregnancies. Inorganic chromium is absorbed at the rate of 1 percent or less, but an organically bound chromium compound, known as glucose tolerance factor (GTF), is absorbed at a rate of 10 to 25 percent.

GTF, which also contains glycine, niacin, cysteine, and glutamic acid, works with insulin to facilitate movement of sugar, fatty acids, and amino acids from cells into tissues, as well as to metabolize other nutrients in the cells.

Chromium also cooperates with other substances to activate trypsin, a digestive enzyme, as well as other enzymes that produce energy from carbohydrates, fats, and protein. It plays a role in stabilizing RNA (nucleic acid) and in stimulating the synthesis of cholesterol and fatty acids in the liver.

How much do I need to consume?

The estimated safe and adequate daily dietary intake levels for chromium are 10 to 60 micrograms for infants, 20 to 120 micrograms for children up to age 6, and 50 to 200 micrograms for people age 7 and up. These recommended rates are based on average intakes rather than definitive requirements.

Because chromium acts with various other nutrients and substances in the body, it is hard to determine if a deficiency exists. Tests used to assess chromium levels include hair analysis, glucose tolerance (blood sugar) test, and urine analysis.

People with diabetic and hypoglycemic symptoms may find that increased dietary chromium may benefit their health. Chromium can also lower cholesterol; chromium was found to be absent in the aortas of people who died from atherosclerosis (heart attack) but not in those who died in accidents. Cataracts—cloudy spots on eye lenses—may also indicate a lack of chromium. (Could sparkly eyes indicate abundant reserves of this shiny metal?) It is generally advised that treatment of suspected chromium deficiency be under medical supervision rather than self-administered.

Chromium toxicity from dietary sources is unlikely, but ingestion of inorganic chromium salts could prove hazardous, as they reduce absorption of other trace elements and may disrupt the balance of insulin and GTF. Chromium contamination from some industrial areas pollutes air, food, and water and may injure body tissues.

FOODS HIGH IN CHROMIUM

Apple peel
Beef
Beer
Bran
Cheese
Chicken
Dolomite tablets
Eggs
Liver
Molasses (blackstrap)
Oysters
Potatoes
Wheat (whole grain)
Wheat germ
Yeast—brewer's and torula

COBALT

What is it?

Cobalt is a hard gray metal whose name holds the story of a sixteenth-century tragedy in the Harz Mountains of central Europe. Silver miners there found an ore thought to be copper but that actually contained both cobalt and arsenic. Upon heating the rocks, a toxic vapor (arsenic trioxide) was released, injuring the workers. That vapor spirit was deemed a goblin, or, in the Germanic language, *Kobold*.

Cobalt has long been used in pottery and glass to make blue dishes and drinking vessels. It was first isolated in 1742 by the Swedish chemist George Brandt. In 1948, cobalt was found to be a small but essential component of vitamin B_{12}.

Cobalt is present in soil but is deficient in some areas, notably Florida, parts of North and South Carolina, western Canada, and Australia. Low cobalt levels are also found in southeastern Minnesota, northern Iowa, southeastern Kansas, northern Michigan, northern and southern parts of New York state, southern Maine, and all the New England states.

How does my body use it?

Cobalt is ingested as part of the vitamin B_{12} molecule (see page 211). It is also present in various foods but is apparently not absorbed in any other form than as a constituent of B_{12}.

Most of the cobalt absorbed by the body is excreted in the feces or urine; a small reserve (0.2 ppm) is stored in the liver and kidneys. Blood concentrations are 80 to 300 micrograms per milliliter.

Cobalt, as a constituent of cobalamin, plays a role in activating enzymes and may substitute for manganese or replace zinc for certain functions.

How much do I need to consume?

Cobalt makes up only about 4 percent of the vitamin B_{12} molecule. The estimated daily intake of cobalt is 1 to 8 micrograms. No adequate or safe levels nor Recommended Daily Allowances have been established for cobalt.

Sheep and cattle that graze on cobalt-deficient lands may show signs of anemia or emaciation. In humans, a deficiency is usually attributed to low levels of vitamin B_{12} rather than to cobalt itself.

Excessive cobalt could be toxic, with symptoms including polycythemia (a high level of red blood cells), nausea, vomiting, appetite loss, and in serious instances deafness and death in children.

FOODS KNOWN TO CONTAIN COBALT*

Beet greens
Buckwheat
Cabbage
Figs
Lettuce
Spinach
Watercress

*Also see the list for vitamin B_{12}, page 212.

COPPER

What is it?

Copper, a metal more commonly known for its use in pipes and kettles, is also an essential trace element for human nutrition. Our bodies contain 75 to 125 milligrams of copper, stored mainly in the liver and brain but also in tissues and other organs.

Copper gets its name from *cuprum,* the Roman word for Cyprian metal. People in the Mediterranean Sea region historically obtained copper from the island of Cyprus. The metal has been used since the late Stone Age but wasn't considered a dietary necessity until tests in the 1920s and 1930s demonstrated the role copper played in preventing anemia.

How does my body use it?

Copper aids in iron absorption for hemoglobin production. It activates cytochrome oxidase, an enzyme that helps release energy to cells and thus enables us to think and have nerve responses. Other enzymes rely on copper for their functioning; these include spermine oxidase, dopamine, tryptophan pyrolase, and superoxide dismutase.

Copper works with vitamin C to synthesize phospholipids (such as lecithin) and is also needed for collagen formation for bones, tendons, and connective tissue.

Copper is absorbed in the stomach and upper small intestine. About 30 percent of ingested copper is absorbed; the rest is excreted in feces. Cobalt, iron, molybdenum, and zinc are needed for copper absorption, which is also enhanced by acids but inhibited by cadmium, calcium, lead, silver, sulfur, oral contraceptives, and excessive intake of molybdenum and zinc.

How much do I need to consume?

The estimated safe and adequate daily dietary intake levels for copper are .4 to .7 milligram for infants, .7 to 2.0 milligrams for children, and 1.5 to 3.0 milligrams for people age 11 and up. We generally consume 2.5 to 5 milligrams of copper every day.

Because of widespread availability of copper in foods, deficiency is rare in the United States. Symptoms include anemia, impaired growth and respiration, and weakness. Copper deficiency can also cause bone demineralization, defects in pigmentation and structure of hair, poor iron utilization, re-

productive failure, and impairment of the central nervous system.

Copper poisoning is also rare but may result from extended intake of 20 to 30 milligrams or more per day, either through supplementation or consumption of water or beverages from pipes or tanks that leach copper. Symptoms of toxicity include a genetic disorder called Wilson's disease, which results in hepatitis (caused by excessive deposits of copper in the liver), neurologic disorders, and renal malfunction. The disease reportedly can be reversed by administration of chelating agents that bind excess copper and eliminate it in the urine, as well as by monitoring dietary intake of copper.

FOODS HIGH IN COPPER

Black pepper
Cocoa
Eggs
Fruits (fresh and dried)
Grains (whole)
Liver
Lobster
Molasses (blackstrap)
Nuts, especially Brazil nuts
Olives, green
Oysters (raw)
Soybean flour
Vegetables, especially green leafy

FOODS LOW IN COPPER

Dairy products
Fats and oils
Sugar

IODINE

What is it?

Iodine is a crystalline nonmetallic trace element unevenly distributed in soil. Its name is from the Greek *iodes,* a word for violet, the color of iodine fumes.

This element is considered to be the first recognized essential nutrient. Chinese treatment of goiter with seaweeds and burnt sponge dates back to 3,000 B.C., and the Greek Hippocrates, known as the father of medicine, prescribed seaweeds to patients with enlarged thyroid glands.

Various regions of the world have low levels of iodine in the soil. In the United States these include the inland Pacific Northwest, the Rockies, the Great Lakes area, and a large span above the Arctic Circle in Alaska. In Canada there are iodine-deficient pockets in British Columbia, Alberta, and Saskatchewan.

Iodine-fortified (iodized) salt was introduced in the United States after Edward Kendall, a Nobel Prize winner who worked at the Mayo Clinic in Rochester, Minnesota, isolated thyroxin in 1914, demonstrated its effectiveness in reducing goiters, and showed how iodine was necessary for synthesizing this hormone.

How does my body use it?

Iodine is converted to an iodide, such as potassium iodide, in the small intestine. About 30 percent is absorbed. It then goes to the thyroid gland to synthesize hormones or is excreted in the urine. Those hormones, thyroxine and its precursors, are the prime governors of nutrient metabolism. They regulate the rate of oxidation within cells, thereby influencing physical and mental growth and the functioning of the muscle tissues and nervous and circulatory systems.

Our bodies contain 20 to 50 milligrams of iodine, about half of which is found in muscles. An estimated 10 milligrams is stored in the thyroid gland; less iodine is stored in skin, bones, and other endocrine glands. It is excreted via the kidneys and to a lesser extent by tears, saliva, sweat, and bile.

Iodine may be important for breast development and is thought to be a possible cancer preventive in combination with selenium.

How much do I need to consume?

Iodine is needed in trace amounts. As little as 150 micrograms a day is adequate to prevent goiter in adults. Recommended Daily Allowances for infants are 40 to 50 micrograms; for children 70 to 120 micrograms. Pregnant and lactating women are advised to have a daily intake of 175 to 200 micrograms.

Most dietary iodine is derived from iodized salt, but it can also be obtained from seafood and seaweeds as well as from drinking water in areas where iodine is prevalent in the soil. Iodine is sometimes used as a stabilizer in bread dough and may therefore be found in breads.

A deficiency of iodine, as mentioned above, results in goiter. This disease literally translates as "big throat," and was fairly common in North America before iodized salt was available. Goiters may also be induced or affected by goitrogens, naturally occurring substances found in *Brassicas* (cabbage, cauliflower, mustard seeds, turnips), peanuts, rutabagas, and soybeans. Synthetic goitrogens are present in the drugs sulfanomide, thiourea, and thiouracil.

Cretinism, a congenital disease marked by mental and physical retardation, is due to mothers whose diets were deficient in iodine during adolescence and pregnancy.

FOODS HIGH IN IODINE

Kelp
Mushrooms
Salt (iodized)
Seafoods
Seaweed
Water (certain areas)

IRON

What is it?

Iron is a finicky element, yet it is one of the most important nutrients for bodily health. A cheap and abundant metal, it is found in ores throughout the world. Ironically, it is deficient in the diets of 10 to 50 percent of the population worldwide.

Two forms of dietary iron are found:

- Ferric—Also called nonheme or inorganic, this is the storage and transport form of iron. It is found in beans, vegetables, and fruits. Only 2 to 10 percent of this type of iron is absorbed by the body.
- Ferrous—Also referred to as functional, heme, or organic iron, it is found in meat, particularly liver. About 30 percent of this type of iron is absorbed by the body.

How does my body use it?

Iron's main job is to work with protein to create hemoglobin for red blood cells (heme = iron; globin = protein). It is also necessary for transporting hydrogen to oxygen for energy production and for enzyme processes.

Iron is absorbed in the small intestine, mostly in the duodenum (the upper part of the small intestine). Absorption is controlled by what is known as the ferritin curtain. This little understood inhibitor apparently needs just the right amounts of vitamins B6, C, E, and F, nineteen amino acids, cobalt, and copper in either the blood serum or tissue structures before it lets iron join the bloodstream. Iron absorption may also be impaired by excess intake of calcium, phosphorus, magnesium, and zinc; phytic, oxalic, and tannic acids; coffee; and antacids.

Once it is absorbed, iron is reused in the body. It is stored in the liver but is also excreted in feces. Dark stools may indicate high iron excretion, and constipation may be caused by too much or too little iron. Some iron is lost through shedding of skin and hair. We lose an estimated 1 to 1.5 milligrams of iron every day. Blood donors and people with ulcers or hemorrhages lose significant amounts of iron.

How much do I need to consume?

The Recommended Daily Allowances for iron are 6 to 10 milligrams for infants and children, 12 milligrams for teenage males, 10 milligrams for adult men and postmenopausal women, 15 milligrams for menstruating and lactating women (ages approximately 11 to 50), and 30 milligrams for pregnant women.

As mentioned above, iron is not readily absorbed, and people who take iron supplements may find that their deficiency symptoms persist. Some nutritionists recommend increased intake of foods or supplements containing vitamin C, B6, B12, and folic acid to aid in iron absorption.

The most prevalent sign of iron deficiency is anemia, indicated by fatigue, lethargy, poor skin color, apathy, headaches, brittle or spoon-shaped nails, and reduced brain function. Other signs of iron shortage include dark circles under the eyes, poor memory, and loss of hair. Another indicator is an unusual appetite for clay, starch, or ice. Children who are low in iron may exhibit a short attention span, reduced IQ, or hyperactivity.

Iron toxicity, known as siderosis or hemochromatosis, may result from excess iron injections or transfusions or long-term excess consumption of iron-fortified foods. It is indicated by the presence of iron in soft tissues, which may cause hyperpigmentation of skin, cirrhosis of the liver, and diabetes. Iron poisoning also occurs when children consume their parents' medicinal iron supplements. Lethal doses of ferrous sulfate are about 3 grams for a two-year-old child and between 200 and 250 milligrams per kilogram of body weight for an adult. Ferrous fumarate is considered to be the safest form of iron supplement.

FOODS HIGH IN IRON

Almonds
Asparagus
Beans and peas
Eggplant
Eggs
Fish and shellfish
Fruits (dried)
Grains (whole)
Herbs—thyme, parsley, marjoram, etc.
Liver and other organ meats
Meat (lean)
Molasses (blackstrap)
Potatoes
Prune juice
Sunflower seeds
Teff
Vegetables, especially green leafy
Wheat germ

MAGNESIUM

What is it?

Magnesium is a white metal and an essential element. The name is from Magnesia, a district in Greece known for its curative white salts (Latin: *magnesia alba*). Long used as a laxative and mineral bath salt, magnesium was isolated by the British chemist Sir Humphrey Davy in 1808.

Magnesium accounts for 20 to 30 grams (about 2 ounces) of an adult's total body weight. It is found in many foods.

Magnesium compounds are often used therapeutically. These include magnesium sulfate (Epsom salts) and magnesium hydroxide (milk of magnesia).

How does my body use it?

Magnesium is absorbed in the small intestine and conserved or resorbed by the kidneys. Only about 40 percent of the dietary element is absorbed, with the remaining 60 percent excreted in urine or feces. Absorption may be enhanced by adequate levels of protein, vitamins B6, C, and D, and lactose (milk sugar), but may be blocked by oxalic and phytic acids, high calcium intake, or poorly digested fats, as well as oral contraceptives and tetracycline.

The roles of magnesium in the body are many. It helps maintain the body's acid/alkaline balance, assists in bone formation and energy production, relaxes muscles, and helps prevent tooth decay. Magnesium is needed to remove excess ammonia and for formation of urea. It has also been used to treat skin problems and senility.

How much do I need to consume?

The Recommended Daily Allowances for magnesium are 40 to 60 milligrams for infants; 80 to 170 milligrams for children ages 1 to 10; 270 to 280 for teenagers 11 to 14 and females age 19 and up; 400 milligrams for men ages 15 to 18; 350 milligrams for men ages 19 and up; 300 milligrams for women ages 15 to 18 and pregnant women; and 340 to 355 milligrams for lactating women.

Signs of magnesium deficiency include anorexia; anxiety; appetite loss; confusion and disorientation; gastrointestinal disorders; hallucinations (especially in alcoholics); lack of coordination; muscle cramps, spasms, tremors, or twitching; noise sensitivity; nausea; vomiting; and weakness. People prone to becoming easily irritable or angry may have inadequate magnesium intake. Long-term deficiency may also cause lesions of the skin and small arteries, swollen gums, and hair loss.

Too much magnesium affects metabolism of cal-

cium and phosphorus. Excessive use of magnesium laxatives may also deplete other minerals.

Hypermagnesemia (toxic intake of magnesium) is often caused by ingestion of antacids, laxatives, or other drugs that contain magnesium and is frequently found in elderly people who consume those products. Symptoms include lethargy, weakness, drowsiness, and in serious instances depression, coma, and death.

FOODS HIGH IN MAGNESIUM

Chocolate
Coffee
Cottonseed flour
Fish and seafood
Fruit (dried)
Grains (whole)
Meat
Molasses
Nuts
Peanuts
Soybean flour
Vegetables, especially green leafy

MANGANESE

What is it?

Manganese is an essential trace mineral that is used industrially as a metal to toughen steel. Its name is derived from *magnesia,* a Latin word for magnetic stone, and may consequently be confused with magnesium.

Manganese is necessary for plant growth and was deemed to be essential to animal nutrition in 1931 after researchers at the University of Wisconsin found that deficiencies in chickens resulted in a bone disease known as slipped tendon.

Like other minerals, manganese levels in food vary with soil conditions. Reportedly, plants grown in soil to which limestone has been added as a fertilizer and pH balancer have less manganese uptake.

How does my body use it?

Manganese activates several enzymes needed for formation of bones, connective tissue, and urea, and for metabolism or synthesis of carbohydrates, lipids, vitamin E, protein, and nucleic acids (RNA and DNA). The mineral also affects the pituitary, reproductive, and thyroid glands. Like zinc, manganese can displace excess copper but can also be stifled by too much iron. Conversely, an excess of manganese may block iron absorption. Excessive calcium and phosphorus may also affect manganese utilization.

Our bodies contain 10 to 20 milligrams of manganese, stored in small amounts in the bones, kidneys, liver, pancreas, pituitary gland, and tissues. It is excreted through feces or resorbed.

How much do I need to consume?

The estimated safe and adequate daily dietary intake levels for manganese are .3 to 1.0 milligram for infants, 1 to 3 milligrams for children, and 2.0 to 5 milligrams for people age 11 and up.

Signs of manganese deficiency include ear noises, hearing loss, impaired glucose (blood sugar) tolerance, failure of muscle coordination, and elevated blood cholesterol.

Toxic levels of manganese are often found in lungs of miners. Symptoms of toxicity include anorexia, apathy, ataxia, headaches, impotence, leg cramps, and speech impairment, which can advance to a condition similar to Parkinson's disease whereby a person so affected has a monotone voice, blank expression, and rigid muscles.

FOODS HIGH IN MANGANESE

> Bananas
> Beans, especially soybeans
> Blueberries
> Bran
> Buckwheat
> Lettuce
> Molasses
> Nuts
> Potatoes
> Rice (brown)
> Spices
> Sunflower seeds

MOLYBDENUM

What is it?

This silver-gray element gets its name from the Greek *molybdos,* a word for lead (a different substance). Molybdenite ore is mined in the southwestern United States and used for hardening steel.

The availability of dietary molybdenum is influenced by its presence in the soil. Land that has low molybdenum levels is often barren, as this element is needed to support bacteria in root nodules of nitrogen-fixing plants such as beans and peas. Molybdenum is also obtained from drinking water, with hard (high mineral content) water providing up to 41 percent of dietary intake in some areas. People who live in molybdenum-deficient regions have a higher-than-normal incidence of esophagal cancer, which is apparently from formation of nitrosamines due to the lack of molybdenum.

Molybdenum's role as an essential element for plant growth was known before researchers learned of its metabolic functioning in animals. Our bodies contain about 9 milligrams of this element, which is stored in the liver, kidney, and body tissues.

How does my body use it?

Molybdenum is necessary for enzyme functions that affect oxidation of aldehydes and the formation of adenosine triphosphate (ATP), which produces energy in our muscles. The enzyme xanthine oxidase affects uric acid formation and helps convert iron from ferrous to ferric (metabolizable) form.

Our bodies metabolize molybdenum most efficiently from foods that contain micronutrients known as purines, which are in beans, liver, and peas. Some nutritionists have expressed concern that because legumes and organ meats are less commonly eaten than in the past and because food processing removes or destroys many nutrients, widespread molybdenum deficiencies may arise. No clear deficiency symptoms are known, however.

How much do I need to consume?

The estimated safe and adequate daily dietary intake levels for molybdenum are 15 to 40 micrograms for infants, 25 to 75 micrograms for children ages 1 to 6, 50 to 150 micrograms for children ages 7 to 10, and 75 to 250 micrograms for people age 11 and up.

Molybdenum could be toxic at high levels but is affected by the presence of copper, sulfate, and other minerals. At 10 to 15 milligrams a day, molybdenum was shown to promote a goutlike syndrome in people in a province of the former Soviet Union.

FOODS HIGH IN MOLYBDENUM

Barley
Beans—green and lima
Buckwheat
Eggs
Liver
Poultry
Wheat germ and flour
Vegetables—cabbage, greens, spinach, potatoes

NICKEL

What is it?

Nickel is a metal and trace mineral about which little is known in terms of human nutrition. It was identified by Cronstedt in 1751 who named it after the demon known as Old Nick. The element is used for the five-cent coin in the United States and in rechargeable batteries (with cadmium).

How does my body use it?

Nickel is thought to play a role in nucleic acid (RNA) stabilization and in membrane metabolism. A deficiency in test animals resulted in dermatitis, impaired liver function, thickened legs, pigment alterations, and poor reproductive performance.

How much do I need to consume?

Since nickel is not regarded as an essential trace element, no Recommended Daily Allowance levels have been established. The estimated daily intake is between 0.17 and 0.7 milligram.

Nickel carbonyl (nickel and carbon monoxide) is emitted from cigarette smoke and is considered deadly. The level of nickel in the blood is reported to rise sharply in persons who have suffered a heart attack, but it is not known why this occurs.

FOODS HIGH IN NICKEL

Cocoa
Gelatin
Grains (unrefined)
Kidney beans
Tea

PHOSPHORUS

What is it?

Phosphorus is a nonmetallic mineral second only to calcium in terms of its presence in the body (one to two pounds in an adult). Like calcium, phosphorus is stored primarily in bones and teeth, but it is also present in every cell of the body.

This element was first identified by a German alchemist, Hennig Brand, in 1669, who found it in urine. The term phosphorus is from the Greek word *phosphoros,* which means "light bearing." In its unnatural free form, phosphorus glows in the dark and can also spontaneously catch fire. Phosphorus occurs in nature in rock form as calcium phosphate, phosphoric acid, and other compounds.

How does my body use it?

Potassium and calcium work together for tooth and bone formation, so a stable ratio of these two minerals is recommended (1.5 calcium to 1 phosphorus for infants, gradually balancing to 1:1 for adults). A ratio range of 2:1 or 1:2 is considered satisfactory.

Phosphorus is also important for growth, maintenance, and repair of all cells and body tissues. It is needed for protein synthesis and energy production and transfer, as it activates enzymes and B-complex vitamins and aids in the oxidation of fats and carbohydrates.

Phosphorus is absorbed in the duodenum (the

upper small intestine) and relies on adequate levels of calcium, vitamins A and D, iron, fat, and other minerals for proper utilization. Too much iron in the body may inhibit intake of phosphorus, however. Phosphorus absorption may also be blocked by aluminum, inorganic magnesium (milk of magnesia and other antacids), phytic acid, and excessive consumption of white sugar.

How much do I need to consume?

The average North American has a more than adequate dietary intake of phosphorus. The Recommended Daily Allowances are 300 to 500 milligrams for infants and 800 to 1,200 milligrams for children and adults. There is no known toxicity level, but it is possible to consume too much phosphorus in relation to calcium and thereby develop hypocalcemia (low blood calcium).

Signs of phosphorus deficiency, which could manifest in people who adhere to strict vegan diets, include nervous disorders, pain in bones, muscle weakness, loss of appetite or weight, irregular breathing, poor teeth, anemia, and stunted growth.

FOODS HIGH IN PHOSPHORUS

Beef
Bran—rice and wheat
Cocoa powder
Cottonseed flour
Fish and seafood
Lamb
Liver
Nuts
Peanut butter and flour
Pumpkin seeds
Sea vegetables
Soybean flour
Sunflower seeds
Wheat germ

FOODS LOW IN PHOSPHORUS

Fruits
Vegetables

POTASSIUM

What is it?

Potassium is a silver-white metallic mineral found not as a pure element but combined with other substances. It is the third most abundant mineral in the body, constituting about 3 ounces of a 150-pound person, or 5 percent of the total mineral content of the body. Potassium is considered a macromineral, along with calcium and phosphorus. It is water soluble and therefore found mainly in the cells of body fluids but also in muscle tissue.

The name potassium was given to this metal by the English chemist Sir Humphrey Davy in 1807. He also gave it the chemical symbol K, from the Arabic word alkali, which in Latin is *kalium*. Potassium is sometimes called potash, a word that literally means pot ashes (ashes from wood used as a cooking fuel contain potassium carbonate). Potash is used as a soil builder and pH balancer in gardens and croplands.

How does my body use it?

Potassium and sodium work together to balance the volume of body fluids. Both elements are regulated by the kidneys and excreted primarily in the urine and skin pores.

Potassium is also important for nerve transmission, muscle contraction, and relaxation. It aids in metabolism of protein and carbohydrates, as well as in the formation of glycogen and the secretion of insulin by the pancreas.

There is no known toxicity of potassium, and people rarely have dietary deficiencies of this element. It can, however, become depleted by fasting, vomiting, diarrhea, excessive urination (from diuretics), intense or prolonged sweating, and chronic use of laxatives. Deficiency symptoms include muscle weakness, continuous thirst, insomnia, constipation, salt retention and edema, dry skin, impaired growth, rapid and irregular heartbeats, and irritability. In severe cases a depletion or deficiency of potassium can lead to fragile bones, sterility, paralysis, and even death.

How much do I need to consume?

Recommended ranges for daily potassium intake are 350 to 1,275 milligrams for infants, 550 to 3,000 grams for children, and 1,875 to 5,625 grams for adults. The estimated minimum requirements for daily potassium intake are 65 milligrams for infants, 15 to 20 milligrams for children, and 35 milligrams for adolescents. Most foods contain potassium, so dietary intake is usually more than adequate.

People who exercise frequently may need to be aware of their body fluid loss through perspiration and therefore pay attention to potassium, salt, and water consumption to maintain a proper balance of electrolytes.

FOODS HIGH IN POTASSIUM

Beans (dried cooked)
Fruits (fresh and dried)—especially apricots, bananas, citrus fruits, dates, figs, peaches, and raisins
Milk products
Molasses, especially blackstrap
Nuts—peanuts, sunflower seeds
Seafood
Tofu
Vegetables—beet greens, broccoli, Brussels sprouts, Chinese cabbage, potatoes, spinach, sprouts, tomatoes

SELENIUM

What is it?

Selenium is a reddish or gray nonmetallic mineral found in trace amounts in soils, and therefore in plants and animals that graze on them. It is found in levels ranging from less than .05 parts per million (ppm) in soils of the Pacific Northwest, Florida, and northeastern United States to more than 0.1 ppm in western, central, and southeastern United States.

Selenium was discovered in 1817 when a Swedish chemist tested residue of sulfur that had been burned to make sulfuric acid. The chemical and physical properties of selenium and sulfur are very similar.

Research in the 1950s showed that selenium, in cooperation with sulfur-containing amino acids and vitamin E, could prevent liver damage, muscle diseases, and other disorders in poultry and livestock. Thereafter, the United States Food and Drug Administration recognized selenium as an essential element.

How does my body use it?

Selenium is absorbed in the intestines, bound to proteins (amino acids), and transported throughout the body via the bloodstream. It works in tandem with antioxidants (vitamins A, C, and E) and iron to protect membranes and cells and to prevent peroxidation of fats. Selenium helps to maintain elastic tissues and a balanced immune system.

Selenium is believed to be important for prevention of cancer and cardiac disorders. It also affects sexual functioning and reproduction, as well as how much light the retina receives. (Cataracts are affected by selenium levels.) Selenium may also reduce mercury toxicity and slow aging pigmentation.

The body stores organic (plant-derived) selenium in the liver, pancreas, kidneys, and muscles. Inorganic selenium (sodium selenite) may be toxic at levels higher than 500 micrograms and may also bind with mercury. Some plants that grow in the Rockies and Great Plains accumulate so much selenium that animals that eat them may be poisoned. Symptoms include blind staggers (blindness, muscle paralysis, respiratory failure) and alkali disease (sore hoofs, hair loss, and dull, dry coat) and other ailments. Symptoms of toxicity in humans include yellow skin color (in light-skinned people), garlic odor on breath when no garlic has been consumed, skin eruptions, abnormal hair or nails, and higher than average tooth decay.

How much do I need to consume?

The Recommended Daily Allowances for selenium are 10 to 15 micrograms for infants, 20 to 30 micrograms for children ages 1 to 10, and 40 to 75 micrograms for people ages 11 and up (the higher numbers for adult men and pregnant and lactating women).

Consuming 10 micrograms per day is considered adequate to prevent deficiencies.

Selenium from plants is more biologically available than that from animal sources. The availability of selenium from tuna and herring, for example, is about one-third of that from wheat. The body absorbs about 90 percent of plant-derived selenium.

Because selenium works so closely with sulfur-containing amino acids and vitamin E, it is hard to determine whether a symptom is due to a deficiency of this mineral or the other nutrients. A blood test may reveal half as much selenium in the red blood cells of a malnourished person (.2 micrograms per milliliter) than that of a healthy person (.4 mcg/ml). Research suggests that the more stress a person or animal is subjected to, the lower the levels of selenium will be in the body, and consequently the higher need for it in their diet.

FOODS HIGH IN SELENIUM

  Beer
  Bran
  Brazil nuts
  Butter
  Eggs
  Fish and seafood
  Meat, especially organs
  Molasses (blackstrap)
  Mushrooms
  Onions
  Spices
  Swiss chard
  Tomatoes
  Turnips
  Vinegar (cider)
  Wheat germ
  Whole grains
  Yeast—brewer's and torula

SILICON

What is it?
If you've ever played in the sand, you know what silicon feels like.

Silicon is one of the most abundant elements on earth, not in its pure form but as the oxide silica (sand, quartz, agate, and other rocks), or silicates (granites, asbestos, mica, clay). The name is derived from *silex* or *silicis,* Latin terms for flint. A Swedish man named Jons J. Berzilius, the scientist who discovered selenium, is also credited with discovering silicon in 1823.

Besides the mineral forms of silicon, this substance is found in all plant and animal tissue, particularly in skin, hair or feathers, bones, and lungs.

How does my body use it?
Silicon, in its biologically active forms, is absorbed by the body and maintained at a fairly constant level of not more than 1 milligram per 100 milliliters. The body excretes it through urine and feces. Studies of laboratory chicks and rats show that silicon is necessary for skeletal growth and bone calcification. Silicon and calcium levels are regulated by the parathyroid glands. No toxicity or deficiency symptoms of dietary silicon are known, although inhalation of silicon oxide dust causes brown lung disease, also known as silicosis.

How much do I need to consume?
The average daily dietary intake of silicon is 1 gram. No Recommended Daily Allowance has been established. The best sources of silicon are high-fiber foods such as grains, vegetables, fruits, and spices. If your stools float, you are probably absorbing enough silicon fiber.

SODIUM

Sodium is discussed in the section on salt, pages 186–187.

SULFUR

What is it?
Sulfur, from the Latin term *sulphurum,* was also known as burning stone, or brimstone, and used historically for purification of buildings and in ceremonies. As a dietary mineral, it is obtained from foods as a component of three amino acids in protein (cysteine, cystine, and methionine) and two

vitamins (biotin and thiamine). About .25 percent of our body weight is sulfur.

The preserving qualities of sulfur have long been known. Dried fruits, such as golden raisins and apricots, are often exposed to sulfur dioxide gas before drying to inhibit yeast and mold growth as well as to retain color.

How does my body use it?
Sulfur-containing amino acids and vitamins are broken down in the small intestine, and sulfur is absorbed into all the body cells, particularly the hair, nails, and skin.

Sulfur is important for oxidation-reduction reactions which affect protein molecules and keratin in the hair. It also plays a role in metabolizing fat and carbohydrates. Sulfur compounds can also convert toxic phenols and cresols (copper-containing enzymes that cause foods to turn brown and "off" flavored) to a nontoxic substance excreted in the urine. Sulfur with magnesium helps detoxify metabolic sulfuric acid.

Sulfur and molasses reportedly was once prescribed as a spring tonic and laxative. Sulfa drugs (compounds containing sulfur and nitrogen) are used to control certain bacteria. Sulfur has also been used to normalize unwanted fungal flora and yeast, and it has been promoted as a beauty mineral for clear complexion and shiny hair.

How much do I need to consume?
Because dietary sulfur is usually derived from amino acids in protein, no separate Recommended Dietary Allowance levels have been established.

Sulfur deficiencies may occur if protein intake or synthesis is not adequate. Specific symptoms may be dermatitis and irregular development of nails and hair.

No toxicity levels of organic sulfur have been found, although inorganic sulfur (which is not well utilized by humans) could be toxic if a large amount were consumed.

Food analyses generally do not include separate tests for sulfur content. If you are a fan of—or repelled by—onions and garlic, you may be interested to know that their odors are due to sulfur content.

FOODS HIGH IN SULFUR
Beans—lima and navy
Brazil nuts
Brewer's yeast
Cheese
Chicken and turkey
Eggs
Fish—salmon and sardines
Grains—barley, oats, rice, and wheat
Meat—beef, lamb, and pork
Molasses
Peanuts, roasted

TIN

What is it?
Tin is a metal used in cans and other industrial applications. Dietary intake is often due to eating acidic foods that were processed and stored in unlacquered cans, or may be from toothpastes made with stannous fluoride (tin fluoride). It is more often considered as a contaminant than as a necessary element in human diets, and is found in the lungs of people who live in industrial areas with air pollution.

How does my body use it?
Absorption of tin is reportedly poor, and it is unknown whether it functions by itself or with copper and iron in the body. We eat an estimated 1.5 to 3.5 milligrams of tin every day.

Tests on laboratory rats showed that tin was necessary for growth in very small amounts but would stunt growth at higher levels.

Toxicity levels or deficiencies of tin have not been established.

VANADIUM

What is it?
Vanadium is a lustrous silver metallic powder more commonly known in the steel industry than as a nutritional trace element. Named after Vanadis, the

Norse goddess of beauty, it was identified by a Swedish scientist named Nils Sefstrom in 1831.

How does my body use it?

Vanadium is found in teeth, bones, and body tissue. About 90 percent of ingested vanadium is excreted in the urine. It reportedly can lower serum cholesterol and is thought to play a role in metabolizing lipids (fats and sterols) and catecholamines (transmitters of impulses in the nervous system and brain). There are no known toxic levels of vanadium.

Tests on laboratory rats revealed that a deficiency of vanadium could cause impaired growth, increased infant mortality, and reduced fertility that extended into fourth-generation descendants.

How much do I need to consume?

No Recommended Daily Allowance levels have been established for vanadium, as it is not considered an essential element in human nutrition, although an estimated 0.1 to 0.3 milligrams would be required for adults. The average daily intake of vanadium is 4 milligrams. About 20 milligrams of this element is stored in the body.

FOODS HIGH IN VANADIUM

Black pepper
Corn
Fish
Olive oil
Soybeans

ZINC

What is it?

Zinc is a metallic trace element found in the soil as a carbonate or silicate. It is water soluble, so it will, over time, be depleted from most soils by rain. Plants absorb zinc in trace amounts. Humans absorb zinc through ingestion of certain plants or animal products or from supplements. Drinking water has negligible amounts of zinc.

About two grams of zinc are found throughout an adult's body—one of the lowest levels of all min-

erals. Yet it plays a big role in maintaining health. The biological significance of zinc in humans was demonstrated in the early 1960s, and since then our understanding of zinc metabolism and functioning has grown enormously.

How does my body use it?

Zinc, like vitamin A, fosters the growth of bones, hair, and skin. It aids in protein metabolism, wound or burn healing, digestion of carbohydrates, and growth and development or maturity of reproductive and sexual organs. Zinc is a co-factor in more than twenty enzymatic reactions that affect energy production, respiration, synthesis of other nutrients, and DNA. It is needed for transferring carbon dioxide to red blood cells, as well as for maintaining our ability to accurately taste foods or beverages.

Zinc is thought to aid in eliminating deposits of cholesterol and may also be helpful for infertility and prostate problems. Zinc lozenges are sometimes recommended to prevent or relieve symptoms of the common cold. Skin rashes and outbreaks (acne, eczema, and psoriasis) and excessive hair loss or baldness may be eliminated or minimized by an increase in zinc consumption.

How much do I need to consume?

The Recommended Daily Allowances for zinc are 5 milligrams for infants, 10 milligrams for children ages 1 through 10, 15 milligrams for men ages 11 and up, 12 milligrams for women ages 11 and up, and 3 to 7 additional milligrams for pregnant and lactating women.

Unfortunately, zinc is not easily absorbed by the body. Up to 90 percent of the zinc consumed is excreted or blocked by excessive calcium, copper, iron, and/or phytic acid (from plant fibers). Alcohol, oral contraceptives, and diuretics may also deplete zinc reserves stored in the liver. Adequate levels of phosphorus and vitamins A and B6 also need to be present for zinc absorption.

Symptoms of zinc deficiency include white spots on fingernails or brittle nails, slow wound healing, split hairs or dull hair, stunted growth, acne and other skin problems, poor memory or learning ability, and reduced taste sensitivity and appetite. Severe deficiencies may result in dwarfism, hypogonadism, and malformation of fetuses.

Zinc can also be toxic, although it seems unlikely that one could consume too much through foods. Zinc supplementation of more than 15 milligrams per day is generally not recommended. Any amount over 2 grams per day for a prolonged period (several months) could cause toxicity. Symptoms include vomiting, anemia, and gastrointestinal disturbances. Poisoning may also occur if foods are stored in direct contact with galvanized containers.

FOODS HIGH IN ZINC

(about 1 milligram or more per serving)
Beans—cowpeas, lentils, limas
Beef
Bran
Cantaloupe
Cheese—cheddar, gouda, Swiss
Chervil, dried (herb)
Clams
Crab
Duck eggs
Fish—herring, pink salmon, trout
Liver
Milk
Nuts (various, including peanuts)
Octopus
Oysters, raw (exceptionally high)
Pork (ham, tenderloin)
Poultry gizzards and hearts
Sesame seeds
Sprouts (raw)—lentil and mung bean
Wheat germ
Whole grains—oats, rye, triticale, wheat*
Yogurt

* Whole grains are also high in phytic acid, which may block zinc absorption.

APPENDIX

The following food composition tables are from the United States Department of Agriculture *Nutritive Values of Foods.* The data presented is for many, but not all, of the nutrients and constituents of most whole foods. A more comprehensive food compositions table can be found in *Food for Health, A Nutrition Encyclopedia,* by Audrey H. Ensminger, et al. (Second edition. Boca Raton, Florida: CRC Press/Times Mirror Company, 1994). Please keep in mind that nutritional analyses represent data for certain tested foods and that nutritional contents vary due to soil, weather, processing, and storage conditions, as well as individual metabolism.

NUTRITIVE VALUES OF FOODS

(Tr indicates nutrient present in trace amounts)

Item No.	Foods, approximate measures, units, and weight (weight of edible portion only)		Grams	Water (Percent)	Food Energy (Calories)	Protein (Grams)	Fat (Grams)
	DAIRY PRODUCTS						
	Butter. See Fats and Oils (items 99–101).						
	Cheese:						
	Natural						
1	Blue	1 oz	28	42	100	6	8
2	Camembert (3 wedges per 4-oz container)	1 wedge	38	52	115	8	9
	Cheddar						
3	Cut pieces	1 oz	28	37	115	7	9
4		1 in³	17	37	70	4	6
5	Shredded	1 cup	113	37	455	28	37
	Cottage (curd not pressed down):						
	Creamed (cottage cheese, 4% fat):						
6	Large curd	1 cup	255	79	235	28	10
7	Small curd	1 cup	210	79	215	26	9
8	With fruit	1 cup	226	72	280	22	8
9	Lowfat (2%)	1 cup	226	79	205	31	4
10	Uncreamed (cottage cheese, dry curd, less than 1/2% fat)	1 cup	145	80	125	25	1
11	Cream	1 oz	28	54	100	2	10
12	Feta	1 oz	28	55	75	4	6
	Mozzarella, made with:						
13	Whole milk	1 oz	28	54	80	6	6
14	Part skim milk (low moisture)	1 oz	28	49	80	8	5
15	Muenster	1 oz	28	42	105	7	9
	Parmesan, grated:						
16	Cup, not pressed down	1 cup	100	18	455	42	30
17	Tablespoon	1 tbsp	5	18	25	2	2
18	Ounce	1 oz	28	18	130	12	9
19	Provolone	1 oz	28	41	100	7	8
	Ricotta, made with:						
20	Whole milk	1 cup	246	72	430	28	32
21	Part skim milk	1 cup	246	74	340	28	19
22	Swiss	1 oz	28	37	105	8	8
	Pasteurized process cheese:						
23	American	1 oz	28	39	105	6	9
24	Swiss	1 oz	28	42	95	7	7
25	*Pasteurized process cheese food:*						
	American	1 oz	28	43	95	6	7
26	*Pasteurized process cheese spread:*						
	American	1 oz	28	48	80	5	6
	Cream, sweet:						
27	*Half-and-half (cream and milk)*	1 cup	242	81	315	7	28
28		1 tbsp	15	81	20	Tr	2
29	*Light, coffee, or table*	1 cup	240	74	470	6	46
30		1 tbsp	15	74	30	Tr	3

Saturated (Grams)	Monounsaturated (Grams)	Polyunsaturated (Grams)	Cholesterol (Milligrams)	Carbohydrate (Grams)	Calcium (Milligrams)	Phosphorus (Milligrams)	Iron (Milligrams)	Potassium (Milligrams)	Sodium (Milligrams)	(International units)	(Retinol equivalents)	Thiamine (Milligrams)	Riboflavin (Milligrams)	Niacin (Milligrams)	Ascorbic acid (Milligrams)
5.3	2.2	0.2	21	1	150	110	0.1	73	396	200	65	0.01	0.11	0.3	0
5.8	2.7	0.3	27	Tr	147	132	0.1	71	370	350	90	0.10	0.19	0.2	0
6.0	2.7	0.3	30	Tr	204	145	0.2	28	176	300	86	0.01	0.11	Tr	0
3.6	1.6	0.2	18	Tr	123	87	0.1	17	105	180	52	Tr	0.06	Tr	0
23.8	10.6	1.1	119	1	815	579	0.8	111	701	1,200	342	0.03	0.42	0.1	0
6.4	2.9	0.3	34	6	135	297	0.3	190	911	370	108	0.05	0.37	0.3	Tr
6.0	2.7	0.3	31	6	126	277	0.3	177	850	340	101	0.04	0.34	0.3	Tr
4.9	2.2	0.2	25	30	108	236	0.2	151	915	280	81	0.04	0.28	0.2	Tr
2.8	1.2	0.1	19	8	155	340	0.4	217	918	160	45	0.05	0.42	0.3	Tr
0.4	0.2	Tr	10	3	46	151	0.3	47	19	40	12	0.04	0.21	0.2	0
6.2	2.8	0.4	31	1	23	30	0.3	34	84	400	124	Tr	0.06	Tr	0
4.2	1.3	0.2	25	1	140	96	0.2	18	316	130	36	0.04	0.24	0.3	0
3.7	1.9	0.2	22	1	147	105	0.1	19	106	220	68	Tr	0.07	Tr	0
3.1	1.4	0.1	15	1	207	149	0.1	27	150	180	54	0.01	0.10	Tr	0
5.4	2.5	0.2	27	Tr	203	133	0.1	38	178	320	90	Tr	0.09	Tr	0
19.1	8.7	0.7	79	4	1,376	807	1.0	107	1,861	700	173	0.05	0.39	0.3	0
1.0	0.4	Tr	4	Tr	69	40	Tr	5	93	40	9	Tr	0.02	Tr	0
5.4	2.5	0.2	22	1	390	229	0.3	30	528	200	49	0.01	0.11	0.1	0
4.8	2.1	0.2	20	1	214	141	0.1	39	248	230	75	0.01	0.09	Tr	0
20.4	8.9	0.9	124	7	509	389	0.9	257	207	1,210	330	0.03	0.48	0.3	0
12.1	5.7	0.6	76	13	669	449	1.1	307	307	1,060	278	0.05	0.46	0.2	0
5.0	2.1	0.3	26	1	272	171	Tr	31	74	240	72	0.01	0.10	Tr	0
5.6	2.5	0.3	27	Tr	174	211	0.1	46	406	340	82	0.01	0.10	Tr	0
4.5	2.0	0.2	24	1	219	216	0.2	61	388	230	64	Tr	0.08	Tr	0
4.4	2.0	0.2	18	2	163	130	0.2	79	337	260	62	0.01	0.13	Tr	0
3.8	1.8	0.2	16	2	159	202	0.1	69	381	220	54	0.01	0.12	Tr	0
17.3	8.0	1.0	89	10	254	230	0.2	314	98	1,050	259	0.08	0.36	0.2	2
1.1	0.5	0.1	6	1	16	14	Tr	19	6	70	16	0.01	0.02	Tr	Tr
28.8	13.4	1.7	159	9	231	192	0.1	292	95	1,730	437	0.08	0.36	0.1	2
1.8	0.8	0.1	10	1	14	12	Tr	18	6	110	27	Tr	0.02	Tr	Tr

244

Item No.	Foods, approximate measures, units, and weight (weight of edible portion only)		Grams	Water (Percent)	Food Energy (Calories)	Protein (Grams)	Fat (Grams)
	Whipping, unwhipped (volume about double when whipped):						
31	Light	1 cup	239	64	700	5	74
32		1 tbsp	15	64	45	Tr	5
33	Heavy	1 cup	238	58	820	5	88
34		1 tbsp	15	58	50	Tr	6
35	*Whipped topping* (pressurized)	1 cup	60	61	155	2	13
36		1 tbsp	3	61	10	Tr	1
37	**Cream, sour**	1 cup	230	71	495	7	48
38		1 tbsp	12	71	25	Tr	3
	Cream products, imitation (made with vegetable fat):						
	Sweet:						
	Creamers:						
39	Liquid (frozen)	1 tbsp	15	77	20	Tr	1
40	Powdered	1 tsp	2	2	10	Tr	1
	Whipped topping:						
41	Frozen	1 cup	75	50	240	1	19
42		1 tbsp	4	50	15	Tr	1
43	Powdered, made with whole milk	1 cup	80	67	150	3	10
44		1 tbsp	4	67	10	Tr	Tr
45	Pressurized	1 cup	70	60	185	1	16
46		1 tbsp	4	60	10	Tr	1
47	*Sour dressing* (filled cream-type product, nonbutterfat)	1 cup	235	75	415	8	39
48		1 tbsp	12	75	20	Tr	2
	Ice cream. See Milk desserts, frozen (items 77–82).						
	Ice milk. See Milk desserts, frozen (items 83–85).						
	Milk:						
	Fluid:						
49	Whole (3.3% fat)	1 cup	244	88	150	8	8
	Lowfat (2%):						
50	No milk solids added	1 cup	244	89	120	8	5
51	Milk solids added, label claims less than 10 g of protein per cup	1 cup	245	89	125	9	5
	Lowfat (1%):						
52	No milk solids added	1 cup	244	90	100	8	3
53	Milk solids added, label claims less than 10 g of protein per cup	1 cup	245	90	105	9	2
	Nonfat (skim):						
54	No milk solids added	1 cup	245	91	85	8	Tr
55	Milk solids added, label claims less than 10 g of protein per cup	1 cup	245	90	90	9	1
56	Buttermilk	1 cup	245	90	100	8	2
	Canned:						
57	Condensed, sweetened	1 cup	306	27	980	24	27

[a] Vitamin A value is largely from beta-carotene used for coloring.

FATTY ACIDS

VITAMIN A VALUE
(IU)   (RE)

Saturated (Grams)	Monounsaturated (Grams)	Polyunsaturated (Grams)	Cholesterol (Milligrams)	Carbohydrate (Grams)	Calcium (Milligrams)	Phosphorus (Milligrams)	Iron (Milligrams)	Potassium (Milligrams)	Sodium (Milligrams)	(International units)	(Retinol equivalents)	Thiamine (Milligrams)	Riboflavin (Milligrams)	Niacin (Milligrams)	Ascorbic acid (Milligrams)
46.2	21.7	2.1	265	7	166	146	0.1	231	82	2,690	705	0.06	0.30	0.1	1
2.9	1.4	0.1	17	Tr	10	9	Tr	15	5	170	44	Tr	0.02	Tr	Tr
54.8	25.4	3.3	326	7	154	149	0.1	179	89	3,500	1,002	0.05	0.26	0.1	1
3.5	1.6	0.2	21	Tr	10	9	Tr	11	6	220	63	Tr	0.02	Tr	Tr
8.3	3.9	0.5	46	7	61	54	Tr	88	78	550	124	0.02	0.04	Tr	0
0.4	0.2	Tr	2	Tr	3	3	Tr	4	4	30	6	Tr	Tr	Tr	0
30.0	13.9	1.8	102	10	268	195	0.1	331	123	1,820	448	0.08	0.34	0.2	2
1.6	0.7	0.1	5	1	14	10	Tr	17	6	90	23	Tr	0.02	Tr	Tr
1.4	Tr	Tr	0	2	1	10	Tr	29	12	10[a]	1[a]	0.00	0.00	0.0	0
0.7	Tr	Tr	0	1	Tr	8	Tr	16	4	Tr	Tr	0.00	Tr	0.0	0
16.3	1.2	0.4	0	17	5	6	0.1	14	19	650[a]	65[a]	0.00	0.00	0.0	0
0.9	0.1	Tr	0	1	Tr	Tr	Tr	1	1	30[a]	3[a]	0.00	0.00	0.0	0
8.5	0.7	0.2	8	13	72	69	Tr	121	53	290[a]	39[a]	0.02	0.09	Tr	1
0.4	Tr	Tr	Tr	1	4	3	Tr	6	3	10[a]	2[a]	Tr	Tr	Tr	Tr
13.2	1.3	0.2	0	11	4	13	Tr	13	43	330[a]	33[a]	0.00	0.00	0.0	0
0.8	0.1	Tr	0	1	Tr	1	Tr	1	2	20[a]	2[a]	0.00	0.00	0.0	0
31.2	4.6	1.1	13	11	266	205	0.1	380	113	20	5	0.09	0.30	0.2	2
1.6	0.2	0.1	1	1	14	10	Tr	19	6	Tr	Tr	Tr	0.02	Tr	Tr
5.1	2.4	0.3	33	11	291	228	0.1	370	120	310	76	0.09	0.40	0.2	2
2.9	1.4	0.2	18	12	297	232	0.1	277	122	500	139	0.10	0.40	0.2	2
2.9	1.4	0.2	18	12	313	245	0.1	397	128	500	140	0.10	0.42	0.2	2
1.6	0.7	0.1	10	12	300	235	0.1	381	123	500	144	0.10	0.41	0.2	2
1.5	0.7	0.1	10	12	313	245	0.1	397	128	500	145	0.10	0.42	0.2	2
0.3	0.1	Tr	4	12	302	247	0.1	406	126	500	149	0.09	0.34	0.2	2
0.4	0.2	Tr	5	12	316	255	0.1	418	130	500	149	0.10	0.43	0.2	2
1.3	0.6	0.1	9	12	285	219	0.1	371	257	80	20	0.08	0.38	0.1	2
16.8	7.4	1.0	104	166	868	775	0.6	1,136	389	1,000	248	0.28	1.27	0.6	8

Item No.	Foods, approximate measures, units, and weight (weight of edible portion only)		Grams	Water (Percent)	Food Energy (Calories)	Protein (Grams)	Fat (Grams)
	Evaporated:						
58	Whole milk	1 cup	252	74	340	17	19
59	Skim milk	1 cup	255	79	200	19	1
	Dried:						
60	Buttermilk	1 cup	120	3	465	41	7
	Nonfat, instantized:						
61	Envelope, 3.2 oz, net wt.[a]	1 envelope	91	4	325	32	1
62	Cup	1 cup	68	4	245	24	Tr
Milk beverages:							
	Chocolate milk (commercial):						
63	Regular	1 cup	250	82	210	8	8
64	Lowfat (2%)	1 cup	250	84	180	8	5
65	Lowfat (1%)	1 cup	250	85	160	8	3
	Cocoa and chocolate-flavored beverages:						
66	Powder containing nonfat dry milk	1 oz	28	1	100	3	1
67	Prepared (6 oz water plus 1 oz powder)	1 serving	206	86	100	3	1
68	Powder without nonfat dry milk	³/₄ oz	21	1	75	1	1
69	Prepared (8 oz whole milk plus ³/₄ oz powder)	1 serving	265	81	225	9	9
70	*Eggnog* (commercial)	1 cup	254	74	340	10	19
	Malted milk:						
	Chocolate:						
71	Powder	³/₄ oz	21	2	85	1	1
72	Prepared (8 oz whole milk plus ³/₄ oz powder)	1 serving	265	81	235	9	9
	Natural:						
73	Powder	³/₄ oz	21	3	85	3	2
74	Prepared (8 oz whole milk plus ³/₄ oz powder)	1 serving	265	81	235	11	10
	Shakes, thick:						
75	Chocolate	10-oz container	283	72	335	9	8
76	Vanilla	10-oz container	283	74	315	11	9
Milk desserts, frozen:							
	Ice cream, vanilla:						
	Regular (about 11% fat):						
77	Hardened	¹/₂ gal	1,064	61	2,155	38	115
78		1 cup	133	61	270	5	14
79		3 fl oz	50	61	100	2	5
80	Soft serve (frozen custard)	1 cup	173	60	375	7	23
81	Rich (about 16% fat), hardened	¹/₂ gal	1,188	59	2,805	33	190
82		1 cup	148	59	350	4	24
	Ice milk, vanilla:						
83	Hardened (about 4% fat)	¹/₂ gal	1,048	69	1,470	41	45
84		1 cup	131	69	185	5	6

[a] Yields 1 qt of fluid milk when reconstituted according to package directions.
[b] With added vitamin A.

FATTY ACIDS

VITAMIN A VALUE
(IU) (RE)

Saturated (Grams)	Monounsaturated (Grams)	Polyunsaturated (Grams)	Cholesterol (Milligrams)	Carbohydrate (Grams)	Calcium (Milligrams)	Phosphorus (Milligrams)	Iron (Milligrams)	Potassium (Milligrams)	Sodium (Milligrams)	(International units)	(Retinol equivalents)	Thiamine (Milligrams)	Riboflavin (Milligrams)	Niacin (Milligrams)	Ascorbic acid (Milligrams)
11.6	5.9	0.6	74	25	657	510	0.5	764	267	610	136	0.12	0.80	0.5	5
0.3	0.2	Tr	9	29	738	497	0.7	845	293	1,000	298	0.11	0.79	0.4	3
4.3	2.0	0.3	83	59	1,421	1,119	0.4	1,910	621	260	65	0.47	1.89	1.1	7
0.4	0.2	Tr	17	47	1,120	896	0.3	1,552	499	2,160[b]	646[b]	0.38	1.59	0.8	5
0.3	0.1	Tr	12	35	837	670	0.2	1,160	373	1,610[b]	483[b]	0.20	1.19	0.6	4
5.3	2.5	0.3	31	26	280	251	0.6	417	149	300	73	0.09	0.41	0.3	2
3.1	1.5	0.2	17	26	284	254	0.6	422	151	500	143	0.09	0.41	0.3	2
1.5	0.8	0.1	7	26	287	256	0.6	425	152	500	148	0.10	0.42	0.3	2
0.6	0.3	Tr	1	22	90	88	0.3	223	139	Tr	Tr	0.03	0.17	0.2	Tr
0.6	0.3	Tr	1	22	90	88	0.3	223	139	Tr	Tr	0.03	0.17	0.2	Tr
0.3	0.2	Tr	0	19	7	26	0.7	136	56	Tr	Tr	Tr	0.03	0.1	Tr
5.4	2.5	0.3	33	30	298	254	0.9	508	176	310	76	0.10	0.43	0.3	3
11.3	5.7	0.9	149	34	330	278	0.5	420	138	890	203	0.09	0.48	0.3	4
0.5	0.3	0.1	1	18	13	37	0.4	130	49	20	5	0.04	0.04	0.4	1
5.5	2.7	0.4	34	29	304	265	0.5	500	168	330	80	0.14	0.43	0.7	2
0.9	0.5	0.3	4	15	56	79	0.2	159	96	70	17	0.11	0.14	1.1	0
6.0	2.9	0.6	37	27	347	307	0.3	529	215	380	93	0.20	0.54	1.3	2
4.8	2.2	0.3	30	60	374	357	0.9	634	314	240	59	0.13	0.63	0.4	0
5.3	2.5	0.3	33	50	413	326	0.3	517	270	320	79	0.08	0.55	0.4	0
71.3	33.1	4.3	476	254	1,406	1,075	1.0	2,052	929	4,340	1,064	0.42	2.63	1.1	6
8.9	4.1	0.5	59	32	176	134	0.1	257	116	540	133	0.05	0.33	0.1	1
3.4	1.6	0.2	22	12	66	51	Tr	96	44	200	50	0.02	0.12	0.1	Tr
13.5	6.7	1.0	153	38	236	199	0.4	338	153	790	199	0.08	0.45	0.2	1
118.3	54.9	7.1	703	256	1,213	927	0.8	1,771	868	7,200	1,758	0.36	2.27	0.9	5
14.7	6.8	0.9	88	32	151	115	0.1	221	108	900	219	0.04	0.28	0.1	1
28.1	13.0	1.7	146	232	1,409	1,035	1.5	2,117	836	1,710	419	0.61	2.78	0.9	6
3.5	1.6	0.2	18	29	176	129	0.2	265	105	210	52	0.08	0.35	0.1	1

Item No.	Foods, approximate measures, units, and weight (weight of edible portion only)		Grams	Water (Percent)	Food Energy (Calories)	Protein (Grams)	Fat (Grams)
85	Soft serve (about 3% fat)	1 cup	175	70	225	8	5
86	*Sherbet* (about 2% fat)	½ gal	1,542	66	2,160	17	31
		1 cup	193	66	270	2	4
	Yogurt:						
	With added milk solids:						
	Made with lowfat milk:						
88	Fruit-flavored[a]	8-oz container	227	74	230	10	2
89	Plain	8-oz container	227	85	145	12	4
90	Made with nonfat milk	8-oz container	227	85	125	13	Tr
	Without added milk solids:						
91	Made with whole milk	8-oz container	227	88	140	8	7

Eggs

	Eggs, large (24 oz per dozen):						
	Raw:						
92	Whole, without shell	1 egg	50	75	75	6	5
93	White	1 white	33	88	15	4	0
94	Yolk	1 yolk	17	49	60	3	5
	Cooked:						
95	Fried in margarine	1 egg	46	69	90	6	7
96	Hard cooked, shell removed	1 egg	50	75	75	6	5
97	Poached	1 egg	50	75	75	6	5
98	Scrambled (milk added) in margarine	1 egg	61	73	100	7	7

Fats and Oils

	Butter (4 sticks per lb):						
99	*Stick*	½ cup	113	16	810	1	92
100	*Tablespoon* (⅛ stick)	1 tbsp	14	16	100	Tr	11
101	*Pat* (1-in square, ⅓ in high; 90 per lb)	1 pat	5	16	35	Tr	4
102	**Fats,** cooking (vegetable shortenings)	1 cup	205	0	1,810	0	205
103		1 tbsp	13	0	115	0	13
104	**Lard**	1 cup	205	0	1,850	0	205
		1 tbsp	13	0	115	0	13
	Margarine:						
106	*Imitation* (about 40% fat), soft	8-oz container	227	58	785	1	88
107		1 tbsp	14	58	50	Tr	5

[a] Carbohydrate content varies widely because of amount of sugar added and amount and solids content of added flavoring. Consult the label if more precise values for carbohydrates and calories are needed.
[b] For salted butter; unsalted butter contains 12 mg sodium per stick, 2 mg per tbsp, or 1 mg per pat.
[c] Values for vitamin A are year-round average.
[d] For salted margarine.
[e] Based on average vitamin A content of fortified margarine. Federal specifications for fortified margarine require a minimum of 15,000 IU per pound.

FATTY ACIDS   **VITAMIN A VALUE** **(IU) (RE)**

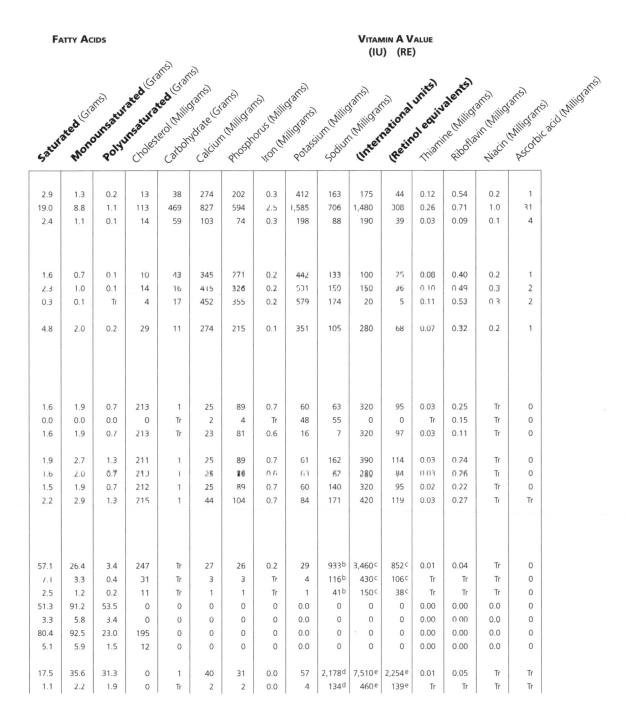

Saturated (Grams)	Monounsaturated (Grams)	Polyunsaturated (Grams)	Cholesterol (Milligrams)	Carbohydrate (Grams)	Calcium (Milligrams)	Phosphorus (Milligrams)	Iron (Milligrams)	Potassium (Milligrams)	Sodium (Milligrams)	(International units)	(Retinol equivalents)	Thiamine (Milligrams)	Riboflavin (Milligrams)	Niacin (Milligrams)	Ascorbic acid (Milligrams)
2.9	1.3	0.2	13	38	274	202	0.3	412	163	175	44	0.12	0.54	0.2	1
19.0	8.8	1.1	113	469	827	594	2.5	1,585	706	1,480	308	0.26	0.71	1.0	31
2.4	1.1	0.1	14	59	103	74	0.3	198	88	190	39	0.03	0.09	0.1	4
1.6	0.7	0.1	10	43	345	271	0.2	442	133	100	25	0.08	0.40	0.2	1
2.3	1.0	0.1	14	16	415	326	0.2	501	150	150	36	0.10	0.49	0.3	2
0.3	0.1	Tr	4	17	452	355	0.2	579	174	20	5	0.11	0.53	0.3	2
4.8	2.0	0.2	29	11	274	215	0.1	351	105	280	68	0.07	0.32	0.2	1
1.6	1.9	0.7	213	1	25	89	0.7	60	63	320	95	0.03	0.25	Tr	0
0.0	0.0	0.0	0	Tr	2	4	Tr	48	55	0	0	Tr	0.15	Tr	0
1.6	1.9	0.7	213	Tr	23	81	0.6	16	7	320	97	0.03	0.11	Tr	0
1.9	2.7	1.3	211	1	25	89	0.7	61	162	390	114	0.03	0.24	Tr	0
1.6	2.0	0.7	210	1	25	86	0.6	60	62	280	84	0.03	0.26	Tr	0
1.5	1.9	0.7	212	1	25	89	0.7	60	140	320	95	0.02	0.22	Tr	0
2.2	2.9	1.3	215	1	44	104	0.7	84	171	420	119	0.03	0.27	Tr	Tr
57.1	26.4	3.4	247	Tr	27	26	0.2	29	933[b]	3,460[c]	852[c]	0.01	0.04	Tr	0
7.1	3.3	0.4	31	Tr	3	3	Tr	4	116[b]	430[c]	106[c]	Tr	Tr	Tr	0
2.5	1.2	0.2	11	Tr	1	1	Tr	1	41[b]	150[c]	38[c]	Tr	Tr	Tr	0
51.3	91.2	53.5	0	0	0	0	0	0.0	0	0	0	0.00	0.00	0.0	0
3.3	5.8	3.4	0	0	0	0	0	0.0	0	0	0	0.00	0.00	0.0	0
80.4	92.5	23.0	195	0	0	0	0	0.0	0	0	0	0.00	0.00	0.0	0
5.1	5.9	1.5	12	0	0	0	0	0.0	0	0	0	0.00	0.00	0.0	0
17.5	35.6	31.3	0	1	40	31	0.0	57	2,178[d]	7,510[e]	2,254[e]	0.01	0.05	Tr	Tr
1.1	2.2	1.9	0	Tr	2	2	0.0	4	134[d]	460[e]	139[e]	Tr	Tr	Tr	Tr

Item No.	Foods, approximate measures, units, and weight (weight of edible portion only)		Grams	Water (Percent)	Food Energy (Calories)	Protein (Grams)	Fat (Grams)
	Regular (about 80% fat):						
	Hard (4 sticks per lb):						
108	Stick	½ cup	113	16	810	1	91
109	Tablespoon (⅛ stick)	1 tbsp	14	16	100	Tr	11
110	Pat (1-in square, ⅓ in high; 90 per lb)	1 pat	5	16	35	Tr	4
111	*Soft*	8-oz container	227	16	1,625	2	183
112		1 tbsp	14	16	100	Tr	11
	Spread (about 60% fat):						
	Hard (4 sticks per lb):						
113	Stick	½ cup	113	37	610	1	69
114	Tablespoon (⅛ stick)	1 tbsp	14	37	75	Tr	9
115	Pat (1-in square, ⅓ in high; 90 per lb)	1 pat	5	37	25	Tr	3
116	Soft	8-oz container	227	37	1,225	1	138
117		1 tbsp	14	37	75	Tr	9
	Oils, salad or cooking:						
118	*Corn*	1 cup	218	0	1,925	0	218
119		1 tbsp	14	0	125	0	14
120	*Olive*	1 cup	216	0	1,910	0	216
121		1 tbsp	14	0	125	0	14
122	*Peanut*	1 cup	216	0	1,910	0	216
123		1 tbsp	14	0	125	0	14
124	*Safflower*	1 cup	218	0	1,925	0	218
125		1 tbsp	14	0	125	0	14
126	*Soybean oil,* hydrogenated (partially hardened)	1 cup	218	0	1,925	0	218
127		1 tbsp	14	0	125	0	14
128	*Soybean-cottonseed oil blend,* hydrogenated	1 cup	218	0	1,925	0	218
129		1 tbsp	14	0	125	0	14
130	*Sunflower*	1 cup	218	0	1,925	0	218
131		1 tbsp	14	0	125	0	14
	FRUITS AND FRUIT JUICES						
	Apples:						
	Raw:						
	Unpeeled, without cores:						
132	2¾-in diam. (about 3 per lb with cores)	1 apple	138	84	80	Tr	Tr
133	3¼-in diam. (about 2 per lb with cores)	1 apple	212	84	125	Tr	1
134	Peeled, sliced	1 cup	110	84	65	Tr	Tr
135	*Dried,* sulfured	10 rings	64	32	155	1	Tr

[a] For salted margarine.

[b] Based on average vitamin A content of fortified margarine. Federal specifications for fortified margarine require a minimum of 15,000 IU per pound.

[c] Sodium bisulfite used to preserve color; unsulfited product would contain less sodium.

| **FATTY ACIDS** | | | | | | | | | | **VITAMIN A VALUE** (IU) (RE) | | | | | |
Saturated (Grams)	Monounsaturated (Grams)	Polyunsaturated (Grams)	Cholesterol (Milligrams)	Carbohydrate (Grams)	Calcium (Milligrams)	Phosphorus (Milligrams)	Iron (Milligrams)	Potassium (Milligrams)	Sodium (Milligrams)	(International units)	(Retinol equivalents)	Thiamine (Milligrams)	Riboflavin (Milligrams)	Niacin (Milligrams)	Ascorbic acid (Milligrams)
17.9	40.5	28.7	0	1	34	26	0.1	48	1,066[a]	3,740[b]	1,122[b]	0.01	0.04	Tr	Tr
2.2	5.0	3.6	0	Tr	4	3	Tr	6	132[a]	460[b]	139[b]	Tr	0.01	Tr	Tr
0.8	1.8	1.3	0	Tr	1	1	Tr	2	47[a]	170[b]	50[b]	Tr	Tr	Tr	Tr
31.3	64.7	78.5	0	1	60	46	0.0	86	2,409[a]	7,510[b]	2,254[b]	0.02	0.07	Tr	Tr
1.9	4.0	4.8	0	Tr	4	3	0.0	5	151[a]	460[b]	139[b]	Tr	Tr	Tr	Tr
15.9	29.4	20.5	0	0	24	18	0.0	34	1,123[a]	3,740[b]	1,122[b]	0.01	0.03	Tr	Tr
2.0	3.6	2.5	0	0	3	2	0.0	4	139[a]	460[b]	139[b]	Tr	Tr	Tr	Tr
0.7	1.3	0.9	0	0	1	1	0.0	1	50[a]	170[b]	50[b]	Tr	Tr	Tr	Tr
29.1	71.5	31.3	0	0	47	37	0.0	68	2,256[a]	7,510[b]	2,254[b]	0.02	0.06	Tr	Tr
1.8	4.4	1.9	0	0	3	2	0.0	4	139[a]	460[b]	139[b]	Tr	Tr	Tr	Tr
27.7	52.8	128.0	0	0	0	0	0.0	0	0	0	0	0.00	0.00	0.0	0
1.8	3.4	8.2	0	0	0	0	0.0	0	0	0	0	0.00	0.00	0.0	0
29.2	159.2	18.1	0	0	0	0	0.0	0	0	0	0	0.00	0.00	0.0	0
1.9	10.3	1.2	0	0	0	0	0.0	0	0	0	0	0.00	0.00	0.0	0
36.5	99.8	69.1	0	0	0	0	0.0	0	0	0	0	0.00	0.00	0.0	0
2.4	6.5	4.5	0	0	0	0	0.0	0	0	0	0	0.00	0.00	0.0	0
19.8	26.4	162.4	0	0	0	0	0.0	0	0	0	0	0.00	0.00	0.0	0
1.3	1.7	10.4	0	0	0	0	0.0	0	0	0	0	0.00	0.00	0.0	0
32.5	93.7	82.0	0	0	0	0	0.0	0	0	0	0	0.00	0.00	0.0	0
2.1	6.0	5.3	0	0	0	0	0.0	0	0	0	0	0.00	0.00	0.0	0
39.2	64.3	104.9	0	0	0	0	0.0	0	0	0	0	0.00	0.00	0.0	0
2.5	4.1	6.7	0	0	0	0	0.0	0	0	0	0	0.00	0.00	0.0	0
22.5	42.5	143.2	0	0	0	0	0.0	0	0	0	0	0.00	0.00	0.0	0
1.4	2.7	9.2	0	0	0	0	0.0	0	0	0	0	0.00	0.00	0.0	0
0.1	Tr	0.1	0	21	10	10	0.2	159	Tr	70	7	0.02	0.02	0.1	8
0.1	Tr	0.2	0	32	15	15	0.4	244	Tr	110	11	0.04	0.03	0.2	12
0.1	Tr	0.1	0	16	4	8	0.1	124	Tr	50	5	0.02	0.01	0.1	4
Tr	Tr	0.1	0	42	9	24	0.9	288	56[c]	0	0	0.00	0.10	0.6	2

Item No.	Foods, approximate measures, units, and weight (weight of edible portion only)		Grams	Water (Percent)	Food Energy (Calories)	Protein (Grams)	Fat (Grams)
136	**Apple juice,** bottled or canned[a]	1 cup	248	88	115	Tr	Tr
	Applesauce, canned:						
137	*Sweetened*	1 cup	255	80	195	Tr	Tr
138	*Unsweetened*	1 cup	244	88	105	Tr	Tr
	Apricots:						
139	*Raw,* without pits (about 12 per lb with pits)	3 apricots	106	86	50	1	Tr
	Canned (fruit and liquid):						
140	Heavy syrup pack	1 cup	258	78	215	1	Tr
141		3 halves	85	78	70	Tr	Tr
142	Juice pack	1 cup	248	87	120	2	Tr
143		3 halves	84	87	40	1	Tr
	Dried:						
144	Uncooked (28 large or 37 medium halves per cup)	1 cup	130	31	310	5	1
145	Cooked, unsweetened, fruit and liquid	1 cup	250	76	210	3	Tr
146	**Apricot nectar,** canned	1 cup	251	85	140	1	Tr
	Avocados, raw, whole, without skin and seed:						
147	*California* (about 2 per lb with skin and seed)	1 avocado	173	73	305	4	30
148	*Florida* (about 1 per lb with skin and seed)	1 avocado	304	80	340	5	27
	Bananas, raw, without peel:						
149	*Whole* (about 2½ per lb with peel)	1 banana	114	74	105	1	1
150	*Sliced*	1 cup	150	74	140	2	1
151	**Blackberries,** raw	1 cup	144	86	75	1	1
	Blueberries:						
152	*Raw*	1 cup	145	85	80	1	1
153	*Frozen,* sweetened	10-oz container	284	77	230	1	Tr
154		1 cup	230	77	185	1	Tr
	Cantaloupe. See Melons (item 185).						
	Cherries:						
155	*Sour,* red, pitted, canned, water pack	1 cup	244	90	90	2	Tr
156	*Sweet,* raw, without pits and stems	10 cherries	68	81	50	1	1
157	**Cranberry juice cocktail,** bottled, sweetened	1 cup	253	85	145	Tr	Tr
158	**Cranberry sauce,** sweetened, canned, strained	1 cup	277	61	420	1	Tr
	Dates:						
159	*Whole,* without pits	10 dates	83	23	230	2	Tr
160	*Chopped*	1 cup	178	23	490	4	1
161	**Figs,** dried	10 figs	187	28	475	6	2
	Fruit cocktail, canned, fruit and liquid:						
162	*Heavy syrup pack*	1 cup	255	80	185	1	Tr
163	*Juice pack*	1 cup	248	87	115	1	Tr
	Grapefruit:						
164	*Raw,* without peel, membrane and seeds (3¾-in diam., 1 lb 1 oz, whole, with refuse)	½ grapefruit	120	91	40	1	Tr

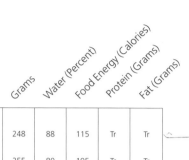

[a] Also applies to pasteurized apple cider.
[b] Without added ascorbic acid. For value with added ascorbic acid, refer to label.
[c] With added ascorbic acid.
[d] For white grapefruit; pink grapefruit have about 310 IU or 31 RE.

| Fatty Acids | | | | | | | | | | Vitamin A Value (IU) (RE) | | | | | |
Saturated (Grams)	Monounsaturated (Grams)	Polyunsaturated (Grams)	Cholesterol (Milligrams)	Carbohydrate (Grams)	Calcium (Milligrams)	Phosphorus (Milligrams)	Iron (Milligrams)	Potassium (Milligrams)	Sodium (Milligrams)	(International units)	(Retinol equivalents)	Thiamine (Milligrams)	Riboflavin (Milligrams)	Niacin (Milligrams)	Ascorbic acid (Milligrams)
Tr	Tr	0.1	0	29	17	17	0.9	295	7	Tr	Tr	0.05	0.04	0.2	2[b]
0.1	Tr	0.1	0	51	10	18	0.9	159	8	30	3	0.03	0.07	0.5	4[b]
Tr	Tr	Tr	0	28	7	17	0.3	183	5	70	7	0.03	0.06	0.5	3[b]
Tr	0.2	0.1	0	12	15	20	0.6	214	1	2,770	277	0.03	0.04	0.6	11
Tr	0.1	Tr	0	55	23	31	0.8	361	10	3,170	317	0.05	0.06	1.0	8
Tr	Tr	Tr	0	18	8	10	0.3	119	3	1,050	105	0.02	0.02	0.3	3
Tr	Tr	Tr	0	31	30	50	0.7	409	10	4,190	419	0.04	0.05	0.9	12
Tr	Tr	Tr	0	10	10	17	0.3	139	3	1,420	142	0.02	0.02	0.3	4
Tr	0.3	0.1	0	80	59	152	6.01	1,791	13	9,410	941	0.01	0.20	3.9	3
Tr	0.2	0.1	0	55	40	103	4.2	1,222	8	5,910	591	0.02	0.08	2.4	4
Tr	0.1	Tr	0	36	18	23	1.0	286	8	3,300	330	0.02	0.04	0.7	2[b]
4.5	19.4	3.5	0	12	19	73	2.0	1,097	21	1,060	106	0.19	0.21	3.3	14
5.3	14.8	4.5	0	27	33	119	1.6	1,484	15	1,860	186	0.33	0.37	5.8	24
0.2	Tr	0.1	0	27	7	23	0.4	451	1	90	9	0.05	0.11	0.6	10
0.3	0.1	0.1	0	35	9	30	0.5	594	2	120	12	0.07	0.15	0.8	14
0.2	0.1	0.1	0	18	46	30	0.8	282	Tr	240	24	0.04	0.06	0.6	30
Tr	0.1	0.3	0	20	9	15	0.2	129	9	150	15	0.07	0.07	0.5	19
Tr	0.1	0.2	0	62	17	20	1.1	170	3	120	12	0.06	0.15	0.7	3
Tr	Tr	0.1	0	50	14	16	0.9	138	2	100	10	0.05	0.12	0.6	2
0.1	0.1	0.1	0	22	27	24	3.3	239	17	1,840	184	0.04	0.10	0.4	5
0.1	0.2	0.2	0	11	10	13	0.3	152	Tr	150	15	0.03	0.04	0.3	5
Tr	Tr	0.1	0	38	8	3	0.4	61	10	10	1	0.01	0.04	0.1	108[c]
Tr	0.1	0.2	0	108	11	17	0.6	72	80	60	6	0.04	0.06	0.3	6
0.1	0.1	Tr	0	61	27	33	1.0	541	2	40	4	0.07	0.08	1.8	0
0.3	0.2	Tr	0	131	57	71	2.0	1,161	5	90	9	0.16	0.18	3.9	0
0.4	0.5	1.0	0	122	269	127	4.2	1,331	21	250	25	0.13	0.16	1.3	1
Tr	Tr	0.1	0	48	15	28	0.7	224	15	520	52	0.05	0.05	1.0	5
Tr	Tr	Tr	0	29	20	35	0.5	236	10	760	76	0.03	0.04	1.0	7
Tr	Tr	Tr	0	10	14	10	0.1	167	Tr	10[d]	1[d]	0.04	0.02	0.3	41

Item No.	Foods, approximate measures, units, and weight (weight of edible portion only)		Grams	Water (Percent)	Food Energy (Calories)	Protein (Grams)	Fat (Grams)
165	*Canned,* sections with syrup	1 cup	254	84	150	1	Tr
	Grapefruit juice:						
166	*Raw*	1 cup	247	90	95	1	Tr
	Canned:						
167	Unsweetened	1 cup	247	90	95	1	Tr
168	Sweetened	1 cup	250	87	115	1	Tr
	Frozen concentrate, unsweetened						
169	Undiluted	6-fl-oz can	207	62	300	4	1
170	Diluted with 3 parts water by volume	1 cup	247	89	100	1	Tr
	Grapes, European type (adherent skin), raw:						
171	*Thompson Seedless*	10 grapes	50	81	35	Tr	Tr
172	*Tokay and Emperor,* seeded types	10 grapes	57	81	40	Tr	Tr
	Grape juice:						
173	*Canned or bottled*	1 cup	253	84	155	1	Tr
	Frozen concentrate, sweetened:						
174	Undiluted	6-fl-oz can	216	54	385	1	1
175	Diluted with 3 parts water by volume	1 cup	250	87	125	Tr	Tr
176	**Kiwifruit,** raw, without skin (about 5 per lb with skin)	1 kiwifruit	76	83	45	1	Tr
177	**Lemons,** raw, without peel and seeds (about 4 per lb with peel and seeds)	1 lemon	58	89	15	1	Tr
	Lemon juice:						
178	*Raw*	1 cup	244	91	60	1	Tr
179	*Canned or bottled,* unsweetened	1 cup	244	92	50	1	1
180		1 tbsp	15	92	5	Tr	Tr
181	*Frozen,* single-strength, unsweetened	6-fl-oz can	244	92	55	1	1
	Lime juice:						
182	*Raw*	1 cup	246	90	65	1	Tr
183	*Canned,* unsweetened	1 cup	246	93	50	1	1
184	**Mangos,** raw, without skin and pit (about 1½ per lb with skin and pit)	1 mango	207	82	135	1	1
	Melons, raw, without rind and cavity contents:						
185	*Cantaloupe,* orange-fleshed (5-in diam., 2⅓ lb, whole, with rind and cavity contents)	½ melon	267	90	95	2	1
186	*Honeydew* (6½-in diam., 5¼ lb, whole, with rind and cavity contents)	1/10 melon	129	90	45	1	Tr
187	**Nectarines,** raw, without pits (about 3 per lb with pits)	1 nectarine	136	86	65	1	1
	Oranges, raw:						
188	*Whole,* without peel and seeds (2¼-in diam., about 2½ per lb, with peel and seeds)	1 orange	131	87	60	1	Tr

[a] Without added ascorbic acid. For value with added ascorbic acid, refer to label.

[b] With added ascorbic acid.

[c] Sodium benzoate and sodium bisulfite added as preservatives.

		FATTY ACIDS										VITAMIN A VALUE (IU) (RE)					
Saturated (Grams)	Monounsaturated (Grams)	Polyunsaturated (Grams)	Cholesterol (Milligrams)	Carbohydrate (Grams)	Calcium (Milligrams)	Phosphorus (Milligrams)	Iron (Milligrams)	Potassium (Milligrams)	Sodium (Milligrams)	(International units)	(Retinol equivalents)	Thiamine (Milligrams)	Riboflavin (Milligrams)	Niacin (Milligrams)	Ascorbic acid (Milligrams)
Tr	Tr	0.1	0	39	36	25	1.0	328	5	Tr	Tr	0.10	0.05	0.6	54
Tr	Tr	0.1	0	23	22	37	0.5	400	2	20	2	0.10	0.05	0.5	94
Tr	Tr	0.1	0	22	17	27	0.5	378	2	20	2	0.10	0.05	0.6	72
Tr	Tr	0.1	0	28	20	28	0.9	405	5	20	2	0.10	0.06	0.8	67
0.1	0.1	0.2	0	72	56	101	1.0	1,002	6	60	6	0.30	0.16	1.6	248
Tr	Tr	0.1	0	24	20	35	0.3	336	2	20	2	0.10	0.05	0.5	83
0.1	Tr	0.1	0	9	6	7	0.1	93	1	40	4	0.05	0.03	0.2	5
0.1	Tr	0.1	0	10	6	7	0.1	105	1	40	4	0.05	0.03	0.2	6
0.1	Tr	0.1	0	38	23	28	0.6	334	8	20	2	0.07	0.09	0.7	Tr[a]
0.2	Tr	0.2	0	96	28	32	0.8	160	15	60	6	0.11	0.20	0.9	179[b]
0.1	Tr	0.1	0	32	10	10	0.3	53	5	20	2	0.04	0.07	0.3	60[b]
Tr	0.1	0.1	0	11	20	30	0.3	252	4	130	13	0.02	0.04	0.4	74
Tr	Tr	0.1	0	5	15	9	0.3	80	1	20	2	0.02	0.01	0.1	31
Tr	Tr	Tr	0	21	17	15	0.1	303	2	50	5	0.07	0.02	0.2	112
0.1	Tr	0.2	0	16	27	22	0.3	249	51[c]	40	4	0.10	0.02	0.5	61
Tr	Tr	Tr	0	1	2	1	Tr	15	3[c]	Tr	Tr	0.01	Tr	Tr	4
0.1	Tr	0.2	0	16	20	20	0.3	217	2	30	3	0.14	0.03	0.3	77
Tr	Tr	0.1	0	22	22	17	0.1	268	2	20	2	0.05	0.02	0.2	72
0.1	0.1	0.2	0	16	30	25	0.6	185	39[c]	40	4	0.08	0.01	0.4	16
0.1	0.2	0.1	0	35	21	23	0.3	323	4	8,060	806	0.12	0.12	1.2	57
0.1	0.1	0.3	0	22	29	45	0.6	825	24	8,610	861	0.10	0.06	1.5	113
Tr	Tr	0.1	0	12	8	13	0.1	350	13	50	5	0.10	0.02	0.8	32
0.1	0.2	0.3	0	16	7	22	0.2	288	Tr	1,000	100	0.02	0.06	1.3	7
Tr	Tr	Tr	0	15	52	18	0.1	237	Tr	270	27	0.11	0.05	0.4	70

Item No.	Foods, approximate measures, units, and weight (weight of edible portion only)		Grams	Water (Percent)	Food Energy (Calories)	Protein (Grams)	Fat (Grams)
189	*Sections,* without membranes	1 cup	180	87	85	2	Tr
	Orange juice:						
190	*Raw,* all varieties	1 cup	248	88	110	2	Tr
191	*Canned,* unsweetened	1 cup	249	89	105	1	Tr
192	*Chilled*	1 cup	249	88	110	2	1
	Frozen concentrate:						
193	Undiluted	6-fl-oz can	213	58	340	5	Tr
194	Diluted with 3 parts water by volume	1 cup	249	88	110	2	Tr
195	**Orange and grapefruit juice,** canned	1 cup	247	89	105	1	Tr
196	**Papayas,** raw, ¹/₂-in cubes	1 cup	140	86	65	1	Tr
	Peaches:						
	Raw:						
197	Whole, 2¹/₂-in diam., peeled, pitted (about 4 per lb with peels and pits)	1 peach	87	88	35	1	Tr
198	Sliced	1 cup	170	88	75	1	Tr
	Canned, fruit and liquid:						
199	Heavy syrup pack	1 cup	256	79	190	1	Tr
200		1 half	81	79	60	Tr	Tr
201	Juice pack	1 cup	248	87	110	2	Tr
202		1 half	77	87	35	Tr	Tr
	Dried:						
203	Uncooked	1 cup	160	32	380	6	1
204	Cooked, unsweetened, fruit and liquid	1 cup	258	78	200	3	1
205	Frozen, sliced, sweetened	10-oz container	284	75	265	2	Tr
206		1 cup	250	75	235	2	Tr
	Pears:						
	Raw, with skin, cored:						
207	Bartlett, 2¹/₂-in diam. (about 2¹/₂ per lb with cores and stems)	1 pear	166	84	100	1	1
208	Bosc, 2¹/₂-in diam. (about 3 per lb with cores and stems)	1 pear	141	84	85	1	1
209	D'Anjou, 3-in diam. (about 2 per lb with cores and stems)	1 pear	200	84	120	1	1
	Canned, fruit and liquid:						
210	Heavy syrup pack	1 cup	255	80	190	1	Tr
211		1 half	79	80	60	Tr	Tr
212	Juice pack	1 cup	248	86	125	1	Tr
213		1 half	77	86	40	Tr	Tr
	Pineapple:						
214	*Raw,* diced	1 cup	155	87	75	1	1
	Canned, fruit and liquid:						
	Heavy syrup pack:						
215	Crushed, chunks, tidbits	1 cup	255	79	200	1	Tr

[a] With added ascorbic acid.

	FATTY ACIDS									VITAMIN A VALUE (IU) (RE)					
Saturated (Grams)	Monounsaturated (Grams)	Polyunsaturated (Grams)	Cholesterol (Milligrams)	Carbohydrate (Grams)	Calcium (Milligrams)	Phosphorus (Milligrams)	Iron (Milligrams)	Potassium (Milligrams)	Sodium (Milligrams)	(International units)	(Retinol equivalents)	Thiamine (Milligrams)	Riboflavin (Milligrams)	Niacin (Milligrams)	Ascorbic acid (Milligrams)
Tr	Tr	Tr	0	21	72	25	0.2	326	Tr	370	37	0.16	0.07	0.5	96
0.1	0.1	0.1	0	26	27	42	0.5	496	2	500	50	0.22	0.07	1.0	124
Tr	0.1	0.1	0	25	20	35	1.1	436	5	440	44	0.15	0.07	0.8	86
0.1	0.1	0.2	0	25	25	27	0.4	473	2	190	19	0.28	0.05	0.7	82
0.1	0.1	0.1	0	81	68	121	0.7	1,430	6	590	59	0.60	0.14	1.5	294
Tr	Tr	Tr	0	27	22	40	0.2	473	2	190	19	0.20	0.04	0.5	97
Tr	Tr	Tr	0	25	20	35	1.1	390	7	290	29	0.14	0.07	0.8	72
0.1	0.1	Tr	0	17	35	12	0.3	247	9	400	40	0.04	0.04	0.5	92
Tr	Tr	Tr	0	10	4	10	0.1	171	Tr	470	47	0.01	0.04	0.9	6
Tr	0.1	0.1	0	19	9	20	0.2	335	Tr	910	91	0.03	0.07	1.7	11
Tr	0.1	0.1	0	51	8	28	0.7	236	15	850	85	0.03	0.06	1.6	7
Tr	Tr	Tr	0	16	2	9	0.2	75	5	270	27	0.01	0.02	0.5	2
Tr	Tr	Tr	0	29	15	42	0.7	317	10	940	94	0.02	0.04	1.4	9
Tr	Tr	Tr	0	9	5	13	0.2	99	3	290	29	0.01	0.01	0.4	3
0.1	0.4	0.6	0	98	45	190	6.5	1,594	11	3,460	346	Tr	0.34	7.0	8
0.1	0.2	0.3	0	51	23	98	3.4	826	5	510	51	0.01	0.05	3.9	10
Tr	0.1	0.2	0	68	9	31	1.1	369	17	810	81	0.04	0.10	1.9	268[a]
Tr	0.1	0.2	0	60	8	28	0.9	325	15	710	71	0.03	0.09	1.6	236[a]
Tr	0.1	0.2	0	75	18	18	0.4	208	Tr	30	3	0.03	0.07	0.2	7
Tr	0.1	0.1	0	21	16	16	0.4	176	Tr	30	3	0.03	0.06	0.1	6
Tr	0.2	0.2	0	30	22	22	0.5	250	Tr	40	4	0.04	0.08	0.2	8
Tr	0.1	0.1	0	49	13	18	0.6	166	13	10	1	0.03	0.06	0.6	3
Tr	Tr	Tr	0	15	4	6	0.2	51	4	Tr	Tr	0.01	0.02	0.2	1
Tr	Tr	Tr	0	32	22	30	0.7	238	10	10	1	0.03	0.03	0.5	4
Tr	Tr	Tr	0	10	7	9	0.2	74	3	Tr	Tr	0.01	0.01	0.2	1
Tr	0.1	0.2	0	19	11	11	0.6	175	2	40	4	0.14	0.06	0.7	24
Tr	Tr	0.1	0	52	36	18	1.0	265	3	40	4	0.23	0.06	0.7	19

258

Item No.	Foods, approximate measures, units, and weight (weight of edible portion only)		Grams	Water (Percent)	Food Energy (Calories)	Protein (Grams)	Fat (Grams)
216	Slices	1 slice	58	79	45	Tr	Tr
	Juice pack:						
217	Chunks or tidbits	1 cup	250	84	150	1	Tr
218	Slices	1 slice	58	84	35	Tr	Tr
219	**Pineapple juice,** unsweetened						
	Canned	1 cup	250	86	140	1	Tr
	Plantains, without peel:						
220	*Raw*	1 plantain	179	65	220	2	1
221	*Cooked,* boiled, sliced	1 cup	154	67	180	1	Tr
	Plums, without pits:						
	Raw:						
222	2¹⁄₈-in diam. (about 6¹⁄₂ per lb with pits)	1 plum	66	85	35	1	Tr
223	1¹⁄₂-in diam. (about 15 per lb with pits)	1 plum	28	85	15	Tr	Tr
	Canned, purple, fruit and liquid:						
224	Heavy syrup pack	1 cup	258	76	230	1	Tr
225		3 plums	133	76	120	Tr	Tr
226	Juice pack	1 cup	252	74	145	1	Tr
227		3 plums	95	84	55	Tr	Tr
	Prunes, dried:						
228	*Uncooked*	4 extra large or 5 large prunes	49	32	115	1	Tr
229	*Cooked,* unsweetened, fruit and liquid	1 cup	212	70	225	2	Tr
230	**Prune juice,** canned or bottled	1 cup	256	81	180	2	Tr
	Raisins, seedless:						
231	*Cup,* not pressed down	1 cup	145	15	435	5	1
232	*Packet,* ¹⁄₂ oz (1¹⁄₂ tbsp)	1 packet	14	15	40	Tr	Tr
	Raspberries:						
233	*Raw*	1 cup	123	87	60	1	1
234	*Frozen,* sweetened	10-oz container	284	73	295	2	Tr
235		1 cup	250	73	255	2	Tr
236	**Rhubarb,** cooked, sugar added	1 cup	240	68	280	1	Tr
	Strawberries:						
237	*Raw,* capped, whole	1 cup	149	92	45	1	1
238	*Frozen,* sweetened, sliced	10-oz container	284	73	275	2	Tr
239		1 cup	255	73	245	1	Tr
	Tangerines:						
240	*Raw,* without peel and seeds (2³⁄₈-in diam., about 4 per lb with peel and seeds)	1 tangerine	84	88	35	1	Tr
241	*Canned,* light syrup, fruit and liquid	1 cup	252	83	155	1	Tr
242	**Tangerine juice,** canned, sweetened	1 cup	249	87	125	1	Tr
	Watermelon, raw, without rind and seeds:						
243	*Piece* (4-by-8-in wedge with rind and seeds; ¹⁄₁₆ of 32²⁄₃-lb melon, 10 by 16 in)	1 piece	482	92	155	3	2
244	*Diced*	1 cup	160	92	50	1	1

	FATTY ACIDS										**VITAMIN A VALUE** (IU) (RE)					
Saturated (Grams)	Monounsaturated (Grams)	Polyunsaturated (Grams)	Cholesterol (Milligrams)	Carbohydrate (Grams)	Calcium (Milligrams)	Phosphorus (Milligrams)	Iron (Milligrams)	Potassium (Milligrams)	Sodium (Milligrams)	(International units)	(Retinol equivalents)	Thiamine (Milligrams)	Riboflavin (Milligrams)	Niacin (Milligrams)	Ascorbic acid (Milligrams)
Tr	Tr	Tr	0	12	8	4	0.2	60	1	10	1	0.05	0.01	0.2	4
Tr	Tr	0.1	0	39	35	15	0.7	305	3	100	10	0.24	0.05	0.7	24
Tr	Tr	Tr	0	9	8	3	0.2	71	1	20	2	0.06	0.01	0.2	6
Tr	Tr	0.1	0	34	43	20	0.7	335	3	10	1	0.14	0.06	0.6	27
0.3	0.1	0.1	0	57	5	61	1.1	893	7	2,020	202	0.09	0.10	1.2	33
0.1	Tr	0.1	0	48	3	43	0.9	716	8	1,400	140	0.07	0.08	1.2	17
Tr	0.3	0.1	0	9	3	7	0.1	114	Tr	210	21	0.03	0.06	0.3	6
Tr	0.1	Tr	0	4	1	3	Tr	48	Tr	90	9	0.01	0.03	0.1	3
Tr	0.2	0.1	0	60	23	34	2.2	235	49	670	67	0.04	0.10	0.8	1
Tr	0.1	Tr	0	31	12	17	1.1	121	25	340	34	0.02	0.05	0.4	1
Tr	Tr	Tr	0	38	25	38	0.9	388	3	2,540	254	0.06	0.15	1.2	7
Tr	Tr	Tr	0	14	10	14	0.3	146	1	960	96	0.02	0.06	0.4	3
Tr	0.2	0.1	0	31	25	39	1.2	365	2	970	97	0.04	0.08	1.0	2
Tr	0.3	0.1	0	60	49	74	2.4	708	4	650	65	0.05	0.21	1.5	6
Tr	0.1	Tr	0	45	31	64	3.0	707	10	10	1	0.04	0.18	2.0	10
0.2	Tr	0.2	0	115	71	141	3.0	1,089	17	10	1	0.23	0.13	1.2	5
Tr	Tr	Tr	0	11	7	14	0.3	105	2	Tr	Tr	0.02	0.01	0.1	Tr
Tr	0.1	0.4	0	14	27	15	0.7	187	Tr	160	16	0.04	0.11	1.1	31
Tr	Tr	0.3	0	74	43	48	1.8	3,224	3	170	17	0.05	0.13	0.7	47
Tr	Tr	0.2	0	65	38	43	1.6	285	3	150	15	0.05	0.11	0.6	41
Tr	Tr	0.1	0	75	348	19	0.5	230	2	170	17	0.04	0.06	0.5	8
Tr	0.1	0.3	0	10	21	28	0.6	247	1	40	4	0.03	0.10	0.3	84
Tr	0.1	0.2	0	74	31	37	1.7	278	9	70	7	0.05	0.14	1.1	118
Tr	Tr	0.2	0	66	28	33	1.5	250	8	60	6	0.04	0.13	1.0	106
Tr	Tr	Tr	0	9	12	8	0.1	132	1	770	77	0.09	0.02	0.1	26
Tr	Tr	0.1	0	41	18	25	0.9	197	15	2,120	212	0.13	0.11	1.1	50
Tr	Tr	0.1	0	30	45	35	0.5	443	2	1,050	105	0.15	0.05	0.2	55
0.3	0.2	1.0	0	35	39	43	0.8	559	10	1,760	176	0.39	0.10	1.0	46
0.1	0.1	0.3	0	11	13	14	0.3	186	3	590	59	0.13	0.03	0.3	15

Item No.	Foods, approximate measures, units, and weight (weight of edible portion only)		Grams	Water (Percent)	Food Energy (Calories)	Protein (Grams)	Fat (Grams)
GRAIN PRODUCTS							
245	**Barley,** pearled, light						
	Uncooked	1 cup	200	11	700	16	2
	Breakfast cereals, hot, cooked:						
	Corn (hominy) grits:						
246	Regular and quick, enriched	1 cup	242	85	145	3	Tr
247	Instant, plain	1 pkt	137	85	80	2	Tr
	Oatmeal or rolled oats:						
248	Regular, quick, instant, nonfortified	1 cup	234	85	145	6	2
	Instant, fortified:						
249	Plain	1 pkt	117	86	105	4	2
250	Flavored	1 pkt	164	76	160	5	2
251	**Buckwheat flour,** light, sifted	1 cup	98	12	340	6	1
252	**Bulgur,** uncooked	1 cup	170	10	600	19	3
	Cornmeal:						
253	*Whole-ground,* unbolted, dry form	1 cup	122	12	435	11	5
254	*Bolted* (nearly whole-grain), dry form	1 cup	112	12	440	11	4
	Degermed, enriched:						
255	Dry form	1 cup	138	12	500	1	2
256	Cooked	1 cup	240	88	120	3	Tr
	Macaroni, enriched, cooked (cut lengths, elbows, shells):						
257	*Firm stage* (hot)	1 cup	130	64	190	7	1
	Tender stage:						
258	Cold	1 cup	105	72	115	4	Tr
259	Hot	1 cup	140	72	155	5	1
260	**Noodles (egg noodles),** enriched, cooked	1 cup	160	70	200	7	2
261	**Noodles,** chow mein, canned	1 cup	45	11	220	6	11
	Popcorn, popped:						
262	*Air-popped,* unsalted	1 cup	8	4	30	1	Tr
263	*Popped in vegetable oil,* salted	1 cup	11	3	55	1	3
264	*Sugar syrup coated*	1 cup	35	4	135	2	1
	Rice:						
265	*Brown,* cooked, served hot	1 cup	195	70	230	5	1
	White, enriched:						
	Commercial varieties, all types:						
266	Raw	1 cup	185	12	670	12	1
267	Cooked, served hot	1 cup	205	73	225	4	Tr

a Nutrient added.

b Cooked without salt. If salt is added according to label recommendations, sodium content is 540 mg.

c For white corn grits. Cooked yellow grits contain 145 IU or 14 RE.

d Cooked without salt. If salt is added according to label recommendations, sodium content is 374 mg.

FATTY ACIDS

VITAMIN A VALUE
(IU) (RE)

Saturated (Grams)	Monounsaturated (Grams)	Polyunsaturated (Grams)	Cholesterol (Milligrams)	Carbohydrate (Grams)	Calcium (Milligrams)	Phosphorus (Milligrams)	Iron (Milligrams)	Potassium (Milligrams)	Sodium (Milligrams)	(International units)	(Retinol equivalents)	Thiamine (Milligrams)	Riboflavin (Milligrams)	Niacin (Milligrams)	Ascorbic acid (Milligrams)
0.3	0.2	0.9	0	150	32	378	4.2	320	6	0	0	0.24	0.10	6.2	0
Tr	0.1	0.2	0	31	0	29	1.5[a]	53	0[b]	0[c]	0[c]	0.24[a]	0.15[a]	2.0[a]	0
Tr	Tr	0.1	0	18	7	16	1.0[a]	29	343	0	0	0.18[a]	0.08[a]	1.3[n]	0
0.4	0.8	0.1	0	25	19	178	1.6	131	2[d]	40	4	0.26	0.05	0.3	0
0.3	0.6	0.7	0	18	163[a]	133	6.3	99	285[a]	1,510[a]	453[a]	0.53[a]	0.28[a]	5.5[a]	0
0.3	0.7	0.8	0	31	168[a]	148	6.7	137	254[a]	1,530[a]	460[a]	0.53[a]	0.38[a]	5.9[a]	Tr
0.21	0.4	0.4	0	78	11	86	1.0	314	2	0	0	0.08	0.04	0.4	0
1.2	0.3	1.2	0	129	49	575	9.5	389	7	0	0	0.48	0.24	7.7	0
0.5	1.1	2.5	0	90	24	312	2.2	346	1	629	62	0.46	0.13	2.4	0
0.5	0.9	2.2	0	91	21	272	2.2	303	1	590	59	0.37	0.10	2.3	0
0.2	0.4	0.9	0	108	8	137	5.9	166	1	610	61	0.61	0.36	4.8	0
Tr	0.1	0.2	0	26	2	34	1.4	38	0	140	14	0.14	0.10	1.2	0
0.1	0.1	0.3	0	39	14	85	2.1	103	1	0	0	0.23	0.13	1.8	0
0.1	0.1	0.2	0	24	8	53	1.3	64	1	0	0	0.15	0.08	1.2	0
0.1	0.1	0.2	0	32	11	70	1.7	85	1	0	0	0.20	0.11	1.5	0
0.5	0.6	0.6	50	37	16	94	2.6	70	3	110	34	0.22	0.13	1.9	0
2.1	7.3	0.4	5	26	14	41	0.4	33	450	0	0	0.05	0.03	0.6	0
Tr	0.1	0.2	0	6	1	22	0.2	70	Tr	10	1	0.03	0.01	0.2	0
0.5	1.4	1.2	0	6	3	31	0.3	19	86	20	2	0.01	0.02	0.1	0
0.1	0.3	0.6	0	30	2	47	0.5	90	Tr	30	3	0.13	0.02	0.4	0
0.3	0.3	0.4	0	50	23	142	1.0	137	0	0	0	0.18	0.04	2.7	0
0.2	0.2	0.3	0	149	44	174	5.4	170	9	0	0	0.81	0.06	6.5	0
0.1	0.1	0.1	0	50	21	57	1.8	57	0	0	0	0.23	0.02	2.1	0

Item No.	Foods, approximate measures, units, and weight (weight of edible portion only)		Grams	Water (Percent)	Food Energy (Calories)	Protein (Grams)	Fat (Grams)
268	*Instant, ready-to-serve,* hot	1 cup	165	73	180	4	0
	Parboiled:						
269	Raw	1 cup	185	10	685	14	1
270	Cooked, served hot	1 cup	175	73	185	4	Tr
271	**Tortillas,** corn	1 tortilla	30	45	65	2	1
	Wheat flours:						
	All-purpose or family flour, enriched:						
272	Sifted, spooned	1 cup	115	12	420	12	1
273	Unsifted, spooned	1 cup	125	12	455	13	1
274	*Cake or pastry flour,* enriched, sifted, spooned	1 cup	96	12	350	7	1
275	*Self-rising,* enriched, unsifted, spooned	1 cup	125	12	440	12	1
276	*Whole-wheat,* from hard wheats, stirred	1 cup	120	12	400	16	2

LEGUMES, NUTS, AND SEEDS

Item No.	Foods, approximate measures, units, and weight		Grams	Water (Percent)	Food Energy (Calories)	Protein (Grams)	Fat (Grams)
	Almonds, shelled:						
277	*Slivered,* packed	1 cup	135	4	795	27	70
278	*Whole*	1 oz	28	4	165	6	15
	Beans, dry:						
	Cooked, drained:						
279	Black	1 cup	171	66	225	15	1
280	Great Northern	1 cup	180	69	210	14	1
281	Lima	1 cup	190	64	260	16	1
282	Pea (navy)	1 cup	190	69	225	15	1
283	Pinto	1 cup	180	65	265	15	1
	Canned, solids and liquid:						
	White with:						
284	Frankfurters (sliced)	1 cup	255	71	365	19	18
285	Pork and tomato sauce	1 cup	255	71	310	16	7
286	Pork and sweet sauce	1 cup	255	66	385	16	12
287	Red kidney	1 cup	255	76	230	15	1
288	**Blackeyed peas,** dry, cooked (with residual cooking liquid)	1 cup	250	80	190	13	1
289	**Brazil nuts,** shelled	1 oz	28	3	185	4	19
290	**Carob flour**	1 cup	140	3	255	6	Tr
	Cashew nuts, salted:						
291	*Dry roasted*	1 cup	137	2	785	21	63
292		1 oz	28	2	165	4	13
293	*Roasted in oil*	1 cup	130	4	750	21	63
294		1 oz	28	4	165	5	14
295	**Chestnuts,** European (Italian), roasted, shelled	1 cup	143	40	350	5	3

[a] Cashews without salt contain 21 mg sodium per cup or 4 mg per oz.

[b] Cashews without salt contain 22 mg sodium per cup or 5 mg per oz.

FATTY ACIDS　　　　　　　　　　　　　**VITAMIN A VALUE**
　　　　　　　　　　　　　　　　　　　　　　(IU)　(RE)

Saturated (Grams)	Monounsaturated (Grams)	Polyunsaturated (Grams)	Cholesterol (Milligrams)	Carbohydrate (Grams)	Calcium (Milligrams)	Phosphorus (Milligrams)	Iron (Milligrams)	Potassium (Milligrams)	Sodium (Milligrams)	(International units)	(Retinol equivalents)	Thiamine (Milligrams)	Riboflavin (Milligrams)	Niacin (Milligrams)	Ascorbic acid (Milligrams)
0.1	0.1	0.1	0	40	5	31	1.3	0	0	0	0	0.21	0.02	1.7	0
0.1	0.1	0.2	0	150	111	370	5.4	278	17	0	0	0.81	0.07	6.5	0
Tr	Tr	0.1	0	41	33	100	1.4	75	0	0	0	0.19	0.02	2.1	0
0.1	0.3	0.6	0	13	42	55	0.6	43	1	80	8	0.05	0.03	0.1	0
0.2	0.1	0.5	0	88	18	100	5.1	109	2	0	0	0.73	0.46	6.1	0
0.2	0.1	0.5	0	95	20	109	5.5	119	3	0	0	0.80	0.50	6.6	0
0.1	0.1	0.3	0	76	16	70	4.2	91	2	0	0	0.58	0.38	5.1	0
0.2	0.1	0.5	0	93	331	583	5.5	113	1,349	0	0	0.80	0.50	6.6	0
0.3	0.3	1.1	0	85	49	446	5.2	444	4	0	0	0.66	0.14	5.2	0
6.7	45.8	14.8	0	28	359	702	4.9	988	15	0	0	0.28	1.05	4.5	1
1.4	9.6	3.1	0	6	75	147	1.0	208	3	0	0	0.06	0.22	1.0	Tr
0.1	0.1	0.5	0	41	47	239	2.9	608	1	Tr	Tr	0.43	0.05	0.9	0
0.1	0.1	0.6	0	38	90	266	4.9	749	13	0	0	0.25	0.13	1.3	0
0.2	0.1	0.5	0	40	55	293	5.9	1,163	4	0	0	0.25	0.11	1.3	0
0.1	0.1	0.7	0	40	95	281	5.1	790	13	0	0	0.27	0.13	1.3	0
0.1	0.1	0.5	0	49	86	296	5.4	882	3	Tr	Tr	0.33	0.16	0.7	0
7.4	8.8	0.7	30	32	94	303	4.8	668	1,374	330	33	0.18	0.15	3.3	Tr
2.4	2.7	0.7	10	48	138	235	4.6	536	1,181	330	33	0.20	0.08	1.5	5
4.3	4.9	1.2	10	54	161	291	5.9	536	969	330	33	0.15	0.10	1.3	5
0.1	0.1	0.6	0	42	74	278	4.6	673	968	10	1	0.13	0.10	1.5	0
0.2	Tr	0.3	0	35	43	238	3.3	573	20	30	3	0.40	0.10	1.0	0
4.6	6.5	6.8	0	4	50	170	1.0	170	1	Tr	Tr	0.28	0.03	0.5	Tr
Tr	0.1	0.1	0	126	390	102	5.7	1,275	24	Tr	Tr	0.07	0.07	2.2	Tr
12.5	37.4	10.7	0	45	62	671	8.2	774	877 [a]	0	0	0.27	0.27	1.9	0
2.6	7.7	2.2	0	9	13	139	1.7	160	181 [a]	0	0	0.06	0.06	0.4	0
12.4	36.9	10.6	0	37	53	554	5.3	689	814 [b]	0	0	0.55	0.23	2.3	0
2.7	8.1	2.3	0	8	12	121	1.2	150	177 [b]	0	0	0.12	0.05	0.5	0
0.6	1.1	1.2	0	76	41	153	1.3	847	3	30	3	0.35	0.25	1.9	37

264

Item No.	Foods, approximate measures, units, and weight (weight of edible portion only)		Grams	Water (Percent)	Food Energy (Calories)	Protein (Grams)	Fat (Grams)
296	**Chickpeas,** cooked, drained	1 cup	163	60	270	15	4
	Coconut:						
	Raw:						
297	Piece, about 2 by 2 by ½ in	1 piece	45	47	160	1	15
298	Shredded or grated	1 cup	80	47	285	3	27
299	*Dried,* sweetened, shredded	1 cup	93	13	470	3	33
300	**Filberts (hazelnuts),** chopped	1 cup	115	5	725	15	72
301		1 oz	28	5	180	4	18
302	**Lentils,** dry, cooked	1 cup	200	72	215	16	1
303	**Macadamia nuts,** roasted in oil, salted	1 cup	134	2	960	10	103
304		1 oz	28	2	205	2	22
	Mixed nuts, with peanuts, salted:						
305	*Dry roasted*	1 oz	28	2	170	5	15
306	*Roasted in oil*	1 oz	28	2	175	5	16
307	**Peanuts,** roasted in oil, salted	1 cup	145	2	840	39	71
308		1 oz	28	2	165	8	14
309	**Peanut butter**	1 tbsp	16	1	95	5	8
310	**Peas,** split, dry, cooked	1 cup	200	70	230	16	1
311	**Pecans,** halves	1 cup	108	5	720	8	73
312		1 oz	28	5	190	2	19
313	**Pine nuts (pinyons),** shelled	1 oz	28	6	160	3	17
314	**Pistachio nuts,** dried, shelled	1 oz	28	4	165	6	14
315	**Pumpkin and squash kernels,** dry, hulled	1 oz	28	7	155	7	13
316	**Refried beans,** canned	1 cup	290	72	295	18	3
317	**Sesame seeds,** dry, hulled	1 tbsp	8	5	45	2	4
318	**Soybeans,** dry, cooked, drained	1 cup	180	71	235	20	10
	Soy products:						
319	*Miso*	1 cup	276	53	470	29	13
320	*Tofu,* piece, 2½ by 2¾ by 1 in	1 piece	120	85	85	9	5
321	**Sunflower seeds,** dry, hulled	1 oz	28	5	160	6	14
322	**Tahini**	1 tbsp	15	3	90	3	8
	Walnuts:						
323	*Black,* chopped	1 cup	125	4	760	30	71
324		1 oz	28	4	170	7	16
325	*English or Persian,* pieces or chips	1 cup	120	4	770	17	74
326		1 oz	28	4	180	4	18
	SUGARS AND SWEETS						
	Chocolate:						
327	*Semisweet,* small pieces (60 per oz)	1 cup or 6 oz	170	1	860	7	61
328	*Sweet* (dark)	1 oz	28	1	150	1	10

[a] Macadamia nuts without salt contain 9 mg sodium per cup or 2 mg per oz.

[b] Mixed nuts without salt contain 3 mg sodium per oz.

[c] Peanuts without salt contain 22 mg sodium per cup or 4 mg per oz.

FATTY ACIDS

VITAMIN A VALUE
(IU)   (RE)

Saturated (Grams)	Monounsaturated (Grams)	Polyunsaturated (Grams)	Cholesterol (Milligrams)	Carbohydrate (Grams)	Calcium (Milligrams)	Phosphorus (Milligrams)	Iron (Milligrams)	Potassium (Milligrams)	Sodium (Milligrams)	(International units)	(Retinol equivalents)	Thiamine (Milligrams)	Riboflavin (Milligrams)	Niacin (Milligrams)	Ascorbic acid (Milligrams)
0.4	0.9	1.9	0	45	80	273	4.9	475	11	Tr	Tr	0.18	0.09	0.9	0
13.4	0.6	0.2	0	7	6	51	1.1	160	9	0	0	0.03	0.01	0.2	1
23.8	1.1	0.3	0	12	11	90	1.9	285	16	0	0	0.05	0.02	0.4	3
29.3	1.4	0.4	0	44	14	99	1.8	313	244	0	0	0.03	0.02	0.4	1
5.3	56.5	6.9	0	18	216	359	3.8	512	3	80	8	0.58	0.13	1.3	1
1.3	13.9	1.7	0	4	53	88	0.9	126	1	20	2	0.14	0.03	0.3	Tr
0.1	0.2	0.5	0	38	50	238	4.2	498	26	40	4	0.14	0.12	1.2	0
15.4	80.9	1.8	0	17	60	268	2.4	441	348[a]	10	1	0.29	0.15	2.7	0
3.2	17.1	0.4	0	4	13	57	0.5	93	74[a]	Tr	Tr	0.06	0.03	0.6	0
2.0	8.9	3.1	0	7	20	123	1.0	169	190[b]	Tr	Tr	0.06	0.06	1.3	0
2.5	9.0	3.8	0	6	31	131	0.9	165	185[b]	10	1	0.14	0.06	1.4	Tr
9.9	35.5	22.6	0	27	125	734	2.8	1,019	626[c]	0	0	0.42	0.15	21.5	0
1.9	6.9	4.4	0	5	24	143	0.5	199	122[c]	0	0	0.08	0.03	4.2	0
1.4	4.0	2.5	0	3	5	60	0.3	110	75	0	0	0.02	0.02	2.2	0
0.1	0.1	0.3	0	42	22	178	3.4	592	26	80	8	0.30	0.18	1.8	0
5.9	45.5	18.1	0	20	39	314	2.3	423	1	140	14	0.92	0.14	1.0	2
1.5	12.0	4.7	0	5	10	83	0.6	11	Tr	40	4	0.24	0.04	0.3	1
7.7	6.5	7.3	0	5	2	10	0.9	178	20	10	1	0.35	0.06	1.2	1
1.7	9.3	2.1	0	7	38	143	1.9	310	2	70	7	0.23	0.05	0.5	Tr
2.5	4.0	5.9	0	5	12	333	4.2	229	5	110	11	0.06	0.09	0.5	Tr
0.4	0.6	1.4	0	51	141	245	5.1	1,141	1,228	0	0	0.14	0.16	1.4	17
0.6	1.7	1.9	0	1	11	62	0.6	33	3	10	1	0.06	0.01	0.4	0
1.3	1.9	5.3	0	19	131	322	4.9	972	4	50	5	0.38	0.16	1.1	0
1.8	2.6	7.3	0	65	188	853	4.7	922	8,142	110	11	0.17	0.28	0.8	0
0.7	0.1	2.9	0	3	108	151	2.3	50	8	0	0	0.07	0.04	0.1	0
1.5	2.7	9.3	0	5	33	200	1.9	195	1	10	1	0.65	0.07	1.3	Tr
1.1	3.0	3.5	0	3	21	119	0.7	69	5	10	1	0.24	0.02	0.8	1
4.5	15.9	46.9	0	15	73	580	3.8	655	1	370	37	0.27	0.14	0.9	Tr
0.1	3.6	10.6	0	3	16	132	0.9	149	Tr	80	8	0.06	0.03	0.2	Tr
6.7	17.0	47.0	0	22	113	380	2.9	602	12	150	15	0.46	0.18	1.3	4
1.6	4.0	11.1	0	5	27	90	0.7	142	3	40	4	0.11	0.04	0.3	1
36.2	19.9	1.9	0	97	51	178	5.8	593	24	30	3	0.10	0.14	0.9	Tr
5.9	3.3	0.3	0	16	7	41	0.6	86	5	10	1	0.01	0.04	0.1	Tr

Item No.	Foods, approximate measures, units, and weight (weight of edible portion only)		Grams	Water (Percent)	Food Energy (Calories)	Protein (Grams)	Fat (Grams)
329	**Honey,** strained or extracted	1 cup	339	17	1,030	1	0
330		1 tbsp	21	17	65	Tr	0
	Sugars:						
331	*Brown,* pressed down	1 cup	220	2	820	0	0
	White:						
332	*Granulated*	1 cup	200	1	770	0	0
333		1 tbsp	12	1	45	0	0
334		1 packet	6	1	25	0	0
335	*Powdered,* sifted, spooned into cup	1 cup	100	1	385	0	0
336	**Molasses,** cane, blackstrap	2 tbsp	40	24	85	0	0
337	**Table syrup** (corn and maple)	2 tbsp	42	25	122	0	0

Vegetables and Vegetable Products

Item No.	Foods, approximate measures, units, and weight		Grams	Water (Percent)	Food Energy (Calories)	Protein (Grams)	Fat (Grams)
338	**Alfalfa seeds,** sprouted, raw	1 cup	33	91	10	1	Tr
339	**Artichokes,** globe or French, cooked, drained	1 artichoke	120	87	55	3	Tr
	Asparagus, green, cooked, drained:						
	From raw:						
340	Cuts and tips	1 cup	180	92	45	5	1
341	Spears, 1/2-in diam. at base	4 spears	60	92	15	2	Tr
	From frozen:						
342	Cuts and tips	1 cup	180	91	50	5	1
343	Spears, 1/2-in diam. at base	4 spears	60	91	15	2	Tr
344	*Canned,* spears, 1/2-in diam. at base	4 spears	80	95	10	1	Tr
345	**Bamboo shoots,** canned, drained	1 cup	131	94	25	2	1
	Beans:						
	Lima, immature seeds, frozen, cooked, drained:						
346	Thick-seeded types (Fordhooks)	1 cup	170	74	170	10	1
347	Thin-seeded types (baby limas)	1 cup	180	72	190	12	1
	Snap:						
	Cooked, drained:						
348	From raw (cut and French style)	1 cup	125	89	45	2	Tr
349	From frozen (cut)	1 cup	135	92	35	2	Tr
350	*Canned,* drained solids (cut)	1 cup	135	93	25	2	Tr
	Beans, mature. See Beans, dry (items 279–287) and Blackeyed peas, dry (item 288).						
	Bean sprouts (mung):						
351	*Raw*	1 cup	104	90	30	3	Tr
352	*Cooked,* drained	1 cup	124	93	25	3	Tr

[a] For regular pack; special dietary pack contains 3 mg sodium.

[b] For green varieties; yellow varieties contain 101 IU or 10 RE.

[c] For green varieties; yellow varieties contain 151 IU or 15 RE.

[d] For regular pack; special dietary pack contains 3 mg sodium.

[e] For green varieties; yellow varieties contain 142 IU or 14 RE.

FATTY ACIDS

VITAMIN A VALUE
(IU) (RE)

Saturated (Grams)	Monounsaturated (Grams)	Polyunsaturated (Grams)	Cholesterol (Milligrams)	Carbohydrate (Grams)	Calcium (Milligrams)	Phosphorus (Milligrams)	Iron (Milligrams)	Potassium (Milligrams)	Sodium (Milligrams)	(International units)	(Retinol equivalents)	Thiamine (Milligrams)	Riboflavin (Milligrams)	Niacin (Milligrams)	Ascorbic acid (Milligrams)
0.0	0.0	0.0	0	279	17	20	1.7	173	17	0	0	0.02	0.14	1.0	3
0.0	0.0	0.0	0	17	1	1	0.1	11	1	0	0	Tr	0.01	0.1	Tr
0.0	0.0	0.0	0	212	187	56	4.8	757	97	0	0	0.02	0.07	0.2	0
0.0	0.0	0.0	0	199	3	Tr	0.1	7	5	0	0	0.00	0.00	0.0	0
0.0	0.0	0.0	0	12	Tr	Tr	Tr	Tr	Tr	0	0	0.00	0.00	0.0	0
0.0	0.0	0.0	0	6	Tr	Tr	Tr	Tr	Tr	0	0	0.00	0.00	0.0	0
0.0	0.0	0.0	0	100	1	Tr	Tr	4	2	0	0	0.00	0.00	0.0	0
0.0	0.0	0.0	0	22	274	34	10.1	1,171	38	0	0	0.04	0.08	0.8	0
0.0	0.0	0.0	0	32	1	4	Tr	7	19	0	0	0.00	0.00	0.0	0
Tr	Tr	0.1	0	1	11	23	0.3	26	2	50	5	0.03	0.04	0.2	3
Tr	Tr	0.1	0	12	47	72	1.6	316	79	170	17	0.07	0.06	0.7	9
0.1	Tr	0.2	0	8	43	110	1.2	558	7	1,490	149	0.18	0.22	1.9	49
Tr	Tr	0.1	0	3	14	37	0.4	186	2	500	50	0.06	0.07	0.6	16
0.2	Tr	0.3	0	9	41	99	1.2	392	7	1,470	147	0.12	0.19	1.9	44
0.1	Tr	0.1	0	3	14	33	0.4	131	2	490	49	0.04	0.06	0.6	15
Tr	Tr	0.1	0	2	11	30	0.5	122	278[a]	380	38	0.04	0.07	0.7	13
0.1	Tr	0.2	0	4	10	33	0.4	105	9	10	1	0.03	0.03	0.2	1
0.1	Tr	0.3	0	32	37	107	2.3	694	90	320	32	0.13	0.10	1.8	22
0.1	Tr	0.3	0	35	50	202	3.5	740	52	300	30	0.13	0.10	1.4	10
0.1	Tr	0.2	0	10	58	49	1.6	374	4	830[b]	83[b]	0.09	0.12	0.8	12
Tr	Tr	0.1	0	8	61	32	1.1	151	18	710[c]	71[c]	0.06	0.10	0.6	11
Tr	Tr	0.1	0	6	35	26	1.2	147	339[d]	470[e]	47[e]	0.02	0.08	0.3	6
Tr	Tr	0.1	0	6	14	56	0.9	155	6	20	2	0.09	0.13	0.8	14
Tr	Tr	Tr	0	5	15	35	0.8	125	12	20	2	0.06	0.13	1.0	14

Item No.	Foods, approximate measures, units, and weight (weight of edible portion only)		Grams	Water (Percent)	Food Energy (Calories)	Protein (Grams)	Fat (Grams)
	Beets, cooked, drained:						
353	*Diced or sliced*	1 cup	170	91	55	2	Tr
354	*Whole beets,* 2-in diam.	2 beets	100	91	30	1	Tr
355	*Canned,* drained solids, diced or sliced	1 cup	170	91	55	2	Tr
356	**Beet greens,** leaves and stems, cooked, drained	1 cup	144	89	40	4	Tr
	Blackeyed peas, immature seeds, cooked and drained:						
357	*From raw*	1 cup	165	72	180	13	1
358	*From frozen*	1 cup	170	66	225	14	1
	Broccoli:						
359	*Raw*	1 spear	151	91	40	4	1
	Cooked, drained:						
	From raw:						
360	Spear, medium	1 spear	180	90	50	5	1
361	Spears, cut into 1/2-in pieces	1 cup	155	90	45	5	Tr
	From frozen:						
362	Piece, 4 1/2 to 5 in long	1 piece	30	91	10	1	Tr
363	Chopped	1 cup	185	91	50	6	Tr
	Brussels sprouts, cooked, drained:						
364	*From raw,* 7–8 sprouts, 1 1/4- to 1 1/2-in diam.	1 cup	155	87	60	4	1
365	*From frozen*	1 cup	155	87	65	6	1
	Cabbage, common varieties:						
366	*Raw,* coarsely shredded or sliced	1 cup	70	93	15	1	Tr
367	*Cooked,* drained	1 cup	150	94	30	1	Tr
	Cabbage, Chinese:						
368	*Pak-choi,* cooked, drained	1 cup	170	96	20	3	Tr
369	*Pe-tsai,* raw, 1-in pieces	1 cup	76	94	10	1	Tr
370	**Cabbage,** red, raw, coarsely shredded or sliced	1 cup	70	92	20	1	Tr
371	**Cabbage,** savoy, raw, coarsely shredded or sliced	1 cup	70	91	20	1	Tr
	Carrots:						
	Raw, without crowns and tips, scraped:						
372	Whole, 7 1/2 by 1 1/8 in, or strips, 2 1/2 to 3 in long	1 carrot or 18 strips	72	88	30	1	Tr
373	Grated	1 cup	110	88	45	1	Tr
	Cooked, sliced, drained:						
374	From raw	1 cup	156	87	70	2	Tr
375	From frozen	1 cup	146	90	55	2	Tr
376	*Canned,* sliced, drained solids	1 cup	146	93	35	1	Tr
	Cauliflower:						
377	*Raw,* (flowerets)	1 cup	100	92	25	2	Tr
	Cooked, drained:						
378	From raw (flowerets)	1 cup	125	93	30	2	Tr
379	From frozen (flowerets)	1 cup	180	94	35	3	Tr

[a] For regular pack; special dietary pack contains 78 mg sodium.

[b] For regular pack; special dietary pack contains 61 mg sodium.

FATTY ACIDS

VITAMIN A VALUE
(IU)   (RE)

Saturated (Grams)	Monounsaturated (Grams)	Polyunsaturated (Grams)	Cholesterol (Milligrams)	Carbohydrate (Grams)	Calcium (Milligrams)	Phosphorus (Milligrams)	Iron (Milligrams)	Potassium (Milligrams)	Sodium (Milligrams)	(International units)	(Retinol equivalents)	Thiamine (Milligrams)	Riboflavin (Milligrams)	Niacin (Milligrams)	Ascorbic acid (Milligrams)
Tr	Tr	Tr	0	11	19	53	1.1	530	83	20	2	0.05	0.02	0.5	9
Tr	Tr	Tr	0	7	11	31	0.6	312	49	10	1	0.03	0.01	0.3	6
Tr	Tr	0.1	0	12	26	29	3.1	252	466[a]	20	2	0.02	0.07	0.3	7
Tr	0.1	0.1	0	8	164	59	2.7	1,309	347	7,340	734	0.17	0.42	0.7	36
0.3	0.1	0.6	0	30	46	196	2.4	693	7	1,050	105	0.11	0.18	1.8	3
0.3	0.1	0.5	0	40	39	207	3.6	638	9	130	13	0.44	0.11	1.2	4
0.1	Tr	0.3	0	8	72	100	1.3	491	41	2,330	233	0.10	0.18	1.0	141
0.1	Tr	0.2	0	10	82	86	2.1	293	20	2,540	254	0.15	0.37	1.4	113
0.1	Tr	0.2	0	9	71	74	1.8	253	17	2,180	218	0.13	0.32	1.2	97
Tr	Tr	Tr	0	2	15	17	0.2	54	7	570	57	0.02	0.02	0.1	12
Tr	Tr	0.1	0	10	94	102	1.1	333	44	3,500	350	0.10	0.15	0.8	74
0.2	0.1	0.4	0	13	56	87	1.9	491	33	1,110	111	0.17	0.12	0.9	96
0.1	Tr	0.3	0	13	37	84	1.1	504	36	910	91	0.16	0.18	0.8	71
Tr	Tr	0.1	0	4	33	16	0.4	172	13	90	9	0.04	0.02	0.2	33
Tr	Tr	0.2	0	7	50	38	0.6	308	29	130	13	0.09	0.08	0.3	36
Tr	Tr	0.1	0	3	158	49	1.8	631	58	4,370	437	0.05	0.11	0.7	44
Tr	Tr	0.1	0	2	59	22	0.2	181	7	910	91	0.03	0.04	0.3	21
Tr	Tr	0.1	0	4	36	29	0.3	144	8	30	3	0.04	0.02	0.2	40
Tr	Tr	Tr	0	4	25	29	0.3	161	20	700	70	0.05	0.02	0.2	22
Tr	Tr	0.1	0	7	19	32	0.4	233	25	20,250	2,025	0.07	0.04	0.7	7
Tr	Tr	0.1	0	11	30	48	0.6	355	39	30,940	3,094	0.11	0.06	1.0	10
0.1	Tr	0.1	0	16	48	47	1.0	354	103	38,300	3,830	0.05	0.09	0.8	4
Tr	Tr	0.1	0	12	41	38	0.7	231	86	25,850	2,585	0.04	0.05	0.6	4
0.1	Tr	0.1	0	8	37	35	0.9	261	352[b]	20,110	2,011	0.03	0.04	0.8	4
Tr	Tr	0.1	0	5	29	46	0.6	355	15	20	2	0.08	0.06	0.6	72
Tr	Tr	0.1	0	6	34	44	0.5	404	8	20	2	0.08	0.07	0.7	69
0.1	Tr	0.2	0	7	31	43	0.7	250	32	40	4	0.07	0.10	0.6	56

Item No.	Foods, approximate measures, units, and weight (weight of edible portion only)		Grams	Water (Percent)	Food Energy (Calories)	Protein (Grams)	Fat (Grams)
	Celery, pascal type, raw:						
380	*Stalk,* large outer, 8 by 1½ in (at root end)	1 stalk	40	95	5	Tr	Tr
381	*Pieces,* diced	1 cup	120	95	20	1	Tr
	Collards, cooked, drained:						
382	*From raw* (leaves without stems)	1 cup	190	96	25	2	Tr
383	*From frozen,* chopped	1 cup	170	88	60	5	1
	Corn, sweet:						
	Cooked, drained:						
384	From raw, ear, 5 by 1¾ in	1 ear	77	70	85	3	1
	From frozen:						
385	Ear, trimmed to about 3½ in long	1 ear	63	73	60	2	Tr
386	Kernels	1 cup	165	76	135	5	Tr
	Canned:						
387	Cream style	1 cup	256	79	185	4	1
388	Whole kernel, vacuum pack	1 cup	210	77	165	5	1
	Cowpeas. See Blackeyed peas, immature (items 357, 358), mature (item 288).						
389	**Cucumber,** with peel, slices, ⅛ in thick (large, 2⅛-in diam.; small, 1¾-in diam.)	6 large or 8 small slices	28	96	5	Tr	Tr
390	**Dandelion greens,** cooked, drained	1 cup	105	90	35	2	1
391	**Eggplant,** cooked, steamed	1 cup	96	92	25	1	Tr
392	**Endive,** curly (including escarole), raw, small pieces	1 cup	50	94	10	1	Tr
393	**Jerusalem artichoke,** raw, sliced	1 cup	150	78	115	3	Tr
	Kale, cooked, drained:						
394	*From raw,* chopped	1 cup	130	91	40	2	1
395	*From frozen,* chopped	1 cup	130	91	40	4	1
396	**Kohlrabi,** thickened bulblike stems, cooked, drained, diced	1 cup	165	90	50	3	Tr
	Lettuce, raw:						
	Butterhead, as Boston types:						
397	Head, 5-in diam.	1 head	163	96	20	2	Tr
398	Leaves	1 outer or 2 inner	15	96	Tr	Tr	Tr
	Crisphead, as iceberg:						
399	Head, 6-in diam.	1 head	539	96	70	5	1
400	Wedge, ¼ of head	1 wedge	135	96	20	1	Tr
401	Pieces, chopped or shredded	1 cup	55	96	5	1	Tr
402	*Leaf* (bunching varieties including romaine or cos), chopped or shredded pieces	1 cup	56	94	10	1	Tr
	Mushrooms:						
403	*Raw,* sliced or chopped	1 cup	70	92	20	1	Tr
404	*Cooked,* drained	1 cup	156	91	40	3	1

[a] For yellow varieties; white varieties contain only a trace of vitamin A.

[b] For regular pack; special dietary pack contains 8 mg sodium.

[c] For regular pack; special dietary pack contains 6 mg sodium.

| FATTY ACIDS | | | | | | | | | | VITAMIN A VALUE (IU) (RE) | | | | | |
Saturated (Grams)	Monounsaturated (Grams)	Polyunsaturated (Grams)	Cholesterol (Milligrams)	Carbohydrate (Grams)	Calcium (Milligrams)	Phosphorus (Milligrams)	Iron (Milligrams)	Potassium (Milligrams)	Sodium (Milligrams)	(International units)	(Retinol equivalents)	Thiamine (Milligrams)	Riboflavin (Milligrams)	Niacin (Milligrams)	Ascorbic acid (Milligrams)
Tr	Tr	Tr	0	1	14	10	0.2	114	35	50	5	0.01	0.01	0.1	3
Tr	Tr	0.1	0	4	43	31	0.6	341	106	150	15	0.04	0.04	0.4	8
0.1	Tr	0.2	0	5	148	19	0.8	177	36	4,220	422	0.03	0.08	0.4	19
0.1	0.1	0.4	0	12	357	46	1.9	427	85	10,170	1,017	0.08	0.20	1.1	45
0.2	0.3	0.5	0	19	2	79	0.5	192	13	170[d]	17[a]	0.17	0.056	1.2	5
0.1	0.1	0.2	0	14	2	47	0.4	158	3	130[a]	13[a]	0.11	0.4	1.0	3
Tr	Tr	0.1	0	34	3	78	0.5	229	8	410[a]	41[a]	0.11	0.12	2.1	4
0.2	0.3	0.5	0	46	8	131	1.0	343	730[b]	250[a]	25[a]	0.06	0.14	2.5	12
0.2	0.3	0.5	0	41	11	134	0.9	391	571[c]	510[a]	51[a]	0.09	0.15	2.5	17
Tr	Tr	Tr	0	1	4	5	0.1	42	1	10	1	0.01	0.01	0.1	1
0.1	Tr	0.3	0	7	147	44	1.9	244	46	12,290	1,229	0.14	0.18	0.5	19
Tr	Tr	0.1	0	6	6	21	0.3	238	3	60	6	0.07	0.02	0.6	1
Tr	Tr	Tr	0	2	26	14	0.4	157	11	1,030	103	0.04	0.04	0.2	3
0.0	Tr	Tr	0	26	21	117	5.1	644	6	30	3	0.30	0.09	2.0	6
0.1	Tr	0.3	0	7	94	36	1.2	296	30	9,620	962	0.07	0.09	0.7	53
0.1	Tr	0.3	0	7	179	36	1.2	417	20	8,260	826	0.06	0.15	0.9	33
Tr	Tr	0.1	0	11	41	74	0.7	561	35	60	6	0.07	0.03	0.6	89
Tr	Tr	0.2	0	4	52	38	0.5	419	8	1,580	158	0.10	0.10	0.5	13
Tr	Tr	Tr	0	Tr	5	3	Tr	39	1	150	15	0.01	0.01	Tr	1
0.1	Tr	0.5	0	11	102	108	2.7	852	49	1,780	178	0.25	0.16	1.0	21
Tr	Tr	0.1	0	3	26	27	0.7	213	12	450	45	0.06	0.04	0.3	5
Tr	Tr	0.1	0	1	10	11	0.3	87	5	180	18	0.03	0.02	0.1	2
Tr	Tr	0.1	0	2	38	14	0.8	148	5	1,060	106	0.03	0.04	0.2	10
Tr	Tr	0.1	0	3	4	73	0.9	259	3	0	0	0.07	0.31	2.9	2
0.1	Tr	0.3	0	8	9	136	2.7	555	3	0	0	0.11	0.47	7.0	6

Item No.	Foods, approximate measures, units, and weight (weight of edible portion only)		Grams	Water (Percent)	Food Energy (Calories)	Protein (Grams)	Fat (Grams)
405	*Canned,* drained solids	1 cup	156	91	35	3	Tr
406	**Mustard greens,** without stems and midribs, cooked, drained	1 cup	140	94	20	3	Tr
407	**Okra pods,** 3 by ⅝ in, cooked	8 pods	85	90	25	2	Tr
	Onions:						
	Raw:						
408	Chopped	1 cup	160	91	55	2	Tr
409	Sliced	1 cup	115	91	40	1	Tr
410	*Cooked* (whole or sliced), drained	1 cup	210	92	60	2	Tr
411	**Onions,** spring, raw, bulb (⅜-in diam.) and white portion of top	6 onions	30	92	10	1	Tr
412	**Onion rings,** breaded, par-fried, frozen, prepared	2 rings	20	29	80	1	5
	Parsley:						
413	*Raw*	10 sprigs	10	88	5	Tr	Tr
414	*Freeze-dried*	1 tbsp	0.4	2	Tr	Tr	Tr
415	**Parsnips,** cooked, (diced or 2-in lengths), drained	1 cup	156	78	125	2	Tr
416	**Peas,** edible pod, cooked, drained	1 cup	160	89	65	5	Tr
	Peas, green:						
417	*Canned,* drained solids	1 cup	170	82	115	8	1
418	*Frozen,* cooked, drained	1 cup	160	80	125	8	Tr
	Peppers:						
419	*Hot chili,* raw	1 pepper	45	88	20	1	Tr
	Sweet (about 5 per lb, whole), stem and seeds removed:						
420	Raw	1 pepper	74	93	20	1	Tr
421	Cooked, drained	1 pepper	73	95	15	Tr	Tr
	Potatoes, cooked:						
	Baked (about 2 per lb, raw):						
422	With skin	1 potato	202	71	220	5	Tr
423	Flesh only	1 potato	156	75	145	3	Tr
	Boiled (about 3 per lb, raw):						
424	Peeled after boiling	1 potato	136	77	120	3	Tr
425	Peeled before boiling	1 potato	135	77	115	2	Tr
	French-fried, strip, 2 to 3½ in long, frozen:						
426	Oven heated	10 strips	50	53	110	2	4
427	Fried in vegetable oil	10 strips	50	38	160	2	8
428	**Potato chips**	10 chips	20	3	105	1	7
	Pumpkin:						
429	*Cooked from raw,* mashed	1 cup	245	94	50	2	Tr
430	*Canned*	1 cup	245	90	85	3	1
431	**Radishes,** raw, stem ends, rootlets cut off	4 radishes	18	95	5	Tr	Tr

[a] For regular pack; special dietary pack contains 3 mg sodium.

[b] For red peppers; green peppers contain 350 IU or 35 RE.

[c] For green peppers; red peppers contain 4,220 IU or 422 RE.

[d] For green peppers; red peppers contain 141 mg ascorbic acid.

[e] For green peppers; red peppers contain 2,740 IU or 274 RE.

[f] For green peppers; red peppers contain 121 mg ascorbic acid.

| Fatty Acids | | | | | | | | | | Vitamin A Value | | | | | |
Saturated (Grams)	Monounsaturated (Grams)	Polyunsaturated (Grams)	Cholesterol (Milligrams)	Carbohydrate (Grams)	Calcium (Milligrams)	Phosphorus (Milligrams)	Iron (Milligrams)	Potassium (Milligrams)	Sodium (Milligrams)	(International units)	(Retinol equivalents)	Thiamine (Milligrams)	Riboflavin (Milligrams)	Niacin (Milligrams)	Ascorbic acid (Milligrams)
0.1	Tr	0.2	0	8	17	103	1.2	201	663	0	0	0.13	0.03	2.5	0
Tr	0.2	0.1	0	3	104	57	1.0	283	22	4,240	424	0.06	0.09	0.6	35
Tr	Tr	Tr	0	6	54	48	0.4	274	4	490	49	0.11	0.05	0.7	14
0.1	0.1	0.2	0	12	40	46	0.6	248	3	0	0	0.10	0.02	0.2	13
0.1	Tr	0.1	0	8	29	33	0.4	178	2	0	0	0.07	0.01	0.1	10
0.1	Tr	0.1	0	13	57	48	0.4	319	17	0	0	0.09	0.02	0.2	12
Tr	Tr	Tr	0	2	18	10	0.6	77	1	1,500	150	0.02	0.04	0.1	14
1.7	2.2	1.0	0	8	6	16	0.3	26	75	50	5	0.06	0.03	0.7	Tr
Tr	Tr	Tr	0	1	13	4	0.6	54	4	520	52	0.01	0.01	0.1	9
Tr	Tr	Tr	0	Tr	1	2	0.2	25	2	250	25	Tr	0.01	Tr	1
0.1	0.2	0.1	0	30	58	108	0.9	573	16	0	0	0.13	0.08	1.1	20
0.1	Tr	0.2	0	11	67	88	3.2	384	6	210	21	0.20	0.12	0.9	77
0.1	0.1	0.3	0	21	34	114	1.6	294	372[a]	1,310	131	0.21	0.13	1.2	16
0.1	Tr	0.2	0	23	38	144	2.5	269	139	1,070	107	0.45	0.16	2.4	16
Tr	Tr	Tr	0	4	8	21	0.5	153	3	4,840[b]	484[b]	0.04	0.04	0.4	109
Tr	Tr	0.2	0	4	4	16	0.9	144	2	390[c]	39[c]	0.06	0.04	0.4	95[d]
Tr	Tr	0.1	0	3	3	11	0.6	94	1	280[e]	28[e]	0.04	0.03	0.3	81[f]
0.1	Tr	0.1	0	51	20	115	2.7	844	16	0	0	0.22	0.07	3.3	26
Tr	Tr	0.1	0	34	8	78	0.5	610	8	0	0	0.16	0.03	2.2	20
Tr	Tr	0.1	0	27	7	60	0.4	515	5	0	0	0.14	0.03	2.0	18
Tr	Tr	0.1	0	27	11	54	0.4	443	7	0	0	0.13	0.03	1.8	10
2.1	1.8	0.3	0	17	5	43	0.7	229	16	0	0	0.06	0.02	1.2	5
2.5	1.6	3.8	0	20	10	47	0.4	366	108	0	0	0.09	0.01	1.6	5
1.8	1.2	3.6	0	10	5	31	0.2	260	94	0	0	0.03	Tr	0.8	8
0.1	Tr	Tr	0	12	37	74	1.4	564	2	2,650	265	0.08	0.19	1.0	12
0.4	0.1	Tr	0	20	64	86	3.4	505	12	54,040	5,404	0.06	0.13	0.9	10
Tr	Tr	Tr	0	1	4	3	0.1	42	4	Tr	Tr	Tr	0.01	0.1	4

274

Item No.	Foods, approximate measures, units, and weight (weight of edible portion only)		Grams	Water (Percent)	Food Energy (Calories)	Protein (Grams)	Fat (Grams)
432	**Sauerkraut,** canned, solids and liquid	1 cup	236	93	45	2	Tr
	Seaweed:						
433	*Kelp,* raw	1 oz	28	82	10	Tr	Tr
434	*Spirulina,* dried	1 oz	28	5	80	16	2
	Southern peas. See Blackeyed peas, immature (items 357, 358), mature (item 288).						
	Spinach:						
435	*Raw,* chopped	1 cup	55	92	10	2	Tr
	Cooked, drained:						
436	From raw	1 cup	180	91	40	5	Tr
437	From frozen (leaf)	1 cup	190	90	55	6	Tr
438	*Canned,* drained solids	1 cup	214	92	50	6	1
439	**Spinach souffle**	1 cup	136	74	220	11	18
	Squash, cooked:						
440	*Summer* (all varieties), sliced, drained	1 cup	180	94	35	2	1
441	*Winter* (all varieties), baked, cubes	1 cup	205	89	80	2	1
	Sunchoke. See Jerusalem artichoke (item 393).						
	Sweet potatoes:						
	Cooked (raw, 5 by 2 in; about 2½ per lb):						
442	Baked in skin, peeled	1 potato	114	73	115	2	Tr
443	Boiled, without skin	1 potato	151	73	160	2	Tr
444	*Candied,* 2½-by-2-in piece	1 piece	105	67	146	1	3
	Canned:						
445	Solid pack (mashed)	1 cup	255	74	260	5	1
446	Vacuum pack, 2½-by-1-in piece	1 piece	40	76	35	1	Tr
	Tomatoes:						
447	*Raw,* 2½-in diam. (3 per 12-oz pkg)	1 tomato	123	94	25	1	Tr
448	*Canned,* solids and liquid	1 cup	240	94	50	2	1
449	**Tomato juice,** canned	1 cup	244	94	40	2	Tr
	Tomato products, canned:						
450	*Paste*	1 cup	262	74	220	10	2
451	*Puree*	1 cup	250	87	105	4	Tr
452	*Sauce*	1 cup	245	89	75	3	Tr
453	**Turnips,** cooked, diced	1 cup	156	94	30	1	Tr
	Turnip greens, cooked, drained:						
454	*From raw* (leaves and stems)	1 cup	144	93	30	2	Tr
455	*From frozen* (chopped)	1 cup	164	90	50	5	1
456	**Vegetable juice cocktail,** canned	1 cup	242	94	45	2	Tr

[a] Value not determined.
[b] With added salt; if none is added, sodium content is 58 mg.
[c] For regular pack; special dietary pack contains 31 mg sodium.
[d] With added salt; if none is added, sodium content is 24 mg.
[e] With no added salt; if salt is added, sodium content is 2,070 mg.
[f] With no added salt; if salt is added, sodium content is 998 mg.
[g] With salt added.

Fatty Acids Saturated (Grams)	Monounsaturated (Grams)	Polyunsaturated (Grams)	Cholesterol (Milligrams)	Carbohydrate (Grams)	Calcium (Milligrams)	Phosphorus (Milligrams)	Iron (Milligrams)	Potassium (Milligrams)	Sodium (Milligrams)	Vitamin A Value (IU) (International units)	(RE) (Retinol equivalents)	Thiamine (Milligrams)	Riboflavin (Milligrams)	Niacin (Milligrams)	Ascorbic acid (Milligrams)
0.1	Tr	0.1	0	10	71	47	3.5	401	1,560	40	4	0.05	0.05	0.3	35
0.1	Tr	Tr	0	3	48	12	0.8	25	66	30	3	0.01	0.04	0.1	(a)
0.8	0.2	0.6	0	7	34	33	8.1	386	297	160	16	0.67	1.04	3.6	3
Tr	Tr	0.1	0	2	54	27	1.5	307	43	3,690	369	0.04	0.10	0.4	15
0.1	Tr	0.2	0	7	245	101	6.4	839	126	14,740	1,474	0.17	0.42	0.9	18
0.1	Tr	0.2	0	10	277	91	2.9	566	163	14,790	1,479	0.11	0.32	0.8	23
0.2	Tr	0.4	0	7	272	94	4.0	740	683 h	18,780	1,878	0.03	0.30	0.8	31
7.1	6.8	3.1	184	3	230	231	1.3	201	763	3,460	675	0.09	0.30	0.5	3
0.1	Tr	0.2	0	8	49	70	0.6	346	2	520	52	0.08	0.07	0.9	10
0.3	0.1	0.5	0	18	29	41	0.7	896	2	7,290	729	0.17	0.05	1.4	20
Tr	Tr	0.1	0	28	32	63	0.5	397	11	24,880	2,488	0.08	0.14	0.7	28
0.1	Tr	0.2	0	37	32	41	0.8	278	20	25,750	2,575	0.08	0.21	1.0	26
1.4	0.7	0.2	8	29	27	27	1.2	198	74	4,400	440	0.02	0.04	0.4	7
0.1	Tr	0.2	0	59	77	133	3.4	536	191	38,570	3,857	0.07	0.23	2.4	13
Tr	Tr	Tr	0	8	9	20	0.4	125	21	3,190	319	0.01	0.02	0.3	11
Tr	Tr	0.1	0	5	9	28	0.6	255	10	1,390	139	0.07	0.06	0.7	22
0.1	0.1	0.2	0	10	62	46	1.5	530	391 c	1,450	145	0.11	0.07	1.8	36
Tr	Tr	0.1	0	10	22	46	1.4	537	881 d	1,360	136	0.11	0.08	1.6	45
0.3	0.4	0.9	0	49	92	207	7.8	2,442	170 e	6,470	647	0.41	0.50	8.4	111
Tr	Tr	0.1	0	25	38	100	2.3	1,050	50 f	3,400	340	0.18	0.14	4.3	88
0.1	0.1	0.2	0	18	34	78	1.9	909	1,482 g	2,400	240	0.16	0.14	2.8	32
Tr	Tr	0.1	0	8	34	30	0.3	211	78	0	0	0.04	0.04	0.5	18
0.1	Tr	0.1	0	6	197	42	1.2	292	42	7,920	792	0.06	0.10	0.6	39
0.2	Tr	0.3	0	8	249	56	3.2	367	25	13,080	1,308	0.09	0.12	0.8	36
Tr	Tr	0.1	0	11	27	41	1.0	467	883	2,830	283	0.10	0.07	1.8	67

Item No.	Foods, approximate measures, units, and weight (weight of edible portion only)		Grams	Water (Percent)	Food Energy (Calories)	Protein (Grams)	Fat (Grams)
	Vegetables, mixed:						
457	*Canned,* drained solids	1 cup	163	87	75	4	Tr
458	*Frozen,* cooked, drained	1 cup	182	83	105	5	Tr
459	**Water chestnuts,** canned	1 cup	140	86	70	1	Tr

MISCELLANEOUS ITEMS

Item No.	Foods, approximate measures, units, and weight (weight of edible portion only)		Grams	Water (Percent)	Food Energy (Calories)	Protein (Grams)	Fat (Grams)
	Chocolate: See also Semisweet (item 327) and Sweet (item 328).						
460	*Bitter or baking*	1 oz	28	2	145	3	15
461	**Salt**	1 tsp	5.5	0	0	0	0.0
462	**Vinegar,** cider	1 tbsp	15	94	Tr	Tr	0
	Yeast:						
463	*Baker's,* dry, active	1 pkg	7	5	20	3	Tr
464	*Brewer's,* dry	1 tbsp	8	5	25	3	Tr
465	**Sesame oil**	1 tbsp	14	0	120	Tr	14
466	**Apples,** dried	½ cup	42.5	24	117	.45	0.7
467	**Carambola** (Star Fruit), raw	100 grams	100	90.4	35	7	5
468	**Cranberries,** whole	1 cup	100	87.9	45	.4	—
469	**Currants,** raw, red & white	100 grams	100	85.7	50	1.4	0.2
470	**Figs,** fresh	2 large	100	77.5	80	1.2	0.3
471	**Gooseberries,** raw	100	88.9	39	.8	.2	
472	**Guavas**	1 medium	100	83.0	62	.8	0.8
473	**Passion fruit,** raw	3.5 oz	100	75.1	90	2.2	0.7
474	**Persimmons,** kaki	1 medium	100	78.8	77	.7	0.4
475	**Pomegranates**	1 large	275	82.3	97	.8	0.5
476	**Buckwheat,** whole	1 cup	100	11.0	355	11.7	2.4
477	**Buckwheat flour,** dark	1 cup	100	12	333	11.7	2.5
478	**Millet,** raw	¼ cup	58	11.8	190	5.7	1.7
479	**Rye flour,** dark	1 cup	128	11	419	20.9	3.3
480	**Rye flour,** light, sifted	1 cup	80	11	286	7.5	0.8
481	**Wheat bran,** raw	2 tbsp	33	4	21	1.5	0.43
482	**Wheat germ,** raw	¼ cup	25	11.5	91	8.8	2.72
483	**Wild rice,** raw	100 grams	100	8.5	353	14.1	0.7
484	**Fava (Broad) beans,** dry	¼ pound	117	11.9	383	28.5	1.9
485	**Lentil sprouts**	1 cup	100	90	104	8.4	0.3
486	**Soybean sprouts**	1 cup	105	85.3	48	6.5	1.9
	Soybean flour:						
487	*Full-fat*	1 cup	72	8	303	26.4	14.2
488	*Low-fat*	1 cup	100	8	356	43.4	6.7
489	*Defatted*	1 cup	138	8	450	64.9	2.76
490	**Soybean grits**	1 cup	152	8	480	75	8
491	**Soy sauce**	1 tbsp	18	62.8	12	1	0.2

[a] Value may vary from 6 to 60 mg.

FATTY ACIDS

VITAMIN A VALUE (IU) (RE)

Saturated (Grams)	Monounsaturated (Grams)	Polyunsaturated (Grams)	Cholesterol (Milligrams)	Carbohydrate (Grams)	Calcium (Milligrams)	Phosphorus (Milligrams)	Iron (Milligrams)	Potassium (Milligrams)	Sodium (Milligrams)	(International units)	(Retinol equivalents)	Thiamine (Milligrams)	Riboflavin (Milligrams)	Niacin (Milligrams)	Ascorbic acid (Milligrams)
0.1	Tr	0.2	0	15	44	68	1.7	474	243	18,990	1,899	0.08	0.08	0.9	8
0.1	Tr	0.1	0	24	46	93	1.5	308	64	7,780	778	0.13	0.22	1.5	6
Tr	Tr	Tr	0	17	6	27	1.2	165	11	10	1	0.02	0.03	0.5	2
9.0	4.9	0.5	0	8	22	109	1.9	235	1	10	1	0.01	0.07	0.4	0
0.0	0.0	0.0	0	0	14	3	Tr		2,132	0	0	0.00	0.00	0.0	0
0.0	0.0	0.0	1	1	1	1	0.1	15	Tr	0	0	0.00	0.00	0.0	0
Tr	0.1	Tr	0	3	3	90	1.1	140	4	Tr	Tr	0.16	0.38	2.6	Ir
Tr	Tr	0.0	0	3	17[a]	140	1.4	152	10	Tr	Tr	1.25	0.34	3.0	Tr
1.9	5.3	5.9	Tr	Tr	0	0	0		0	0		0	0	0	0
—	—	—		1.3	13	22	.7	242		—		.025	.05	.2	4.5
—	—	—		8.0	4	17	.1.5	192		1,200		.04	.02	.3	35
—	—	—		10.8	14	10	.5	82		40		.03	.02	.1	11
				12.1	32	23	1.0	257		120		.04	.05	.01	41
—	—	—		20.3	35	22	.5	194		80		.06	.05	.4	2
			9.7	18	15	5	155			290		—	—	1.1	
—	—	—		15	23	42	.9	289		280		.05	.05	1.2	242
—	—	—		21.2	13	84	1.5	348		700		Tr	.13	1.5	30
—	—	—		19.7	5	25	.3	174		2,710		.03	.02	.1	11
—	—	—		25.3	5	12	.5	399		Tr		.05	.05	.5	5
—	—	—		72.9	114	282	3.1	448		0		.5	—	4.4	0
—	—	—		72	33	347	2.8	656		0		.58	.15	2.9	0
.40	—	—		42	12	180	3.9	250		0		.42	.22	1.3	0
.42	—	—		87.2	59	686	5.8	1,101		—		.78	.26	3.5	0
—	—	—		62.3	18	148	.9	125		—		.12	.05	.5	0
.07	—	—		54	11	121	1.42	105		0		.07	.03	2.0	0
.47	—	—		11.7	18	279	2.35	207		0		.5	.17	1.05	0
—	—	—		75.3	19	330	4.2	220		0		.45	.63	5.2	25
—	—	—		65	115	443	8.05	—		80		.57	.34	2.83	0
—	—	—			12	—	3.0	—		—		.21	.09	1.1	24
—	—	—		5.6	50	70	1.1	—		80		.24	.21	.8	14
2.6	—	—		2.5	143	402	5.0	1,195		79		.51	.22	1.5	0
1.02	—	—		38.3	263	834	9.1	1,895		80		.83	.35	2.6	0
1.17	—	—		52.5	356	904	15.3	2,512		55		1.5	.47	3.6	0
—	—	—		48	240	—	10.8	—		Tr		2.4	.58	1.6	Tr
—	—	—		1.7	15	19	.9	66		0		Tr	.05	.1	0

Item No.	Foods, approximate measures, units, and weight (weight of edible portion only)		Grams	Water (Percent)	Food Energy (Calories)	Protein (Grams)	Fat (Grams)
492	**Almonds,** roasted	1 cup	157	.7	964	29.2	90.6
493	**Butternuts**		100	3.8	629	23.7	61.2
	Chestnuts						
494	*Dried*		100	8.4	377	6.7	4.1
495	*Fresh*		100	52.5	194	2.9	1.5
496	**Hickory nuts**		100	3.3	673	13.2	68.7
497	**Peanuts,** raw, w/ skins	⅔ cup	100	5.6	564	26.0	47.5
498	**Eggplant,** raw	½ cup	100	92.4	25	1.2	.2
499	**Garlic,** raw	1 clove	3	61.3	4	—	Tr
500	**Kohlrabi,** sliced, raw	½ cup	75	90.3	21.5	1.5	Tr
501	**Rutabagas,** cooked, boiled, drained		100	90.2	35	.9	.1
	Seaweeds:						
502	*Agar-agar*		100	18.3	—	—	.3
503	*Dulse*		100	16.6	—	2.3	3.2
504	*Hijiki*		100	16	—	5.5	.8
505	*Kombu*		100	16	—	7.3	1.1
506	*Nori*		100	17	—	35.6	.8
507	*Wakame*		100	16	—	12.7	1.5
508	**Teff,** whole grain, red	1 oz	28	12.5	91.8	2.7	.7
509	**Yeast,** torula	1 oz	28	6.0	79	10.9	.3

FATTY ACIDS

VITAMIN A VALUE
(IU)   (RE)

Saturated (Grams)	Monounsaturated (Grams)	Polyunsaturated (Grams)	Cholesterol (Milligrams)	Carbohydrate (Grams)	Calcium (Milligrams)	Phosphorus (Milligrams)	Iron (Milligrams)	Potassium (Milligrams)	Sodium (Milligrams)	(International units)	(Retinol equivalents)	Thiamine (Milligrams)	Riboflavin (Milligrams)	Niacin (Milligrams)	Ascorbic acid (Milligrams)
7.3	—	—		30.6	369	791	7.4	1,214		0		0.8	1.44	5.5	0
—	—	—		8.4	—	—	6.8	—		—		—	—	—	—
—	—	—		78.8	52	162	3.3	875		—		.32	.38	1.2	0
—	—	—		42.1	27	88	1.7	454		—		.22	.22	.6	0
6	17	12		178	If	360	2.4	—		—		—	—	—	—
10	20	14		18.0	69	401	2.1	674		0		1.14	.13	17.2	0
—	—	—		5.8	12	28	.7	214		10		.05	.05	.6	5
—	—	—		.9	1	6	Tr	16		Tr		.01	Tr	Tr	Tr
—	—	—		5	30.5	37.5	.275	279		15		.045	.03	.227	49
—	—	—		8.2	59	31	.3	167		550		.06	.06	.8	0
—	—	—		—	567	22	6.3	—		—		—	—	—	—
—	—	—		—	296	287	—	8,060		—		—	—	—	—
—	—	—		42.8	1,400	58	29	—		150		.01	.2	4	0
—	—	—		54.0	900	150	10	—		430		.08	.32	1.8	11
—	—	—		44.3	260	510	12	—		11,000		.25	1.24	10	10
—	—	—		51.4	1,300	260	13	—		140		.11	.14	1	15
—	—	—		20.2	48	88	21.1	—		2		.04	.03	.39	—
—	—	—		10.5	120	486	5.5	580		Tr		3.97	1.43	12.6	Tr

SUGGESTED READING

Listed below are books that were particularly useful in providing information for *Whole Food Facts*. There are many other references from which I obtained interesting tidbits about foods, particularly magazine articles, company literature, and individuals too numerous to list here.

Adams, Ruth, and Frank Murray. *The Good Seeds, the Rich Grains, the Hard Nuts for a Healthier, Happier Life.* New York: Larchmont Books, 1977.

Atlas, Nava. *Vegetariana: A Rich Harvest of Wit, Lore and Recipes.* Garden City, NY: The Dial Press/Doubleday & Company, Inc., 1984.

Axler, Bruce H. *The Cheese Handbook.* New York: Ginger Books/Hastings House, 1968.

Bailey, Alton E. *Industrial Oil and Fat Products.* Second completely revised edition. Interscience Publishers, Inc., New York, 1951.

Ballentine, Rudolph, M.D. *Diet & Nutrition: A Holistic Approach.* Honesdale, PA: Himalayan International Institute, 1978.

Berman, Connie, and Susan Katz. *The Yogurt Book.* New York: Grosset & Dunlap, 1977.

Beyer, Bee. *Food Drying at Home the Natural Way.* Los Angeles, CA: J. P. Tarcher, Inc., 1976.

Bianchini, Francesco, et al. *The Complete Book of Fruits and Vegetables.* New York: Crown Publishers, 1975.

Bianchini, Francesco, and Francesco Corbetta. *Health Plants of the World.* New York: Newsweek Books, 1977.

Black, Helen, ed. *The Berkeley Co-op Food Book.* Palo Alto, CA: Bull Publishing Company, 1980.

Blue Goose Buying Guide for Fresh Fruits, Vegetables, and Nuts. Blue Goose, Inc., Hagerstown, MD.

Brody, Jane. *Jane Brody's Good Food Book: Living the High-Carbohydrate Way.* New York: W. W. Norton & Company, 1985.

————. *Jane Brody's Nutrition Book.* New York: W. W. Norton & Company and Bantam Books, 1981, 1982.

Bumgarner, Marlene Anne. *Book of Whole Grains.* New York: St. Martin's Press, 1976.

Bush, Carroll D. *Nut Grower's Handbook.* New York: Orange Judd Publishing Company, Inc., 1941.

Carcione, Joe, and Bob Lucas, DDS. *The Greengrocer.* San Francisco, CA: Chronicle Books, 1972.

Chen, Philip S., Ph.D., and Helen D. Chung, M.S. *Soybeans for Health and a Longer Life.* New Canaan, CT: Keats Publishing Inc., 1973.

Claiborne, Craig. *Craig Claiborne's The New York Times Food Encyclopedia.* New York: Times Books, 1985.

Coyle, L. Patrick, Jr. *The World Encyclopedia of Food.* New York: Facts on File, 1982.

Davis, Myrna. *The Potato Book.* New York: William Morrow & Co., 1973.

Doyle, Rodger P., and James L. Redding. *The Complete Food Handbook.* New York: Grove Press, Inc., 1976.

Eekhof-Stork, Nancy. *The World Atlas of Cheese.* New York: Paddington Press, 1976.

Encyclopedia of Organic Gardening. Emmaus, PA: Rodale Press, 1976.

Ensminger, Audrey H. *Food for Health: A Nutrition Encyclopedia.* 2d ed. Boca Raton, FL: CRC Press/Times Mirror Co., 1994.

Ewald, Ellen Buchman. *Recipes for a Small Planet.* New York: Ballantine Books, 1973.

Fleur, Henrietta. *Introduction to Nutrition.* 3d ed. New York: Macmillan Publishing Co., 1976.

Froud, Nina. *The World Book of Vegetable, Rice & Pasta Dishes.* London, England: Pelham Books Ltd., 1969.

Garrison, Robert H., Jr., and Elizabeth Somer. *The*

Nutrition Desk Reference. 3d ed. New Canaan, CT: Keats Publishing, 1995.

Gates, J. *Basic Foods.* New York: Holt, Rinehart and Winston, 1976.

Gendel, Evelyn. *Pasta!* New York: Simon & Schuster, 1966.

Goldbeck, Nikki and David. *American Wholefoods Cuisine.* New York: Plume/New American Library, 1983.

———. *The Supermarket Handbook.* New York: Signet/New American Library, 1976.

Hamilton, Eva May Nunnelley, and Eleanor Noss Whitney. *Nutrition Concepts and Controversies.* Saint Paul, MN: West Publishing Company, 1982.

Hays, Wilma, and R. Vernon. *Foods the Indians Gave Us.* New York: Ives Washburn, Inc., 1973.

Hazelton, Nika. *The Unabridged Vegetable Cookbook.* New York: M. Evans & Company, 1976.

Hendrickson, Robert. *The Great American Tomato Book.* Garden City, NY: Doubleday & Company, 1976.

Hertzberg, Ruth, et al. *The New Putting Food By.* Revised edition. Brattleboro, VT: Stephen Greene Press, 1982.

Hunter, Beatrice T. *Consumer Beware!* New York: Touchstone/Simon and Schuster, 1971.

Idyll, C. P., ed. *Exploring the Ocean World.* New York: Thomas Y. Crowell Company, 1969.

———. *Sea Against Hunger.* New York: Thomas Y. Crowell Company, 1970.

Jacobson, Michael F. *Eater's Digest: The Consumer's Factbook of Food Additives.* Garden City, NY: Doubleday & Co., Inc., 1976.

Kadans, Joseph. *Encyclopedia of Fruits, Vegetables, Nuts and Seeds for Healthful Living.* West Nyack, NY: Parker Publishing, 1973.

Kaufman, William I. *The Peanut Butter Cookbook.* New York: Simon and Schuster, 1977.

Kraft, Ken and Pat. *Exotic Vegetables.* New York: Walker & Co., 1979.

Lampert, Lincoln M. *Modern Dairy Products.* New York: Chemical Publishing Co., Inc., 1970.

Lang, Jennifer Harvey, ed. *Larousse Gastronomique: The New American Edition of the World's Greatest Culinary Encyclopedia.* New York: Crown Publishers, 1988.

Lapedes, Daniel N., ed. *McGraw-Hill Encyclopedia of Food, Agriculture, and Nutrition.* New York: McGraw-Hill Books, 1977.

Lappé, Francis Moore. *Diet for a Small Planet.* Tenth anniversary edition. New York: Ballantine Books, 1982.

Mallard, Gwen. *Soy Bean Magic: Delicious Recipes with Soy Beans, Flour, & Grits.* Saanichton, British Columbia: Hancock House Publishers, Ltd., 1976.

Martin, Ruth Marion Somers. *International Dictionary of Food and Cooking.* New York: Hastings House, 1974.

Morse, Roger A. *The Complete Guide to Beekeeping.* Revised edition. New York: E. P. Dutton Co., 1974.

Nantet, Bernard. *Cheeses of the World.* New York: Rizzoli, 1993.

National Research Council. *Recommended Dietary Allowances.* 10th ed. Washington, D.C.: National Academy Press, 1989.

Nutrition Search, Inc. *Nutrition Almanac.* New York: McGraw-Hill Paperbacks, Inc., 1983.

Ogilvy, Susan. *Making Cheese at Home.* New York: Crown Publishers Inc., 1976.

Riotte, Louise. *Nuts for the Food Gardener.* Charlotte, VT: Garden Way Publishing, 1975.

Robertson, Laurel, Carol Flinders, and Brian Ruppenthal. *The New Laurel's Kitchen: A Handbook for Vegetarian Cookery and Nutrition.* Berkeley, CA: Ten Speed Press, 1986.

Rodale's Basic Natural Foods Cookbook. Emmaus, PA: Rodale Press, 1984.

Rosenthal, Sylvia. *Fresh Food.* New York: E. P. Dutton, 1978.

Shannon, Ellen C. *American Dictionary of Culinary Terms.* New York: A. S. Barnes, 1962.

Shurtleff, William, and Akiko Aoyagi. *Book of Miso.* New York: Ballantine Books, 1982.

———. *Book of Tofu.* New York: Ballantine Books, 1983.

Simon, André L. *A Concise Encyclopedia of Gastronomy.* Woodstock, NY: Overlook Press, 1981.

Simon, André L., and Robin Howe. *Dictionary of Gastronomy.* Woodstock, NY: Overlook Press, 1978.

Smith, A. K., et al., eds. *Soybeans: Chemistry and Technology,* Vol. 1. Westport, CT: AVI Publishing Co., 1978.

Street, Len, and Andrew Singer. *Butter, Milk, and Cheese from Your Back Yard.* New York: Sterling Publishing Co., Inc., 1976.

Tannahill, Reay. *Food in History.* New York: Stein and Day, 1973.

Tiedjens, Victor A. *The Vegetable Encyclopedia and Gardener's Guide.* New York: Avenel Books, 1973.

Trager, James. *The Foodbook.* New York: Grossman Publishers, 1970.

United States Department of Agriculture. *Agricultural Statistics.* Washington, D.C.: U.S. Government Printing Office. Annual publication.

Ward, Artemus. *Encyclopedia of Food.* New York: Peter Smith, 1941.

Weiss, Theodore J., Ph.D. *Food Oils and Their Uses.* 2d ed. Westport, CT: AVI Publishing Co., 1982.

Whole Foods Magazine. *Natural Foods Guide.* Berkeley, CA: And/Or Press, 1979.

Winter, Ruth. *Consumer's Dictionary of Food Additives.* New York: Crown Publishers, Inc., 1978.

Wise, Willliam H. and Company, *The Wise Encyclopedia of Cookery.* New York: Wm. H. Wise/Grosset & Dunlap, 1971.

Wood, Rebecca. *The Whole Foods Encyclopedia: A Shopper's Guide.* New York: Prentice Hall, 1988.

INDEX